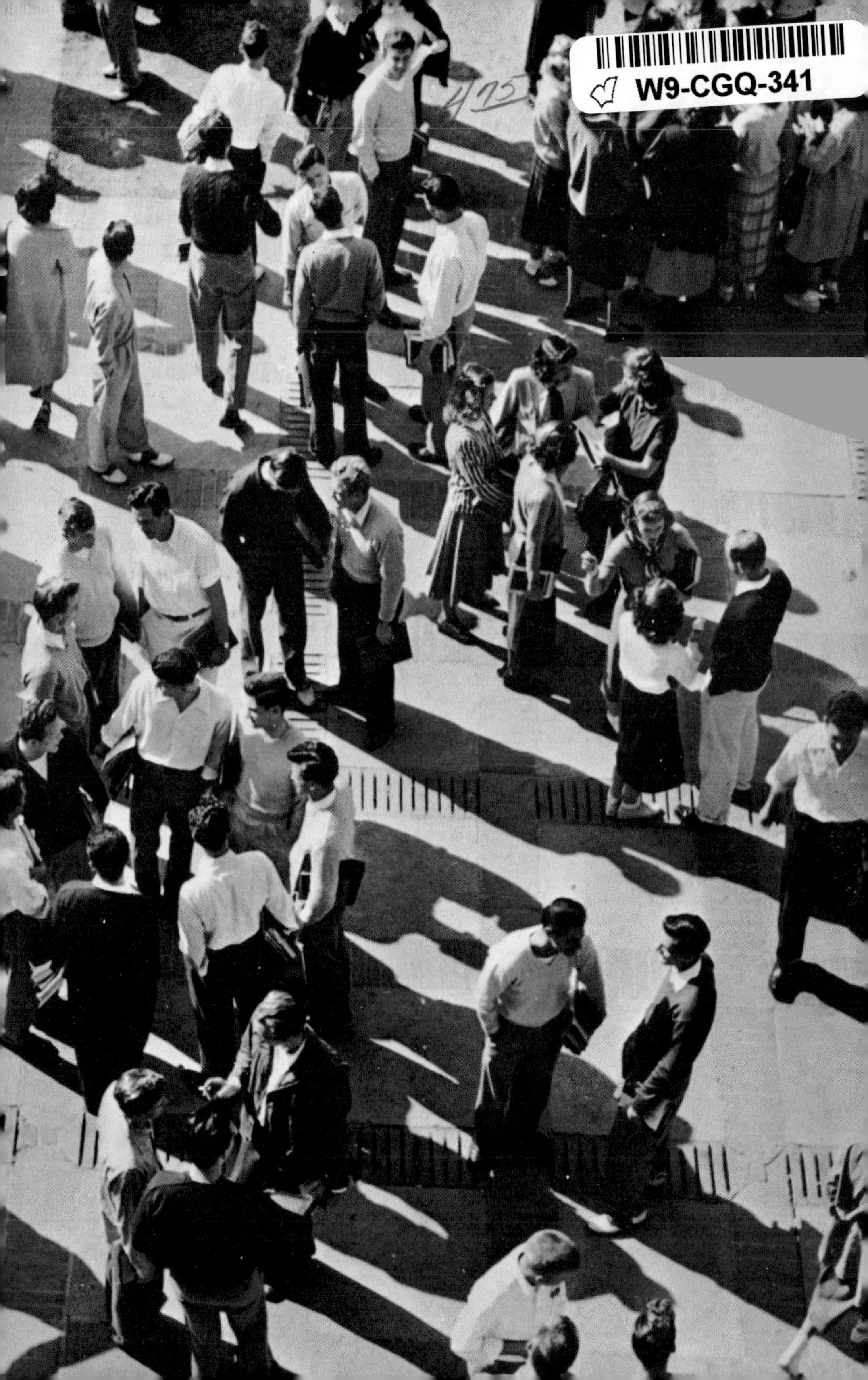

Health for Effective Living

A BASIC HEALTH EDUCATION TEXT FOR COLLEGE STUDENTS

Health for Effective Living

A BASIC HEALTH EDUCATION TEXT
FOR COLLEGE STUDENTS

EDWARD B. JOHNS, Ed.D., F.A.P.H.A.

Associate Professor, School Health Education
University of California, Los Angeles
Formerly a Health Education Consultant
California Community Health Education Project

WILFRED C. SUTTON, Ed.D.

Assistant Supervisor, School Health Education
University of California, Los Angeles

LLOYD E. WEBSTER, M.A.

Director of Health Education, Los Angeles County Schools
Formerly Associate Professor of Health Education
University of Southern California

Adviser and Consultant

WALTER H. BROWN, M.D.

Professor Emeritus, Stanford University
Formerly Professor and Acting Dean
School of Public Health, University of California

Foreword by

BERNICE MOSS, Ed.D.

Professor of Health Education, University of Utah

McGRAW-HILL BOOK COMPANY, INC.

NEW YORK · TORONTO · LONDON · 1954

HEALTH FOR EFFECTIVE LIVING

Library of Congress Catalog Card Number: 54-6721

II

Dedicated to

WALTER H. BROWN, M.D.

family physician, health officer, health foundation executive,
professor, dean, counselor, and friend
for his wise teachings, continual encouragement and inspiration,
constructive criticism, and helpful advice and counsel

Foreword

The maintenance and improvement of the health of its students has long been an accepted objective of the American college or university. Basic to the realization of this objective is the instruction of the students in the principles and practices of healthful living. Freshman or sophomore courses in health education (hygiene) are generally available and frequently required, and some such courses are now organized on the upper-division level, as well.

Health for Effective Living has been written to meet the needs of students enrolled in these courses. The approach of the authors indicates a keen recognition of the present-day needs and interests of college students and of the nature of the college and the wider communities in which students live. The emphasis given to problems of emotional and social adjustment is indicative of the trend toward guidance of young people in the areas of major concern to them. Here is where the text begins—not with cells, organs, tissues, bones, and blood. An honest attempt is made to assist students with their life adjustment problems; to supply them with scientific information; to build improved attitudes; to stimulate effective behavior; and to encourage better all-round living.

While emphasizing the emotional and social adjustment of college youth, the text does not neglect important basic concerns in body maintenance and protection, such as nutrition, balanced daily living, and protection against disease, accidents, and drugs. The inclusion of challenging information and activities in these and other areas makes for balance and for adequate consideration of all important health problems which college students face or in which they indicate a need or an interest.

A third emphasis is noteworthy in the inclusion of chapters concerned with the college health program and with the community, state, and national approaches to group health protection and improvement. The role of the college student as a participating citizen on his campus and in his community is effectively developed. Students who pursue the text, and particularly those who participate in some of the suggested activities, should develop broader understandings and appreciations of the social responsibilities of citizens in the interest of a vigorous and healthy commonwealth. This is a need in the nation today.

This book contains a challenge to students and to their instructors. It represents a new and more functional approach to a basic concern—that of building healthy, happy, effective citizens in a democracy.

BERNICE MOSS

Preface

Health education with its purposeful experiences is a relatively new field within the present-day educational structure. Only a few years ago, the "hygiene" courses taught at the college level were a mixed prescription of unrelated facts in the fields of anatomy, osteology, and physiology. The memorization of such facts resulted in an accumulation of much information but little wisdom.

At present, health education experiences relating to the dynamics of living are planned to meet needs and satisfy interests not only in all aspects of the physical body but in mental, emotional, and social living, as well. These learning experiences are implemented in the classroom by qualified instructors using functional methods and scientifically sound teaching aids.

Such health education experiences, skillfully organized, compose a major part of the educational aspects of the college health program. These experiences are based upon sound principles derived from both the health sciences and the field of education. The fundamental purpose of health education courses is to change favorably the health behavior of students—to enrich their lives. Such purposes can be achieved by providing learning experiences which (1) instill basic scientific information regarding individual and community health, (2) stimulate the development of positive wholesome attitudes, and (3) assist students in developing worthwhile health practices, based on intelligent judgments and purposeful applications of scientific information.

Studies by the authors and others show an extensive lack of scientific health information among college students. Somewhere in the early education of these young people, misconceptions of scientific truths and unwholesome health attitudes and practices were either taught or caught.

The need for guidance in effective living also is apparent when the instructor considers college students entering an enlarged environment with increased stresses or strains. The authors believe that a well-planned college health education program can provide many opportunities for improving the health status of students. This book is written to serve as a basic health education text, a foundation resource in a college health education program.

In so far as possible the materials presented in the book are based on data secured from research studies applying to effective living. The evidence from these studies can be used to open up new areas for discussion and further investigation. Materials have been drawn from the experiences of the authors as they worked with college students in health education classes at the University of Oregon, Stanford University, San Diego State College, University of Hawaii, Columbia College, University of Southern California, and particularly, during the past seven years, at the University of California, Los Angeles.

The book is designed to deal with the student where he is now—in the college environment. First, it attempts to provide him with an understanding of effective living. Second, an opportunity is offered the student to appraise his health needs and interests and study those of other college students. Third, the discussion, consisting of the major portion of the book, is presented with a view to assisting the student in finding ways and means of meeting his health needs and interests now and in the future.

The scope of the book is broad. It is concerned with the total functioning of the individual in the society in which he lives. It integrates personal and civic responsibilities, rather than dividing half the discussion into individual health and the other half into community health concerns. It cuts across all phases of campus and family life and covers domestic and international health problems.

Scientific information is provided the student, and it is organized around the fundamental areas contributing to effective living. The organization of the book is based on a research study of the health needs and interests of college students and upon the teaching experience of the authors. Emphasis is given to the areas of mental health and family life, which head the list of health needs and interests. Because of their importance these areas are given priority at the front of the book rather than at the end, as is the traditional pattern.

In addition to content, learning experiences are suggested in which the student can participate. These experiences are important because participating in them gives meaning and purpose to the content. Some activities may seem inappropriate for certain students; however, if they serve as a challenge to students to develop their own learning activities or to the instructor to point out more vital ones, then they will have been worthwhile. Since the presentation of scientific information is limited by the size of the book, pertinent readings are suggested at the end of each chapter. These readings are recommended for the reader who desires to explore further a topic, problem, or area. Of special note is the suggested list of popular readings which pertain to effective living. These have been included to arouse the interest of the student and widen his concepts of health education.

Health for Effective Living is written as a guide for students and instructors studying together the basic factors producing good health. Sufficient material is available for use in a three-unit semester course or a four-unit year course—two units each semester. Chapters selected on the basis of needs and interests of a particular class make it possible to serve functionally the students in a two-unit or one-unit semester or quarter course. In addition to the organized course, the book is planned to serve as resource material in a core program of instruction and as a personal guide for the student in self-study.

In view of these varied situations, and in keeping with the present trends in health education, this book is designed to assist the student in believing, as well as questioning wisely; to help him understand himself; to stimulate an exploratory and creative attitude toward living; and to help him achieve wholesome behavior.

EDWARD B. JOHNS
WILFRED C. SUTTON
LLOYD E. WEBSTER

Acknowledgments

The authors wish to express their sincere thanks to the many persons who freely gave their intelligent suggestions and constructive criticism during the preparation of this book. These people are in no way responsible for errors which may still be found in the book. The authors take full responsibility for any failure to interpret correctly or properly use criticism and suggestions.

Our special thanks go to the following for encouragement, stimulation, and many helpful suggestions on the total manuscript: Dr. Rosalind Cassidy, University of California, Los Angeles; Dr. Howard S. Hoyman, University of Illinois; Dr. Clifford L. Brownell, Teachers College, Columbia University.

We are indebted to the following for reading and criticizing special parts or making helpful suggestions in the preparation of particular chapters within the parts of the book:

Part One. Orientation in Health Education. Dr. Ruth Abernathy, Dr. Ben Miller, and Donald S. MacKinnon, M.D., University of California, Los Angeles; Alma Nemir, M.D., University of Utah; Dr. Blanche Bobbitt, Los Angeles City Schools; Angela Kitzinger, San Diego State College; Franklin Foote, M.D., National Society for Prevention of Blindness.

Part Two. Developing a Healthy Personality. Dr. James C. Coleman and Dr. George Fitzell, University of California, Los Angeles.

Part Three. Preparing for Effective Family Living. William B. Thompson, M.D., obstetrician and gynecologist, Los Angeles; Dr. George Fitzell, University of California, Los Angeles; Vivian Osborne, Los Angeles City College.

Part Four. Developing and Maintaining Health. Dr. Valerie Hunt, University of California, Los Angeles; George H. Akau, chief, Bureau of Food and Drugs, Department of Public Health, Territory of Hawaii; Donald Billam-Walker, manager, Better Business Bureau of Honolulu.

Part Five. Building Defenses for Effective Living. John M. Chapman, M.D., Director of Communicable Disease Control, Los Angeles City Health Department; Dr. John Beeston, University of California, Los

Angeles; Lewis T. Bullock, M.D., cardiologist, Los Angeles; Dr. Laurence E. Morehouse and Robert Downey, University of Southern California; Alma Nemir, M.D., University of Utah.

Part Six. Effective Living in the Community. J. Allen Davis, Automobile Club of Southern California; Roger Plaisted, Los Angeles Chapter, American Red Cross; Dr. John Beeston, University of California, Los Angeles; Byron Mork, M.D., and Albert Torribio, Los Angeles City Health Department.

We wish to express appreciation to the following instructors and students in colleges and universities using the materials experimentally in health education classes: Vivian Osborne, Los Angeles City College, and her health education students; Patricia Reid and Walter Crowe and their health education students at Long Beach State College; Orsie Thomson, Dr. Ethel Bell, and Dr. Deane Richardson and members of health education classes at the University of California, Los Angeles.

Our special thanks go to Dr. Lester Beck, University of Southern California, David Janison, Los Angeles City Health Department, and Iris Andrews, Bowling Green State University, Bowling Green, Ohio, for assistance and suggestions on illustrations; and to Mrs. Howard C. Ray, Palo Alto, and Charles L. Johns for editorial assistance on Chapters 1 to 8.

We gratefully acknowledge valuable assistance in the preparation of the manuscript on the part of Bertha Johns, Merriom Sutton, and Grace Webster.

We are indebted to the publishing companies indicated in the text for permission to quote and reproduce materials.

E. B. J.
W. C. S.
L. E. W.

Contents

PART THREE. PREPARING FOR EFFECTIVE FAMILY LIVING

PART FOUR. DEVELOPING AND MAINTAINING HEALTH

PART ONE

Orientation in Health Education

1. Understanding Health: A Point of View

What does health mean to you? What are the factors producing health? What are the characteristics of a healthy person? What is health education? What is the goal of health education for you, the college student?

Although college students are interested in themselves, as well as in their own lives, in their families, and in their communities, it is apparent that they are not interested in "health for health's sake." This is only natural and normal. The important fact is that students want to gratify such basic needs as to belong, to be recognized, to be in good standing, to be loved, to eat well, and to play joyously. These are all aspects of good health and fine living. Improvement can be made in the essential factors producing health if there is (1) understanding, (2) desire, and (3) action. Improvement in living then can be made to increase satisfaction from one's work and provide enjoyment, efficiency, and happiness.

The subsequent discussion is organized in an attempt to challenge the college student to develop further his understandings, attitudes, and action patterns relative to healthful, effective living.

What Is Health?

Many misunderstandings and unwholesome attitudes on the part of students, parents, and instructors result from misconceptions and misinterpretations of terms such as "health" and "health education." Lack of complete scientific information, misinterpretation of facts, poor instruction—any one or all three combined are possible reasons for this current confusion. It must be admitted that these terms are difficult to describe, for they are elusive words with relative meanings. Even when described accurately they can be misinterpreted. The word "health" is a good example. It has different meanings and interpretations for different people.

To the man on the street health may mean that he is not sick. The youngster may see it as washing his hands and face or brushing his teeth. To the mother it may connote a happy family. To the coed it may refer to the way she looks, the way she feels, and the dates she gets. To some college men it is closely aligned with body build and athletic skill; to others of this group it is the ability to spend long periods solving an experiment in the laboratory.

To the physiologist it is the product of the normal function of cells, organs, and systems. To the quack doctor health results from the patient's buying that "best bottled health-winning nostrum" or habitually using "organic irrigations" for a fee payable in advance. To the physical culturist it is a "body beautiful," exhibiting rippling muscles gained through performing a set of prescribed systematic exercises. To the family physician it means constant supervision and care utilizing the most modern medical services, including health guidance and periodical examinations, and the best equipment and facilities to ensure happy, zestful living of the total family.

To the person who has lost his health it is the most priceless possession of all. As Sir William Temple wrote: "Health is the soul that animates all the enjoyments of life, which fade and are tasteless without it." To the person who has lost his money, health is his one hope. To quote an old Arabian proverb: "He who has health has hope, and he who has hope has everything." Disraeli once pointed out the significance of health to the state and nation in the statement, "The public health is the foundation upon which reposes the happiness of the people and the strength of the nation."

The World Health Organization [1] defined health as "A state of complete physical, mental and social well-being and not merely the absence of disease or infirmity." This definition is important because some 54 nations reached international agreement on it at the first World Health Assembly in 1948. It is the most widely accepted definition today.

Many of the above concepts or feeling tones about health are fine. Some are only partially true. A few are unscientific but represent common opinion. Such statements, along with the widely accepted but traditional definition by the World Health Organization, lead the authors to attempt a more functional definition of health in the following section.

[1] Constitution of the World Health Organization, p. 3, from *Chronicle of the World Health Organization,* 1:29–43. Geneva: World Health Organization, 1947.

A Point of View about Health

Historically, the term health is derived from an old Anglo-Saxon word "haelth," meaning the condition of being safe and sound or whole. For many years this historical definition was lost because of the common belief that health was in essence freedom from disease. It has been only within recent years that a fuller, richer meaning has evolved. The modern concept of health revives that of the old English term pertaining to the "wholeness" of the individual.

A definition of health. With the foregoing key concept in mind the authors offer the following definition: *Health is the quality, resulting from the total functioning of the individual, that empowers him to achieve a personally satisfying and socially useful life* [1, 7, 8] *. To avoid misinterpretation of this simple definition, several concepts are explained in more detail.

The unity of the individual. This definition expresses health as a dominance of positive or favorable adaptations resulting from the biological equilibrium, that dynamic state, existing between the individual and his environment [9]. Sufficient scientific evidence points to the fact that the individual responds to his environment as a whole, that he lives as a total being. He is made up of cells, organs, and systems, but they are so interrelated and integrated that he functions as a complete unit. That which affects one part brings about changes in others. The concept of psychosomatic medicine is based on the belief in the unity of the organism, which serves as an example of the point. Psychosomatic medicine is not a new field of medicine designed as a cure for man faced with new health problems peculiar to the twentieth century. Actually, "it is simply an approach to the sick patient as a whole person rather than one with a localized disease." [2] This approach unifies the physical, mental, and social factors producing health. All these factors are considered in treating a patient with a disease. Psychiatrists have shown us that a number of bodily disturbances are due to emotional causes. Thus fear of a disease can be so strong as to incapacitate a person from his daily activities when no disease organism is present; or the ideas he builds up about his own body may cause him great disturbance. These disturbances interfering with his quality of living are diseases just as much as are the common cold, influenza, and pneumonia.

* Numbers in brackets refer to items listed in Readings at ends of chapters.

[2] "The ABC's of Psychosomatic Medicine," *Menninger Quarterly*, 4:9–12, October, 1950.

There is no such thing as separate physical, mental, or social health. Each is an aspect of the whole, as the derivation of the term and the definition of health imply. For purposes of discussion or as chapter headings, physical and mental health may be considered separately; but in function they are inseparable. They are interrelated, integrated parts of the total individual, who is a unique personality differing from every other individual.

Health as a quality of life. The "quality of life" resulting from total functioning is a significant aspect of the definition of health for several reasons. First, the phrase denotes a positive outcome of the art of fine living. This is *effective living.* The word effective is used because it is in keeping with the definition of health. According to Webster's *New Collegiate Dictionary,* "effective" means "producing a desired effect and being ready for service or action." Second, the phrase, the quality of life, is important in reference to effective living because it implies that the person utilizes to the fullest his innate powers, all his capacities for living. Third, the product, effective living, results from the individual's functioning in a variety of life activities including physical, mental, social, and spiritual experiences. What he does—his work, his play, his sleep and rest, the food he eats, his loves, his hates, his successes, and his failures—all play a part in determining the quality of life, or how effectively he lives. This means that his daily experiences serve to mold his health. Also, his actions of today assist in building his future health status or, conversely, tend to impair effective living. Today, emphasis is on quantity as well as on quality. Living both a full and a long life is important.

Achievement of a personally satisfying life. Personal achievement means effective action, through daily experiences, in reaching the goals established by the individual. This concept indicates that health is not something given to one but is rather a quality earned through personal actions. Rosalind Cassidy [3] presents a formula for best action: "Believing plus knowing equals 'best' action . . . we know that if we have the facts, and are committed to them by a deep drive of belief in their validity and worth, the 'best' action results."

A personally satisfying life contributes to effective living, that is, to being happy and at the same time useful. A personally satisfying life denotes the ability to adjust to one's own environment—to fulfill individual responsibilities within the family group, to develop wholesome

[3] Rosalind Cassidy, "Effective Action—The Ends for Which We Strive," *California Journal of Secondary Education,* 27:191–192, April, 1952.

attitudes toward life, and to control emotions. A personally satisfying life implies freedom from disease, a part of healthful living. It implies establishing health practices of personal cleanliness, immunization against disease, utilizing competent medical and dental care, and avoiding accidents. It connotes a balanced program of life activities, including work, play, love, and faith.

Achievement of a socially useful life. The culture in which one lives influences effective living. In a democracy health means more than personal satisfaction or pure self-gratification. Each individual has the right to reach his fullest development and live an effective life regardless of race, religion, political belief, or economic situation. Health seen in this cultural setting involves the lives of other people as well as oneself. It is affected by how other people live, how they work, how they eat and sleep, how they think and feel, and how they get along with one another. This concept broadens health to take in the home, the neighborhood, the community, the wider community of the nation, and, since people today know no boundaries, the world.

Democratic group action is illustrated by the fight Americans are waging against such killers as heart disease, cancer, infantile paralysis, venereal disease, blindness, and many other diseases and defects; by a citizens' group working together to assure the building of a community hospital; by the permanent civil defense program in a community; or by the response of college students to the blood bank in time of emergency. Community health endeavors extend from a health committee meeting in the smallest village to the World Health Assembly of the World Health Organization.

In a democracy the individual is responsible for his personal health, but this is only part of his obligation. He also accepts the responsibility to help provide the same right to all others. Whether he knows it or not, the individual changes his behavior as a result of participating in community activities. He changes in the interaction process. Furthermore, he has the opportunity, as well as the responsibility, to help shape his environment. In this respect, the individual's health potential is multiplied when he joins a group endeavor in the interest of health.

Effective living in society implies that the individual makes a contribution to society during his lifetime. It is important to realize, too, that he functions best when he is working for a cause greater than himself. The individual is living more effectively when his attention is directed to others rather than when it is focused entirely on himself [8].

Factors Determining Health

From the previous description of the term health, the essential factors producing effective living are easily identified. They are interrelated factors contributing to the total function of the individual. For the purpose of study, they are categorized as follows: heredity, life activities, personal and social adjustment, proper nutrition, freedom from disease and accidents, and professional health services [5]. Each factor is briefly described below with respect to the possibility of improving healthful, effective living.

Heredity. Heredity is a foundational factor for effective living. It provides the innate endowment for health given by one's parents. Heredity plays an important role in determining the uniqueness of each individual and his particular health status. Good heredity implies a sound constitution, a well-developed body, and normal intelligence. Effective living signifies that the individual is utilizing all his innate capacities to the fullest extent. He cannot change his heredity: no activity of the body cells can affect the germ cells. However, if necessary, guidance from competent counselors can ensure that he is making the most of his endowment.

Life activities. Environment, as well as heredity, is a foundational factor for effective living. Life activities refer to all the experiences engaged in by the individual. These experiences determine the way he lives, which to a large extent produces the quality of life, the degree of effective living. Experiences can be classified as physical, mental, social, and spiritual. They include what the individual does each day—his work, his play, his sleep and rest—all his health practices. The selection of wholesome experiences and participation in a balanced program of life activities exert a positive influence on the quality of life. Usually, improvement in health status can be made by means of the individual's way of life. This fact becomes a challenge both to the individual and to instructors of health education.

Personal and social adjustments. The total integration of the individual results from making intelligent personal and social adjustments while participating in life activities. Personal adjustments include adjustments to one's environment, such as accepting and making the best of one's own body, accepting responsibility and making adjustments within the family group, controlling emotions, and developing wholesome attitudes toward life. Satisfying basic mental health needs, such as those for security and affection, is a specific example.

Social adjustments include adjustments to the physical, social, and cultural environment, for example, cooperating in protecting and promoting public health as a matter of community interest. Improvement in making personal and social adjustments can be made by the individual and the social group.

Proper nutrition. Eating a balanced diet is an essential life activity. Because of the absolute necessity of nutrition to life and health, it is considered here as a separate health-producing factor. A balanced diet provides the cells of the body the essential nutrients for three main purposes: (1) for growth and repair; (2) for regulation of body processes; (3) to yield energy. The right kinds of foods—milk, eggs, vegetables, fruits, meat or fish, cereal, and whole-grain or enriched bread—in proper balance provide the nutritional needs of the body and markedly affect the quality of life. Also, proper foods aid in regular elimination of body wastes.

Proper nutrition is a health problem in the United States. This is not because of lack of food. Rather, a large proportion of our population is undernourished because the food eaten is not of the proper quality and is not in proper balance. Much improvement can be made in the field of nutrition.

Freedom from disease and accidents. This vital factor for health is considered no longer as total health but as merely one aspect of health. Modern control of communicable disease is one of man's great achievements and has done much to increase effective living and longevity. Man's life expectancy at birth in the United States in 1952 was estimated at 68.5 years [3]. Influenza, pneumonia, tuberculosis, and the venereal diseases, to mention several diseases, still remain to be completely eliminated, and there is much yet to be accomplished in disease prevention and control. The chronic degenerative diseases, heart disease, cancer, and other top killers, are still unconquered. Examples of intelligent health practices which increase effective living include building resistance to disease through a balanced program of physical activity, adequate sleep and rest, proper diet, and scientifically proved immunizations; avoiding sources of infection; seeking prompt medical and dental care, including regular medical and dental examinations; and taking plenty of time to recover when disease strikes.

Accidents in the home, on the highways, and in industry constitute one of today's unsolved problems. Learning to live effectively, yet safely, is definitely an art in present-day society.

There is great opportunity for improvement, personally and in the community, with respect to this vital health factor, freedom from disease and accidents, through better health education.

Professional health services. This essential factor contributing to effective living consists of adequate medical and dental care and health education. Health services range from preventive to curative measures, including health guidance, periodic health examinations, recording of health histories, and clinical, surgical, and hospital care. Health education should enable one to (1) understand the role of professional services in effective living, (2) select competent health advisers, (3) discover how to secure continuous medical supervision and care, and (4) determine ways and means to pay for professional services. Great strides in solving the nationwide problem of providing competent professional health services for the individual and the group can and will be made in the near future.

Characteristics of a Healthy Individual

An understanding of health is not complete without considering the characteristics of an individual in a dynamic state of optimum health. The following items [7, 8] are designed to describe either Joe or Josephine College as exemplifying the typical healthy college student in the areas of personal living, personal-social relations, and the wider social relations.

Health in personal living. The student:

1. Is developing a consistent and unified outlook on life.
2. Makes successful adaptation to his environment by participating in life activities.
3. Shows vitality and tone with reserves of energy and power while participating in activities.
4. Is functioning with harmonious integration of his bodily parts at optimum efficiency.
5. Has a feeling of achievement resulting from participation in life activities.
6. Is able to resist disease through personal practices and by taking advantage of competent medical care.
7. Is achieving status as a person through growth in independence, in establishing security, and in developing a sense of belonging.
8. Is freeing himself from adolescent egoism, and evidences growth in social sensitivity and willingness to sublimate personal desires for the larger concerns of the groups to which he belongs.
9. Understands his own health assets and liabilities and is willing to improve

his status when positive changes can be made; does not worry about achieving the impossible.

10. Understands his sex role; both expresses and controls emotions.

Health in personal-social relations. The student:

1. Has status in family relations.
2. Has status with his fellow students of both sexes through his effective participation in several groups.

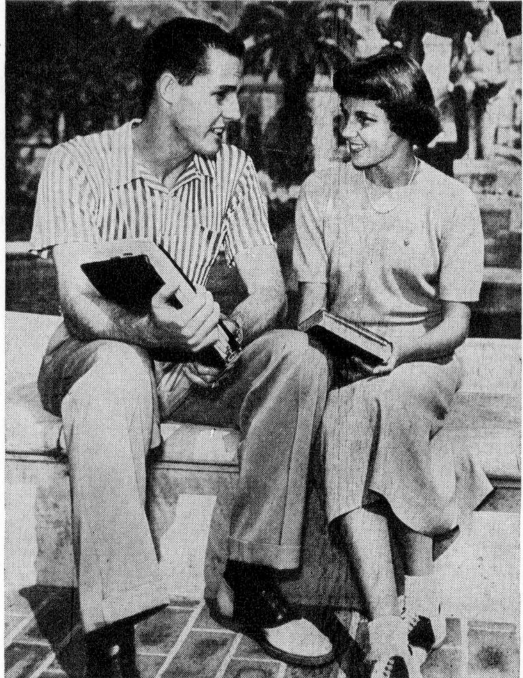

Fig. 1.1. Students typifying characteristics of healthy individuals. (*Photo by Lee Hansen.*)

3. Is frank, communicative, and sociable, entering heartily and with enjoyment into social activities.
4. Is considerate and helpful and is growing in his concerns for other people, their plans, successes, and failures.
5. Makes satisfactory heterosexual adjustments.

Health in the wider social relations. The student:

1. Has interest in promoting better healthful living in his own environment.
2. Is achieving status in society as a contributor to the furthering of more democratic ways of life.

3. Is achieving status in society through increasing economic independence and through social competence.

4. Is beginning to participate effectively in the activities of social institutions —the home, the school, and the community.

What Is Health Education?

Health education, as the term implies, is education for health. The integration of "health" and "education" into the term "health education" provides an educational field for the purpose of improving healthful or effective living. Health denotes its content and education its process. The health content provides scientific information, answering the question, What should be learned about health? The educational process determines how learning takes place.

Health education is concerned with people and their health behavior. Health behavior means what people understand, think, feel, and do about their health. The over-all purpose of health education is to bring about favorable changes in health behavior to improve living.

Health education sometimes is referred to as the applied science of healthful living, and rightfully so. It is not a pure science, for it draws much of its content from the health sciences, such as anatomy, physiology, bacteriology, medicine, and another applied science, public health. Health education is not composed of all these sciences added together; rather it derives from them the purposeful applications that particularly pertain to more effective living. Certainly, health education does not deal with the treatment of disease or defect as does the science of medicine. On the contrary, it is vitally concerned with educating people to live healthfully, to prevent disease, and to take intelligent action when disease or defects occur. Health education then is not synonymous with anatomy, physiology, bacteriology, and the like. These basic sciences form its foundation. More specifically, the content results from what is known about health and the factors that promote, maintain, and improve health. These are the factors that have been discussed previously in this chapter.

Education, psychology, educational psychology, and sociology furnish the understandings, methods, and activities that assist the individual in changing his behavior for more effective living in his environment. Health education is not something done to or for someone. Neither is it the memorizing of health facts. Rather, it is the provision of opportunities for individuals and groups to participate in experiences for healthful living. This means engaging in activities that give meaning and purpose to people's lives, aiding them in achieving personal and social goals through effective action. This is more than knowledge alone. It includes scientific knowledge plus wholesome attitudes and practices leading to improved health behavior.

Health education as a field relates to the individual, the home, the school, and the community. No one person accomplishes all the health education, although persons now are prepared as specialists in this field. Mother, father, brothers and sisters, family physician, dentist, and teacher influence health education in the home. The administrator, the health educator, the various instructors, the school physician, and the school nurse all play their parts in the school and college health education program. Physicians, dentists, public health officers, public health educators, sanitarians, public health nurses, social workers, ministers, and others contribute to health education in the community.

A definition of health education. Ruth Grout [4] defines health education as "the translation of what is known about health into desirable individual and community behavior patterns by means of the educational process." According to her definition there are three components in health education: (1) what is known about health; (2) ultimate health goals in terms of desirable individual and community behavior patterns; (3) the educational process. These components must be present in effective health education.

Examples of health education. A few examples of experiences in health education which lead to intelligent student action may clarify further its meaning. Recently, a student enrolling in a college health education class became interested in the problem of overweight and underweight. After making a study of the subject, he discovered that he had gained rapidly within the past few months without realizing his condition. After conferring with his instructor he made an appointment with his doctor to consider how to solve his problem. The doctor found his condition important but correctable, and a serious overweight problem was avoided.

A second student, after completing a freshman course in health education, returned to his home and found to his surprise that members of his family living in a large metropolitan city were drinking raw milk. Recalling his studies in disease prevention, he set about to educate his parents on the importance of drinking pasteurized milk.

A third student, a year after completing his health education course, came to see his instructor to tell him of a personal problem and how he had solved it. He had contracted gonorrhea and immediately visited

[4] Ruth Grout, *Health Teaching in Schools*, 2d ed., p. 2. Philadelphia: W. B. Saunders Company, 1953.

his physician for treatment. His purpose in talking with his instructor was to inform him how much he appreciated knowing what to do to avoid possible serious health consequences.

A fourth student, a house manager for a fraternity, after his course in nutrition, in which he participated in a diet project, decided that the meals in his house could be much improved. After consultation with his instructor he persuaded a nutritionist from the home economics department to become a consultant. She assisted him in revising his menus to accomplish his goal of providing a balanced diet for his fraternity brothers.

A fifth student participated in a community health project. He studied and worked with health personnel in voluntary agencies and the local health department. Afterward he changed his major to health education so that he could work more effectively for improved health in his community.

A Health Education Objective for the College Student

In 1947 the President of the United States appointed a Commission on Higher Education to investigate problems confronting the colleges and universities. The purpose of the study was to develop a plan of action to solve current instructional problems in the next ten years or more. The primary concern of the Commission was to improve college instruction by making it more relevant to life situations and at the same time more meaningful to students. A significant report was developed which has proved to be a valuable guide to educational leaders responsible for planning and conducting college and university programs.

As one of its first steps in evolving a workable plan, the Commission formulated objectives for general education. These objectives were stated in terms of the needs for college students. The objectives chart the course for general education both for students and faculty. One major goal selected pertained to the health of the individual and the community. An examination of the history of American education shows that this health objective for college students was consistent with that found in the objectives of education prepared by every other distinguished objective-forming body. No doubt these groups charting the course of education relied upon some of the great educational philosophers. It is worthy of note that Herbert Spencer, an exponent of philosophical naturalism, in 1882 expressed what could well be called modern health education concepts. He wrote as follows: [5]

[5] Herbert Spencer, *Education: Intellectual, Moral, and Physical,* pp. 30–31. New York: D. Appleton and Company, 1882.

The function of education is to prepare us for complete living. Complete living involves the right ruling of conduct in all directions under all circumstances. . . . In what way to treat the body; in what way to treat the mind; in what way to manage our affairs; in what way to bring up a family; in what way to behave as a citizen; in what way to utilize all those sources of happiness which nature supplies—how to use all our faculties to the greatest advantage of ourselves and others—how to live completely? And this being the great thing needful for us to learn, is by consequence, the great thing education has to teach.

The Commission's concern for health education, then, is not an original declaration; however, it is fundamental in pointing the direction of general education in the immediate future. The objective for health formulated by the Commission in terms of desirable behavior for the college student [6] is "to maintain and improve his own health and to cooperate actively and intelligently in solving community health problems."

In making its study the Commission found that colleges and universities at present are contributing to the health of individuals and communities; however, much more can and should be done to develop more fully the human resources within our society. In its fact-finding report the Commission made the following recommendation: [7]

What is needed is a course that deals specifically and explicitly with the information, attitudes, and habits the student needs to maintain and improve his own health and that of his community. An important phase of instruction to this end will be emphasis on the fact that health is more than a personal problem, that it has social implications, and that the individual owes it to society no less than to himself to keep his health and energy at their peak.

The Commission's suggestion for such a course is an excellent one. The authors believe that the prescribed course should be an integral part of the total health program of every college or university. Most colleges and universities have such planned, direct health instruction for their students. Evidence from educational research and the experience of instructors and administrators indicates that successful educational programs are those which are constructed on the basis of the needs and interests of the participants. This fact is especially true in health education, concerned with the effective living of people.

[6] *Higher Education for American Democracy: A Report of the President's Commission on Higher Education,* Vol. IV, p. 54. Washington: Government Printing Office, 1947.

[7] *Ibid.*, p. 54.

Summary

The previous discussion has been concerned with developing understandings and appreciations of (1) health—its various meanings and interpretations, its interrelated factors, and the characteristics of a healthy college student; (2) health education, the process through which health behavior may be changed for improved living; and (3) the purpose of health education for the college student, which charts the direction for the educational aspects of the college health program.

Suggested Activities

1. Analyze critically the definitions of health presented by the World Health Organization and the authors of this text. What are the strong and weak points of each definition? Wherein do they differ? To what degree are they similar?
2. Formulate your own definition of health. Justify your basic concepts.
3. Read one of the books listed under Popular Readings. Point out pertinent applications to effective living made by the author of the popular reference. How do they agree with your beliefs?
4. Compare your own characteristics with those outlined for a healthy individual. What are your strong points? What are your weaknesses? How could you make improvements for more effective living?
5. Write a brief account of your previous health education experiences. Were they favorable or unfavorable? Why?
6. How do you think health education can be made more effective today on the college level? Outline your plan.

Suggested Readings

1. A Report of the President's Commission on Higher Education, *Higher Education for American Democracy*, Vol. IV. Washington: Government Printing Office, 1947.
2. Bauer, W. W., and T. G. Hull, *Health Education of the Public*. Philadelphia: W. B. Saunders Company, 1942.
3. Byrd, Oliver E., *Health Instruction Yearbook*. Stanford, Calif.: Stanford University Press, 1943–1952. (Published yearly.)
4. Cassidy, Rosalind, "Effective Action—The Ends for Which We Strive," *California Journal of Secondary Education*, 27:191–192, April, 1952.
5. Joint Committee on Health Problems in Education of the National Education Association and the American Medical Association, *Health Education*, pp. 2–4. Washington: National Education Association, 1948.
6. Oberteuffer, Delbert, *School Health Education*. New York: Harper & Brothers, 1954.

7. Oberteuffer, Delbert, *Physical Education*, pp. 63–68, 127–155. New York: Harper & Brothers, 1951.

8. Williams, J. F., and G. G. Wetherill, *Personal and Community Hygiene, Applied*, pp. 3–18. Philadelphia: W. B. Saunders Company, 1950.

9. Winslow, C. E. A., W. G. Smillie, James A. Doull, and John E. Gordon, *The History of Epidemiology*. St. Louis: The C. V. Mosby Company, Medical Publishers, 1952.

POPULAR READINGS

10. Clendenning, Logan, *The Human Body*. New York: Alfred A. Knopf, Inc., 1941.

11. Dublin, Louis I., *The Facts of Life from Birth to Death*. New York: The Macmillan Company, 1951.

12. Hagman, E. Patricia, *Good Health for You and Your Family*. New York: A. S. Barnes and Company, 1951.

13. Heiser, Victor, *An American Doctor's Odyssey*. New York: W. W. Norton & Company, 1936.

14. Hertzler, Arthur E., *Horse and Buggy Doctor*. New York: Harper & Brothers, 1938.

15. Scheinfeld, Amram, *The New You and Heredity*. Philadelphia: J. B. Lippincott Company, 1950.

16. Yutang, Lin, *The Importance of Living*. New York: The John Day Company, 1937.

2. Appraising Health Needs and Interests

Are you a typical college student with a buoyant feeling of well-being, yet with some feelings of insecurity as you seek the answers to perplexing questions about yourself and your environment? Have you established your goals for college? For later life? Have you ever appraised your health assets and liabilities by means of a thorough personal health inventory? Are you aware of your health needs? How does your college environment assist you in satisfying your health needs and interests? In attaining your goals?

One of the reasons for attending college is to learn how to earn a living. Another equally important purpose of college life is learning how to live [29]. This means living healthfully to the fullest extent through experiences gained from the arts, the sciences, and the humanities. An anonymous writer has suggested that in addition to adding years to an individual's life it is also important to add life to his years. This purpose assumes greater significance in our society as we increase man's life span and also increase the number of hours available for leisure. The advantages of a buoyant state of health apply to both earning a living and learning to live effectively. To a student this precept is expressed in the thought-provoking statement: [1] "Without health, the fruits of education may never mature, or they may perish before they can be enjoyed."

Establishing Goals for College and for Later Life

The individual who has his goals for vocation and healthful living clearly in mind has a distinct advantage over the person who has not yet determined such goals. Immediate goals to strive for in college are most practical if they are formulated in relation to long-term life goals.

[1] *A Health Program for Colleges: Report of the Third National Conference on Health in Colleges,* p. 5. New York: National Tuberculosis Association, 1948.

The student who has not thus established his goals is unable to plan effectively. Because he has no incentive to achieve specific objectives, he offers little resistance to the forces which act upon him. Such an individual drifts through college and fails to accomplish tasks, overcome obstacles, or make good personal and social adjustments. He is likely to continue to drift aimlessly from one job to another and perhaps from one marriage to another. He may also fail to achieve a satisfactory degree of personal security.

The student who has his goals clearly in mind is able to plan his activities in order to achieve them. Personal inadequacies, such as physical, mental, and emotional limitations, may force him to revise his objectives if he discovers that he has set his sights too high. External factors over which he has no control, such as being called for military service, likewise may force a revision of his objectives. But the person who plans effectively is more likely to adjust to modifications in his planning and to achieve alternate goals.

In our democratic society the individual is expected to assume responsibility for his own planning. He has the right to determine his objectives and plan his program for achieving them. However, he must select his goals with due consideration of limiting factors, such as the rights of other individuals. A student's goals must be socially acceptable as well as personally desirable, or their attainment is not conducive to good life adjustment.

Setting goals for college and for later life is a difficult assignment, particularly for some students, but it is one which needs to be faced today and not put off until tomorrow. Every student should answer these questions about himself. Why is he attending college? What does his college have to offer to him? Is he making the most of his opportunities in this college environment? Is he taking steps to provide for effective living for himself, his family group, and his fellow students? Is he doing his part to maintain and improve his college environment? These are a few of the questions to consider as a student sets goals for himself. A mature, well-adjusted student seeks the answers to such questions as he plans and puts into action his decisions for achieving goals for today and tomorrow, and the attaining of immediate goals brings him closer to attaining the objectives set for the future.

Reasons for attending college vary greatly with different individuals in the same school. Colleges differ in what they offer just as widely as do the reasons students have for attending college. Some colleges provide excellent opportunities for the attainment of certain goals, while others provide outstanding opportunities for the attainment of different ones. The two-year college, the teacher-education institution, the small four-year college, and the large university—each has specific contributions to make to students. As a student examines his reasons for being in college, he benefits by considering what his college has to offer him.

Health Needs and Interests

One can take steps to achieve an optimum state of health by knowing, feeling, and doing those things which develop and maintain his health status. An excellent starting point for increasing one's fund of sound, scientific health information, for improving attitudes relating to health, and for establishing and maintaining good health practices is to appraise one's own health needs. This appraisal of health needs involves the determining of one's current health status by such means as medical examinations, psychological tests, motor-fitness tests, and health behavior inventories.

In order to make an accurate appraisal of his health needs and interests, one should have a clear concept of the meaning of these terms.

What are needs? Needs, defined in terms of developmental tasks by some authorities [15], arise as an individual attempts to make adjustments to the environment in which he lives. Most authorities stress the significance of both the personal and the social nature of needs, and they commonly define them as wants or desires of individuals, as well as lacks and inadequacies [11, 15, 27]. These factors are considered in the following definition: *Needs are the demands, both internal and external, made upon an individual as he seeks to adjust to his environment.*

One of the most satisfactory classifications of needs on the basis of their source suggests that they arise as shortcomings of society, as predicated needs, and as psychobiological needs [11]. An example of a need arising from the shortcomings of society is the shortage of hospital facilities in our nation. A student is confronted with many examples of predicated needs. Such needs are the lacks or shortcomings of individuals as foreseen by adults on the basis of their adult experience. The objectives of education have been based to a great extent upon such predicated needs. The psychobiological needs are the basis for all activity, either mental or physical. Such needs include the need for food and for activity.

Some of the demands made upon an individual are obvious. They are referred to as *felt needs.* Most immediate needs fall into this classification. They make themselves known to an individual, and he is motivated to satisfy the demand placed upon him. On the other hand, the individual may have many needs of which he is not aware but which make themselves felt sometime later in life. An example of the difference between immediate and long-term, or remote, needs can be given in relation to nutrition. If a person is hungry, the feeling of hunger immediately brings to focus his desire to satisfy the demand for food. This is an immediate, or felt, need. At the same time, there exists a need for a balanced diet to provide the food essentials for building and repair of body tissues, to supply energy for the body activities, and for the regulation of body processes. Unfortunately, some individuals fail to recognize this long-term need, and as a result their choice of food to satisfy the immediate feeling of hunger does not provide a balanced diet.

What are interests? An interest implies the recognition of a need by an individual. It further implies an expression of a desire on his part to learn more about some particular aspect of living. Older persons frequently discover that students are completely uninterested in an aspect of living which the older person considers to be important. The problems relating to rearing children so that they will be well-adjusted may hold little interest for the college student. He is much more concerned with the task of making his own adjustment to members of the opposite sex. An individual who shows interest in some aspect of living is motivated to improve his own condition in relation to this activity. It is significant that Lantagne in his interest studies found that college students showed a 25 per cent greater interest in health problems than did high school students [21].

Health needs in the United States. In order to appraise one's own health status, it is helpful to understand the health needs of the country in which one lives. It is recommended that each individual consider these needs (1) as they may be of direct concern to him and (2) as to the contribution which he can make toward their fulfillment.

A comprehensive analysis of the health needs of the nation was made in 1948 under the auspices of the National Health Assembly. The summary of committee reports [23] and Oscar Ewing's report of the study to the President [13] provide us with excellent sources of information relative to some of the most outstanding needs.

Ewing's summary includes the following information: (1) each year 325,000 deaths occur which could be prevented by the application of available knowledge and skills; (2) each year 4,300,000 man-years of work are lost through unemployable labor power due to poor health; (3) each year 27 billion dollars in national wealth is lost through sickness and partial and total disability; (4) each year only a little more than

10 per cent of the 1 billion dollars spent on all types of research is spent on medical and related sciences; (5) each year half the patients admitted to our hospitals are victims of mental disease.

Three conclusions may be drawn regarding the key health problems: (1) physicians, dentists, nurses, and supporting personnel are insufficient in number and poorly distributed; (2) there are only about half as many acceptable hospital beds as are required; (3) there is no effective plan for local organization [13].

A March, 1952, report from the United States Public Health Service indicates that the need for hospital beds has not been met [10]. According to this report, existing hospital beds total 1,010,000 plus the 190,000 in Federal government hospitals, while the unmet needs are 874,000 beds.

Mortality figures provide some evidence of health needs, but one must be careful in interpreting the significance of such statistics. On the basis of current information available through the National Office of Vital Statistics, the ten leading causes of death include six which are chronic or degenerative in nature [24]. The six are diseases of the heart, malignant neoplasms (cancer), vascular lesions of the central nervous system (apoplexy or stroke), general arteriosclerosis (hardening of the arteries), chronic nephritis (kidney disorder), and diabetes mellitus. The additional four most frequent causes of death are accidents, diseases of infancy, influenza and pneumonia, and all forms of tuberculosis.

Suicide is high on the list of other causes of death. The 16,000 or more deaths attributed to suicide each year and the tens of thousands of additional attempts at suicide are an indication of the large number of persons who find life too difficult to face [12].

A rapid increase in the number of persons in older age groups has been at least partially responsible for the fact that chronic or degenerative diseases or disorders are high in the list of causes of death. Individuals who survive the diseases characteristic of younger age groups are likely to succumb from the degenerative or chronic diseases as they grow older. Health needs associated with our ever-increasing number of older persons constitute one of the greatest problems in the United States at the present time.

A different type of evidence of health needs is worthy of our attention. On the basis of a survey made by the United States Public Health Service, it is estimated that 16 million American families live in housing that has basic health deficiencies. One-third of the 46 million dwellings in the nation have basic deficiencies such as overcrowding (1 out of 7 dwellings); no decent toilet facilities (12,900,000 dwellings, of which only one-third are in rural areas); no hot and cold running water (1 out of 3 dwellings lacks hot and cold running water); and inadequate bath facilities (1 out of 4 has no tub or shower, and 60 per cent of these are in nonfarm areas). Other deficiencies include poor light and ventilation, no dual means of escape, poor heating, open gas burners, and lack of electricity [17].

In the spring of 1952, President Truman appointed a fifteen-member commission. This Commission on the Health Needs of the Nation undertook the task of determining the total health requirements of the United States and making recommendations for meeting these requirements. The findings of this Commission provide a valuable source of information regarding health needs. The 180 million dollars spent on medical research in 1951 amounts to only three-tenths of 1 per cent of the budget allocated to the nation's defense. The lack of skilled investigators, inadequate salaries for research personnel, and inadequate tenure rights are some of the reasons for an obviously inadequate medical research program. Though chronic disease should be approached on a preventive basis, there is less application of available knowledge in prevention of chronic disease than in any other field. Despite the increased attention of the people to the problem, inadequacy in the care of the mentally ill is reflected in the need for 330,000 additional hospital beds to prevent the overcrowding in state hospitals. Considering the fact that accidents are to some extent preventable, the 9,500,000 disabling accidents occurring in 1951 indicate one of the outstanding health problems confronting the American people at every age level [26].

Health needs and interests of college students. The total educational program offered by a college should be planned with regard to the health needs of the students being served. However, each student is an individual whose needs and interests differ in some respects from those of his fellow students. In spite of such individual differences, every student can benefit by understanding the health needs and interests of college students in general. An understanding of the broader problem assists the individual in determining his own health needs and interests.

Data are presented by many authorities on the needs and interests of college students [1, 9, 18, 20, 21, 22, 25, 28]. The information has been accumulated by such means as using questionnaires to obtain information directly from the students; interviewing students; administering knowledge, attitude, and practice inventories; recording the questions asked by students in health classes; having students evaluate content, methods, and materials of health classes; surveying the reasons why students come to the health service for medical care; studying the health records of students; analyzing the reasons why students seek the assistance of, or are referred to, the counseling services; analyzing the causes of failure in school and reasons for withdrawals; and observing the health practices of students in their college environment.

When the findings are grouped according to the areas of health instruction, they indicate that needs relating primarily to *mental health*—problems of adjustment to self and to others—are most frequent. High on the list of interests in most of the studies one also finds the health needs relating to *family-life education*. The freshman in college is concerned with his adjustment to members of the opposite sex and is beginning to consider the selection of a life partner and the establishing of his own family.

Recent studies note an increase in the needs and interests associated with the use of *stimulants* and *depressants*. The use of alcohol causes problems for some students. In addition, the sleep-inducing drugs and stay-awake pills are a menace to the health of others.

Although mental health, family-life education, and stimulants and depressants cover the areas which seem to provoke the greatest interest in a majority of the college students, interest is high concerning aspects of nutrition, such as eating foods which will maintain a trim figure and neat appearance, specific communicable and chronic or degenerative diseases, consumer health, accidents and how to prevent them, and other personal health problems. An elaboration of needs in the light of their mental and physical health implications may be of assistance to the individual in appraising his own needs.

Needs and interests relating primarily to mental health. College students have some needs and interests which are concerned more specifically with mental health than with physical health. Actually these two facets of health—mental and physical—are so interrelated that it is difficult to separate them even for discussion purposes. Factors which influence one's mental health likewise influence physical health, and vice versa. For discussion purposes those needs which are concerned primarily with the mental health of the student are considered first.

Needs which are related basically to the mental health of the college student may be grouped under such headings as (1) the adjustments associated with home and family relationships, (2) lack of motivation and self-direction, (3) relationships with other individuals, (4) inadequate emotional adjustment, (5) tensions resulting from conflicting moral codes, (6) tensions associated with the academic program, (7) tensions associated with economic adjustments, (8) tensions associated with problems of housing and transportation, (9) tensions associated with the disparity between individual goals and a student's capacity to achieve them, and (10) worry about personal health [3, 7, 9, 14, 28].

The listing of these ten areas does not signify that they are separate and distinct. Many needs arise as a result of a combination of factors, and sometimes one problem may lead to another and in this way involve several of the areas. These adjustment problems are considered in detail in Chapter 5.

Family-life education and the use of stimulants and depressants are high on the interest list. It is significant that these two areas are included in the ten headings considered in relation to mental health. College students are involved in the process of establishing good relationships with members of the opposite sex. Petting and premarital sex relations are immediate problems which many college students have difficulty in solving satisfactorily. Students are confused in some instances because of the lack of accurate information, in others because of conflicting moral codes regarding sex relationships. Most college students are vitally concerned with laying the proper foundation for a successful marriage and a happy home of their own. They feel the need of assistance in reaching this goal.

The use of alcohol is sometimes a problem. Some students, coming from homes where alcohol has not been used and associating now with other students who accept its use, must resolve the conflict between the moral code established in their homes and that practiced by other members of their school group.

The time required for studies, work, and social activities results in the piling up of school assignments unless the student plans carefully. When this happens, some students begin to use stay-awake drugs for long periods of time in order to cram for exams and to complete other work. Occasionally, a student because of emotional tensions finds it difficult to sleep and, as a result, makes use of sleep-inducing drugs. In either case—stay-awake drugs or sleep-inducing compounds—a vicious habit may be started.

Problems associated with the use of stimulants and depressants have serious implications for the physical health of the individual as well as for his mental health.

Needs and interests relating to physical health status. Needs relating primarily to physical health status range from the frequent but usually short-lived annoyance of the common cold to chronic and seriously disabling disorders, such as rheumatic heart disease. The list of specific physical health needs which may be of concern to a college student is extensive, and the degree to which a student is affected varies greatly from person to person. Health needs of this type result in difficult adjustment problems for some.

Ill health is a liability. Therefore it is imperative that each student reduce the number and severity of the conditions which cause ill health.

Information gathered from health service records provides some insight into the problem as it concerns the general college student [9, 28]. Colds and other common respiratory infections are the most frequent cause of students seeking the assistance of health service personnel. Skin disorders resulting either from infections or from dietary inadequacies also cause many to seek treatment through the college health service. Problems associated with vision and with hearing difficulties cause some to call upon the school physician, though there is evidence that more individuals should be under medical care for the prevention and treatment of such troubles.

The increase in the number of students requiring medical care after busy school week ends and holidays and near the end of the semester indicates that chronic fatigue and the resulting poor health are a problem to some. Nutritional insufficiencies are found to be a contributing factor in the poor health status of a number of such cases.

Failure to plan effectively for adequate rest, relaxation, sleep, and leisure-time activities is commonly suggested by students as the reason for a general run-down physical condition. A student who is active in the social life of his college finds that careful planning is necessary in order to provide for adequate rest, along with the time required for studying and for leisure-time activities. A high percentage of students, at some time during college, find that their program is out of balance for one reason or another, and the effect on their general health becomes quite apparent to them.

Of the more serious communicable diseases which attack the college age group, tuberculosis poses the greatest problem at the present time. Medical science and education have been partially successful in reducing the seriousness of this disease. Tuberculosis may be further reduced in prevalence and severity through improved and intensified case finding, development of effective immunization procedures, and the application of specific drug treatment. At the present time it continues to be a threat to the health of many college students.

In the general population, the age group which includes college students has a comparatively high venereal-disease rate. College students as a group do not contract venereal diseases to the extent that the general population does. However, any sexually promiscuous individual is a possible source of venereal infection. Therefore, these diseases are a problem to some college students.

Although the chronic or degenerative diseases do not specifically become a problem to most college students, there are some individuals in this group who have malignant growths, diabetes, nephritis, heart disorders, or rheumatism. In addition, it might be noted that the parents of college students are in the age groups more frequently affected by such disorders. The individual whose parents or relatives have such diseases has a need for accurate information which enables him to clarify his attitudes and beliefs about these diseases. Much false information and many poor attitudes exist in regard to cancer, heart disease, and diabetes. Such information and attitudes create problems for an individual.

College students who eat all their meals at one of the college- or university-regulated food services are likely to be *offered* a well-balanced diet. The offering of well-balanced meals does not ensure, however, that the students select all those foods which are provided. In addition, many students eat their meals in restaurants or other public eating places where they may not be offered foods which provide all the nutrients needed by the body. College students, generally speaking, are well-fed. Few college students show extreme deficiency symptoms. Many students, on the other hand, are operating at a level below their achievement potential because of insufficiencies in their diet.

Because of the impending selection of a mate, the hereditary transmission of characteristics or traits becomes a concern for some students. Evidence about the extent of this need is not abundant. The individual who is concerned should seek help in securing accurate information to solve personal problems of this type.

Accidents continue to play an important role as a cause of disablement or death. Students have accidents in living quarters on and off campus, in vehicles used for transportation to and from school or for recreational purposes, in physical education activities, and in the school buildings. To some degree, partial disablement resulting from an accident affects nearly every student at one time or another during his college career.

The individual student is confronted with the need for selecting competent health services, particularly if the college health services are limited in scope. The influence of advertising makes it difficult to evaluate effectively the many health products which are offered for sale. Some of these products are harmless, and the only ill effect is felt in the pocketbook. In some instances, however, the products are harmful to a particular person. The widespread use of laxatives, painkillers, and vitamin preparations illustrates the need for improved understanding in this area.

Corrective or adaptive programs carried on by the physical education department, working closely with medical personnel, provide evidence of a need for assisting students in overcoming postural problems or difficulties associated with body mechanics. Remediable defects of this type can have a pronounced effect on the individual psychologically as well as physiologically. The detection and correction of such defects are beneficial to many college students.

Poor muscular coordination is a severe health problem for some students because of restricted participation in many group activities. An individual may limit his physical activity to the extent that his health is affected, or he may develop attitudes which destroy many of the benefits to be derived from activities.

The health needs of college students which have been discussed in the preceding pages can be summarized under the following headings: [2]

1. Mental health.
2. Family life.
3. Stimulants and depressants.
4. Nutrition.
5. Communicable and chronic diseases.
6. Consumer health.
7. Accidents and their prevention.
8. Balanced program of physical activity, rest, and relaxation.
9. Social relationships (responsibilities for the health of others).

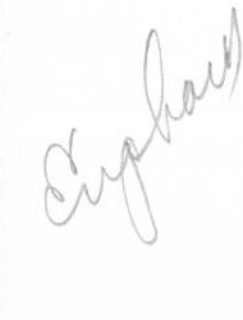

Appraising personal health needs and interests. Techniques for collecting information on the health needs and interests of college students are suggested earlier in the chapter. One can make use of some of these techniques and of others to assemble information for his own health "profile."

Health knowledge tests assist the individual in determining the scope of the accurate health information which he has at his disposal for use in planning everyday activities. In addition to determining what he knows, he discovers facts about which he is misinformed and which, therefore, are the basis for poor health practices.

Because a person knows the answers does not mean that he uses correct

[2] Wilfred C. Sutton, *Determining the Health Needs of College Students.* Unpublished doctoral dissertation, University of California, Los Angeles, 1954.

practices, though the informed individual is more likely to know the correct practices. Knowing what one should eat is important, but selecting and eating proper foods is more important. For this reason practice inventories and check lists can be useful in determining which daily health practices are contributing to good or poor health.

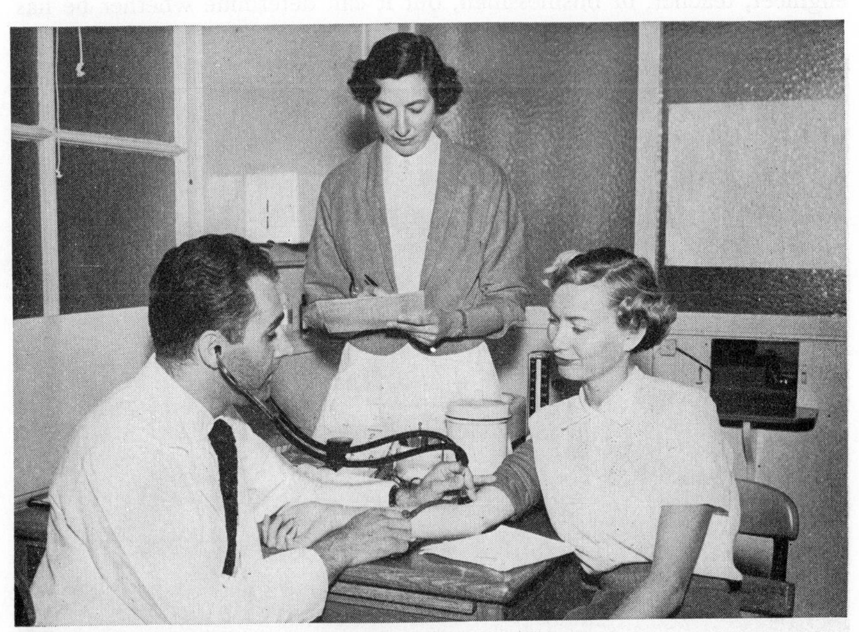

Fig. 2.1. An examination by the college physician provides essential information for determining health status. (*Courtesy of Los Angeles City College. Photo by Lee Hansen.*)

Medical and dental examinations provide information essential in determining health status. The family physician keeps a complete health history with detailed information about the individual and the other members of his family. The function of the medical doctor in treating one who is ill has long been accepted, but his function as an adviser who helps to prevent illness and maintain optimum health is too frequently overlooked. The entrance examination by the college physician provides the health personnel of the college or university with basic information beneficial in health protection and maintenance. It is the individual's responsibility to make the most of the opportunities provided by the health service personnel.

The importance of establishing goals which are personally desirable and socially acceptable is stressed earlier in the chapter. These goals also must be within the realm of possible attainment by the individual. The counseling service on the campus provides an opportunity for determining through appraisal of capacities, aptitudes, and interests whether or not a student is likely to attain certain vocational goals. The counseling service personnel cannot be expected to determine by testing and through interviews that a student will become an outstanding doctor, lawyer, engineer, teacher, or businessman, but it can determine whether he has

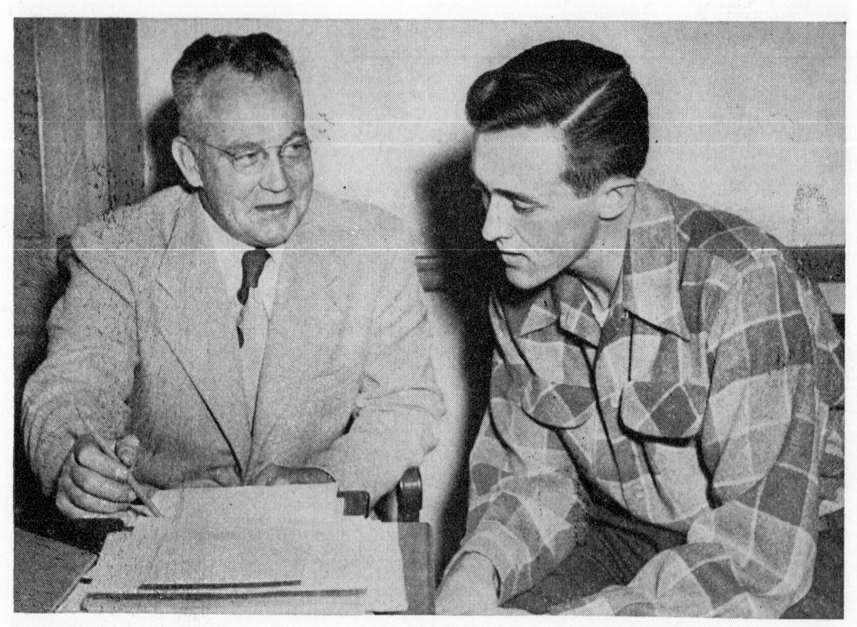

Fig. 2.2. A dean of students, an understanding counselor, provides assistance in clarifying health needs. (*Photo by Stanley Troutman.*)

the qualifications which make for success in a particular field. It is helpful to add information from the counseling services to one's health profile.

Physical education classes should be looked upon as more than periods of physical activity. They should help the student to assess his capabilities in various types of recreational and physical activity according to his individual capacity and likes and dislikes. The function of health service personnel and corrective or adaptive specialists in the physical education department in relation to body mechanics is suggested earlier in the chapter. Information relative to posture and body mechanics is an important aspect of a health profile.

Additional information can be obtained by the individual himself. A diary-type record of one's activities for a period of time provides a good deal of help in appraising personal health status. The balance of activities which shows up in such a record aids in developing and maintaining optimum health. Insufficient periods of rest and sleep, inadequate diet and poor eating habits, too little or too much physical activity, and evidence of inability to get along with other individuals are some of the findings which are of significance to an individual.

The purpose of assembling information to make up a personal health profile is to take advantage of one's assets and to determine one's liabil-

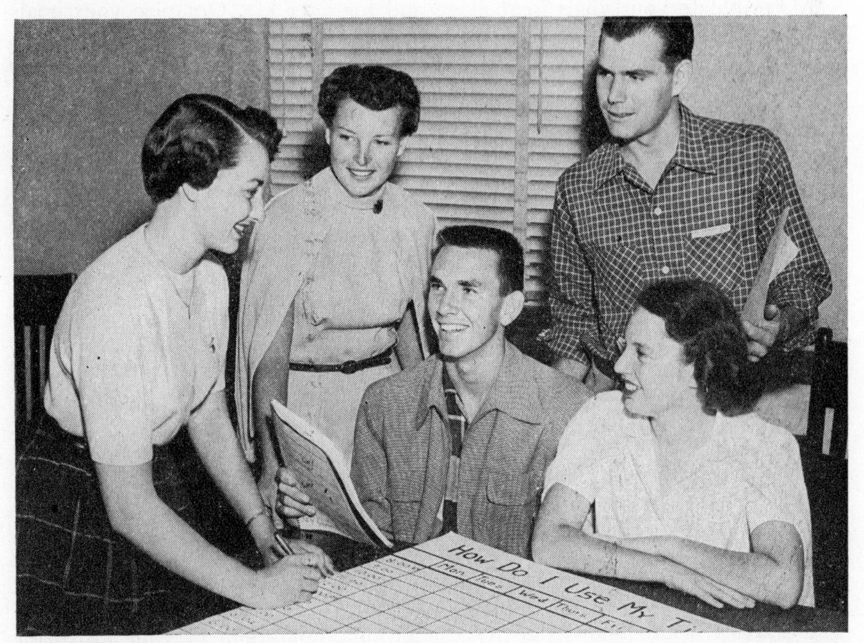

Fig. 2.3. Students discussing health needs and interests as they relate to planning for effective use of time. (*Photo by Lee Hansen.*)

ities. Individual weaknesses should be known in order to concentrate on eliminating them or at least improving them. Gathering information and doing nothing about it is of little value. Individual action is essential.

Before doing additional reading one should appraise his own health potential and plan ways to take advantage of opportunities for developing and maintaining optimum health and for meeting his health needs and interests. The activities listed at the conclusion of the chapter include suggestions regarding some procedures to follow in making this appraisal.

Summary

The individual who clearly understands his own health needs as well as the health needs of the group is more likely to develop and maintain that quality of life which enables him to live most effectively. The preceding discussion of the meaning, identification, and appraisal of health needs and interests of college students provides a basis for the information in the following chapters, which are designed to assist the individual in satisfying his health needs.

Suggested Activities

1. Formulate your goals for college and for later life. Organize your goals for your future vocation and for effective living so that you can refer to them and make revisions as they are needed.

2. Record all your activities for each day for a period of a week or longer. Include sufficient information to show the factors which are influencing your health status. The record should show the time allotted for eating, sleeping, studying, grooming, and recreation; the kind and amount of food which you eat; the type of recreational activity in which you engage; the friends with whom you spend time; and the way in which you solve problems which arise. Analyze the information to determine areas in which you need to improve. Repeat at a later date, and make comparisons.

3. Arrange for an appointment with your personal physician and dentist to discuss the significant information included in your health record. Meet with the physician in the college health service to consider the findings of your medical and dental examination. List health assets and liabilities discovered through these discussions.

4. Make arrangements with the counseling service on your campus to take psychological tests which the counselors consider to be beneficial to you in determining your health needs.

5. Take a health knowledge test under the supervision of your instructor to determine your present understanding of health information. The knowledge tests may be standardized [8, 19], or they may be devised by the instructor to fit the needs of your particular school. Discuss the results with your instructor.

6. Determine your health attitudes by making use of a health attitude inventory [4, 6]. Consider the findings of this inventory with your instructor.

7. Evaluate your health practices by means of a practice inventory [5, 16]. Plan an effective program for improving practices which you find to be poor.

8. Reexamine your goals in light of the information discovered in the appraisal made in the previous activities. Restate goals on the basis of this information.

9. Preview, show, and discuss audio-visual aids pertinent to health needs, such as the following: *Importance of Goals* (sound, 19 minutes), McGraw-Hill Text-Film, 1951.

Suggested Readings

1. Bennett, Bruce L., "Improving College Health Teaching," *Journal of the American Association for Health, Physical Education, and Recreation,* 23:24–26, December, 1952.

2. Bennett, M. C., *College and Life,* 4th ed. New York: McGraw-Hill Book Company, Inc., 1952.

3. Bernard, Harold W., *Toward Better Personal Adjustment.* New York: McGraw-Hill Book Company, Inc., 1951.

4. Byrd, Oliver E., *Health Attitude Scale.* Stanford, Calif.: Stanford University Press, 1940.

5. Cooperative Studies in General Education, "Health Activities," *Health Inventory* I. Princeton, N.J.: Cooperative Test Division, Educational Testing Service, 1950.

6. Cooperative Studies in General Education, "Health Attitudes," *Health Inventory* IV. Princeton, N.J.: Cooperative Test Division, Educational Testing Service, 1950.

7. Crow, Lester D., and Alice Crow, *Mental Hygiene,* 2d ed. New York: McGraw-Hill Book Company, Inc., 1951.

8. Dearborn, Terry H., *College Health Knowledge Test.* Stanford, Calif.: Stanford University Press, 1950.

9. Diehl, Harold S., and Charles E. Shepard, *The Health of College Students.* Washington: American Council on Education, 1939.

10. Division of Hospital Facilities of the Bureau of Medical Services, Public Health Services, "Hospital Beds in the United States," *Public Health Reports,* 67:312–315, March, 1952.

11. Doane, Donald C., "The Needs of Youth: An Evaluation for Curriculum Purposes," *Teachers College Contribution to Education* 848. New York: Teachers College, Columbia University, 1942.

12. Dublin, Louis I., *The Facts of Life from Birth to Death.* New York: The Macmillan Company, 1951.

13. Ewing, Oscar R., *The Nation's Health—A Ten Year Program: A Report to the President.* Washington: Government Printing Office, 1948.

14. Groves, Ernest R., "Mental Hygiene in College and University," *Social Forces,* 8:37–50, September, 1929.

15. Havighurst, Robert J., *Developmental Tasks and Education.* Chicago: University of Chicago Press, 1948.

16. Johns, Edward B., and Warren L. Juhnke, *Health Practice Inventory.* Stanford, Calif.: Stanford University Press, 1952.

17. Johnson, Ralph J., "Health Departments and the Housing Program," *Public Health Reports,* 67:65–72, January, 1952.

18. Kamm, Robert B., "Personalizing the College Experience," *School and Society,* 72:261, Oct. 21, 1950.

19. Kilander, Holger F., *Health Knowledge Test.* Yonkers, N.Y.: World Book Company, 1951.

20. Kitzinger, Angela, "Sans Blood and Bone," *Journal of the American Association for Health, Physical Education, and Recreation,* 21:20–30, September, 1950.

21. Lantagne, Joseph E., "An Analysis of the Health Interests of 1000 Junior College Students in California," *Junior College Journal,* 21:429–433, April, 1952.

22. Metheny, Eleanor, "Some Health Problems of College Women," *Journal of Health and Physical Education,* 17:207–208, April, 1946.

23. National Health Assembly, *America's Health.* New York: Harper & Brothers, 1949.

24. National Office of Vital Statistics, "Leading Causes of Death," *Public Health Reports,* 67:90–95, January, 1952.

25. Oberteuffer, Delbert, "Personal Hygiene for College Students," *Contribution to Education* 407. New York: Teachers College, Columbia University, 1930.

26. President's Commission on Health Needs of the Nation, *Building America's Health,* Vol. 1, *Findings and Recommendations.* Washington: Government Printing Office, 1953.

27. Quillen, I. James, and Lavone A. Hanna, *Education for Social Competence.* Chicago: Scott, Foresman & Company, 1948.

28. Sutton, Wilfred C., *Determining the Health Needs of College Students.* Unpublished doctoral dissertation, University of California, Los Angeles, 1954.

29. Tyler, Harry E. (Ed.), *Learning to Live.* New York: Rinehart & Company, Inc., 1940.

3. Exploring the College Health Program

Are you aware of all the opportunities for healthful living in your college environment? Do you know why there is a planned program of experiences and services for the individual student and the college group? Do you know who is involved in this program? Do you know how these experiences and services are organized into a functional program? Do you know what experiences and services are available for you? Are you sure you know where these experiences and services are found? Do you know when they are available?

The last six questions are the age-old ones of who, what, when, where, why, and how. They have been arranged in a more logical order so that they serve as a framework for presenting health information pertaining to the student's college environment.

Why Healthful Living in the College Environment?

Health today is considered both an individual and a group responsibility. This basic principle must be in operation if the quality of life is to be improved. The college is one segment of society where this health principle is brought clearly into focus. There are other considerations operating today which underlie the development of experiences and services for healthful living in the college environment. These include the objectives of higher education, the legal provisions governing the college or university, and the moral responsibility of the personnel involved. With such considerations in view, the college authorities provide opportunities for developing the maximum potentialities of students and establish procedures for the protection of the total college family, including students, faculty, and other personnel. Thus every college or university has a health program designed to promote, protect, and maintain the health of its students while they are in residence as members of the student body.

Such a program also is planned to develop understandings, attitudes, and practices during one's college career which will carry over into later years to improve individual and community health.

The student-body member, too, has responsibilities for the college health program. Three specific student responsibilities are the following: (1) to determine and explore the experiences and services provided by the college; (2) to utilize fully the services which are available to him; (3) to participate in experiences, such as class projects, individual endeavors, committees, councils, and student-organization activities, to improve and maintain effective living in the college environment.

Who Is Involved?

All persons interacting in the college environment influence healthful living directly or indirectly, that is, every one with whom the student comes in contact, not only fellow members of the student body.

Faculty members play a vital role through their instruction and guidance of students. Certainly, deans and counselors contribute immeasurably to a wholesome environment through their guidance and counseling services. Each faculty member sets the emotional climate in the classroom, which is an important environmental factor. Often, faculty members are aware of health needs of students as a result of keen observation and real interest in their welfare. In addition to imparting information, they are responsible for assisting students in solving their own problems. The whole life of a student may be shaped by the inspiration and guidance given by his professors. Also, some of the best instruction takes place after the class period, in discussions in the corridors or in a professor's office during a conference period.

Other personnel besides the faculty exert their influence. Among these, for example, are the following: laboratory assistants, department secretaries, the girl at the information window at the registrar's office, the admittance nurse at the student health service, custodians, the cashier at the cafeteria, salesgirls at the bookstore, librarians, housemothers, cooks, and a host of others.

The citizens of the surrounding or nearby community also affect the college environment. Particularly is this true of a certain group of citizens, such as doctors, dentists, nurses, health department personnel, voluntary agency representatives, and merchants, including druggists, barbers, beauty-shop operators, and proprietors of eating places.

Naturally, there are a few individuals who play a direct leadership role and who exert a greater influence than the persons mentioned above.

These people, to list a few, include the president of the college or university and his administrative staff; the dean of students; the dean and faculty of the medical school (where a medical school is established); the director or coordinator of the college health program (in some institutions); the director of the student health service and his staff; the director and counselors of the counseling center; health educators who are professors of health education; the campus health officer and his staff of public health personnel, such as sanitarians and nurses; and the director of the department of health, physical education, and recreation.

How Is the College Health Program Organized?

The college health program, composed of activities and services, is organized to meet the health needs of the students in the college environment. The type and extent of the program vary with each educational institution according to its own specific resources. The factors determining the scope include (1) the size, location, and financial resources of the institution; (2) the composition of the student body; (3) the number of day students and dormitory students; (4) the number of married students; (5) the professional health personnel; and (6) the community health resources.

The scope of the college health program. Because of the varying factors determining the make-up of the program no one common pattern of organization exists throughout the country. However, several colleges and universities have established the following administrative divisions: (1) health services; (2) health education (health instruction); (3) healthful college living (a healthful environment); (4) physical education [15]. The activities within these divisions which comprise the program range from minimum first-aid or emergency care and a physical education program during the school hours to a complete array of health education experiences and services, including medical care and hospitalization on a round-the-clock basis. A part of this varied program includes a well-organized counseling and guidance service, along with a diversified program of physical education and recreational activities. The community health resources with their numerous activities supplement and support many of these college functions in a complete program.

Administrative organization. The administrative responsibility for the college health program rests with a director and/or a health committee responsible to the college president, who in turn is responsible to the board of trustees. Some colleges and universities have a coordinator as the administrative officer. In others, the president or a dean coordinates the functions that are performed by several departments. A number of colleges have student members on the health committee or have a separate student health council which makes recommendations for action to the director or faculty committee. The success of the program is enhanced if lines of authority are clarified, if there is coordination of functions among the many departments contributing to the program, if students are permitted to share in the development of the program, and if each faculty member assumes his responsibility for assisting in meeting the health needs of students. Cooperation and support by the administration, faculty, nonacademic personnel, students, and community leaders make possible a functional college health program.

What Activities and Services Compose the College Health Program and Where Are They Found?

The activities comprising the college health program can be understood by a consideration of the specific purposes and functions of each administrative division, along with a description of the contributions of the community health resources.

Health services. A college health service may function as a medical office, an infirmary, a student hospital, or a student health service. Despite the variation in form, the functions are directed to determining student health needs and finding ways and means of meeting them.

Purposes and functions. The health service purposes and functions are as follows:

1. Appraising of the health status of all students (this means assessing the health needs of students through health histories, screening tests for vision and hearing, chest X rays, chest photofluorograms for tuberculosis, medical examinations, including urinalysis, eye, ear, nose, and throat examinations, and dental and psychological examinations).
2. Encouraging and advising the student on ways to correct remediable defects (correcting defects if possible, otherwise referring students to private physicians, local clinics, or other resources as the cases demand).
3. Following up on the correction of defects and the findings of the examinations.
4. Controlling communicable disease, including protection of the student through immunizations, such as those for smallpox and typhoid.
5. Providing medical treatment of ambulatory patients restricted to emergency care only, with limited diagnosis and treatment, or complete diagnosis and treatment (some modern student health services now provide adequate clinical care for the ill as a part of their own function or as a coordinated and

cooperatively conducted function with medical schools and clinical consultants from the local community).

6. Providing dental care (the present trend is to include dental care as well as medical care, at least emergency dentistry).

7. Providing hospitalization for students needing bed care.

8. Providing health education through health guidance—medical counseling for the well.

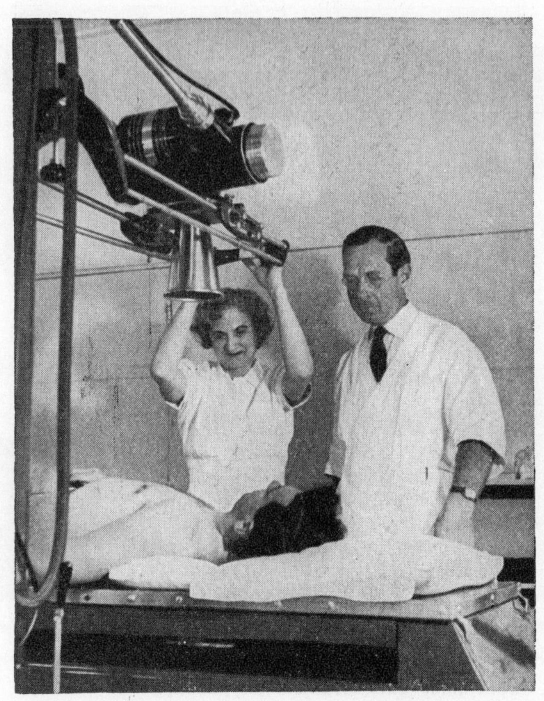

Fig. 3.1. X ray is one of the services offered in many student health services. (*Photo by Stanley Troutman.*)

9. Classifying students with physical and mental defects, recommending the appropriate academic work load and physical activities.

10. Providing mental hygiene and psychiatric care, comprising both prevention and clinical treatment.

11. Cooperating with other departments in providing a safe, healthful environment.

Many of the student health service activities involve health guidance or counseling. More students come to the health service with personal problems such as chronic fatigue, for example, than appear with tuberculosis, anemia, heart disease, glandular disturbance, or other organic disease. Health service doctors often find students attempting to do something which does not interest them or for which they have no aptitude. This calls for vitalized health education on the part of the doctors to the extent of changing a student's course or major. Many students have been saved from dropping out of college by having their load lightened or receiving some valuable advice which relieves worry or anxiety. The

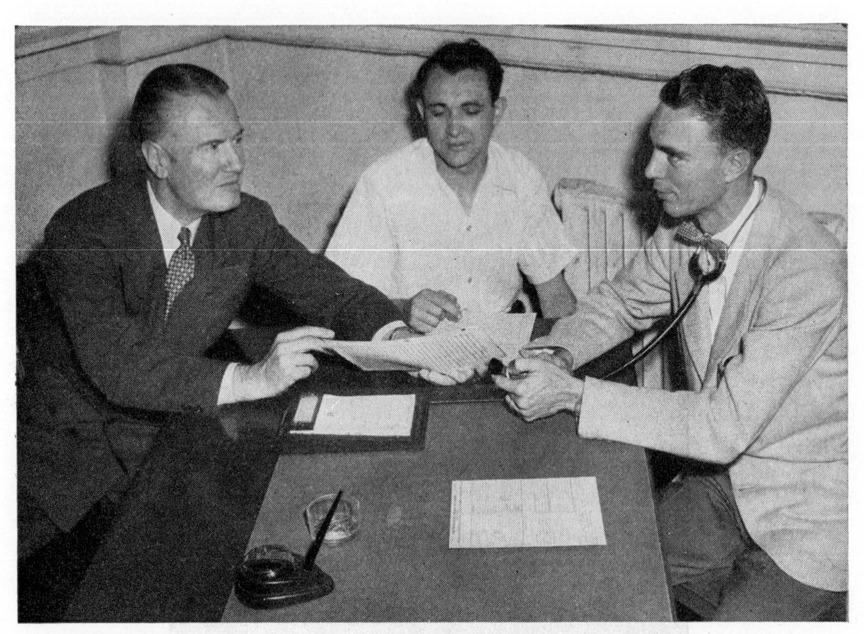

Fig. 3.2. Health guidance on the part of the doctor and the counselor, to assist the student in solving his personal problems, is an important function of student health services. (*Courtesy of Dr. Paul Kinney and Pasadena City College.*)

student who is not sleeping at night may find a consultation with a doctor at the health service most valuable. Proper interpretation of defects found during the entrance or periodic medical examination may relieve needless worry due to lack of understanding of the condition. Advice on premarital and marital health is given students by the staff when it is requested. The student health service is established to benefit the individual student and the total college community.

Method of financing. In some colleges and universities health services are financed entirely by general funds, in others by a special health service or medical fee paid for in tuition fees or included in student fees. Still others use a required insurance plan, plus one of the above-mentioned methods. It is a wise health service policy to provide the student with the experience of participating in a prepayment plan for medical care. This practice, carried over into later years, serves to protect his health and that of his family.

Medical services. Student health services in every college and university may not satisfy all the above objectives adequately; however, the majority of institutions are striving for complete programs and are rendering a high quality of service. The trend throughout American colleges and universities is to give greater significance and attention to student medicine, a medical specialty designed to meet the needs of adolescents and young adults. This new medical group bridges the gap between pediatrics and internal medicine, the latter of which implies the care and treatment of adults [8].

Staff. The staff of the student health service varies considerably with the size of the institution. The staff may consist of (1) one or more nurses; (2) one or more nurses and a part-time physician; (3) one or more nurses and at least one full-time physician. "Over half of the colleges with 6,000 or more students have at least one full-time physician." [1]

The college or university health service is the center around which the effective health program revolves. Its educational activities and medical services contribute immeasurably toward meeting the health needs of students.

Health education. The health education division comprises the learning activities organized for the purpose of changing behavior, that is, favorably influencing knowledge, attitudes, and practices relating to individual and community health [5].

Purpose and functions. The aim of health education is to provide experiences for people which will improve and protect their own health and the health of others. Specifically, health education is designed to enable people to enjoy healthful living, to live scientifically, efficiently, and happily [11].

Health education experiences occur in many situations in the college environment. For example, health education takes place in the student health service office when the doctor discusses the results of the medical examination with the student; in the gymnasium when the physical education instructor discusses with the student the selection of physical activities to suit his needs or considers with him a problem, such as improving his posture; in the classroom when the student is engaged in

[1] F. G. Dickinson and Everett Welker, "Second Survey of University and College Health Services: 1949–1950," Bureau of Medical Economic Research, *Bulletin* 88, p. 5. Chicago: American Medical Association, 1952.

problem-solving situations concerning such subjects as an analysis of his own daily diet or is assigned to a field trip to the local health center to study the protective health services of the community. Health education becomes effective when the student through self-direction applies his learning to everyday living situations. An example of such application is seen in the student living in a fraternity house who rearranges his

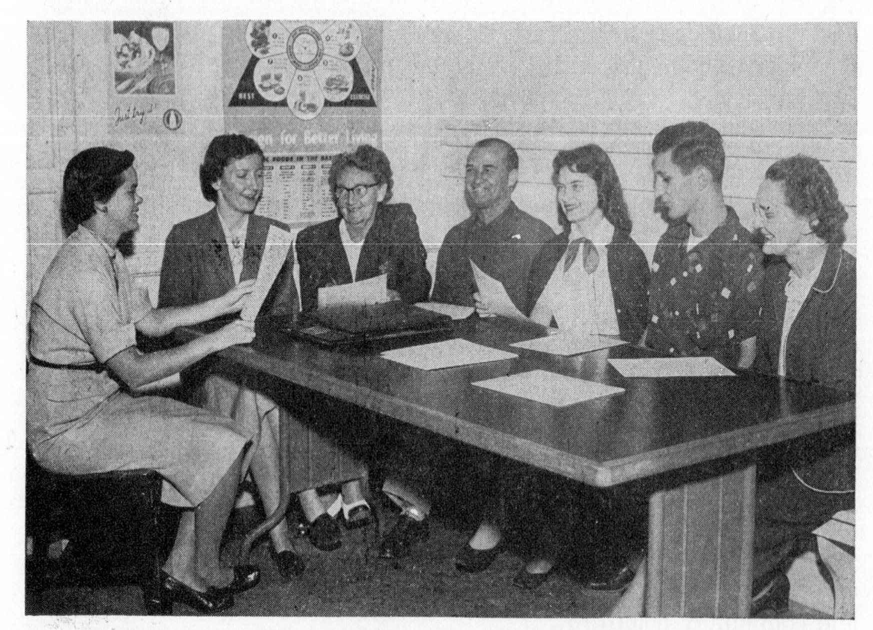

Fig. 3.3. Faculty and students together plan purposeful health education activities. (*Courtesy of Dr. Paul Kinney and Pasadena City College.*)

study desk to receive maximum daylight as well as adequate artificial illumination.

The basic health education course. Since health education is an essential part of the college and university curriculum, the applied science of healthful living is first studied in a foundation course. Common titles for such a course are Personal and Community Health, Principles of Healthful Living, and Personal Hygiene. The content of the course is based on the needs and interests of college students and follows closely the chapter headings of this book.

After completion of the basic course the student is encouraged to enroll in advanced courses, such as Family Relations or Marriage and the Family, Mental Hygiene, Advanced Nutrition, Social Psychology, Culture and Personality, Consumer Education, Community Control of Communicable

Disease, Epidemiology of Chronic Disease, Safety Education, School Health Education, Child Health, Industrial Health, and Rural Health.

Professional preparation. In addition to health education for the general college student, health education experiences are organized in thirty-five or more colleges and universities as a professional major curriculum leading to a career as a health educator. Such curricula leading to bachelor's, master's, and doctoral degrees are designed to prepare school health educators who desire to pursue health teaching in the elementary schools, secondary schools, and colleges. After teaching experience, the graduates may serve as health coordinators and health education supervisors and directors of health education programs. Most schools of public health prepare public health educators with a master of public health degree to work with adults in fostering community health. These public health educators engage in community organization activities, serving as staff members in health departments or centers and in voluntary health agencies. School health educators and public health educators cooperate to develop and improve school and community health programs.

A third category of health education experiences is organized for special professional workers. An example of such a group is the teacher-education group. The individuals composing this group have chosen teaching in the elementary or secondary schools as their profession. In many teacher-education institutions this group is required to complete the basic health education course or a similar one specially designed for them. In addition, they enroll in a course concerned with the school health program and one pertaining to methods and materials of teaching for health. The latter two courses frequently are combined into a core course in school health education.

The experiences in each of the above categories are designed to change the knowledge, attitudes, and practices of people to enable them to live more healthful, productive lives. Health education, then, is an important part of the total college curriculum and is a major administrative division of the college health program. Health education experiences are utilized by each and every division in various ways unique to the divisions themselves.

Healthful college living. This division pertains to those activities, facilities, and interpersonal relationships which provide for a safe and healthful environment. It is the broadest of the four divisions and in many ways is the most difficult to organize and control. Previously, the point was made that all persons involved in the college or university life play a part in the make-up of the environment. Therefore, each person—faculty, student, and nonacademic personnel—shares in the responsibility for providing a healthful environment.

Components of a healthful environment. A healthful school environment encompasses such factors as adequate space, proper lighting, heating, and ventilation, good sanitation, correct seating, regular maintenance, safety, counseling facilities, health services, recreational areas,

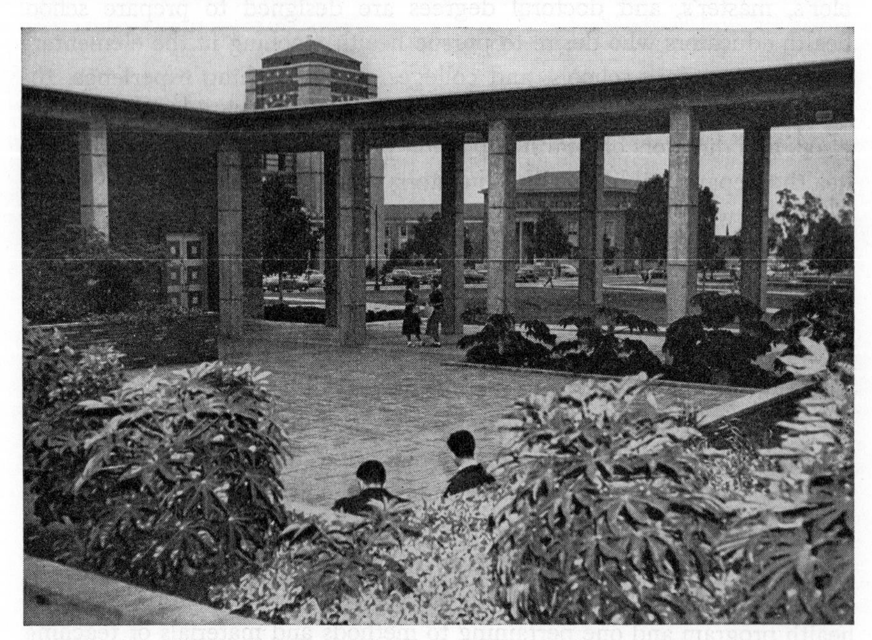

Fig. 3.4. A healthful college environment contributes to effective living. *(Photo by Lee Hansen.)*

eating places, rest rooms, and living quarters. A healthful environment, however, provides more than these physical characteristics. The "emotional climate" is also important if the student is to receive optimum benefits from attendance at college. Some of the factors which exert a profound influence on the emotional climate are the following: (1) the educational qualifications, personality characteristics, and work load of faculty members; (2) the opportunities provided for student-faculty conferences; (3) teaching methods and classroom procedures employed by faculty members; (4) the numbers and demands of the students and the ability of the professor to carry this work load; (5) the attractiveness of the facilities; (6) the adequacy of recreational facilities; (7) the scheduling of time for recreational activities; (8) the nature and extent of school traditions.

The following paragraphs include a consideration of some of the aspects of the environment which make a significant contribution to the health of the student.

Environmental sanitation. Environmental sanitation on the campus involves control of the drinking water and milk supply; the food in eating halls, restaurants, and soda fountains; garbage disposal; water in the swimming pools; health protection of food handlers; housing; building mantenance; and insect and rodent control. Recently added to these functions is the supervision of radiation on the college and university campus. "Radiological monitors" now detect radioactive isotopes and other sources of radiation.

These factors protecting the student and the campus community constitute a major aspect of the college health program. Responsibility for these factors rests with a faculty public health committee, the student health service, a campus health officer, or a campus sanitarian or is assumed by the local public health center in the community. Environmental control standards for these factors are available from the U.S. Public Health Service, Office of Education and Bureau of Standards, Department of Health, Education, and Welfare, Washington, and from the American Public Health Association, the professional association for public health workers.

The student has opportunities to participate in keeping the environment safe and sanitary by taking care of his immediate surroundings. He follows safety precautions, removes unsafe objects, and exercises care in cleaning his room and study area. He properly disposes of leftover food and waste material. He takes part in class and group projects for improving the sanitation and safety of the college or university environment.

Classroom, laboratory, and library aspects. In order to make the most of his opportunities, a college student spends many hours in the classroom, laboratory, and library. An ideal physical environment for learning is provided by a classroom or laboratory which is properly lighted to assure a minimum of eye fatigue, adequately heated and ventilated to promote physical and mental efficiency, correctly equipped with chairs and tables which fit the individual student, and decorated with colors both pleasing and soothing to the eye. The same characteristics are needed in the study rooms in the library, since it is imperative that this facility be conducive to good study habits.

A student under desirable environmental conditions can leave the classroom and laboratory each day with an increased understanding and appreciation of the subject matter, a challenge to discover and understand the significance of topics being discussed, and a feeling of satisfaction with his own contribution to the group. In order to accomplish these objectives the student plans carefully for each class session. He seats himself where he is able to see and hear, in order to receive information, and where he can be seen and heard, in order to contribute to the discussion. If he is assigned a seat by the instructor which is not conducive to hearing and seeing, he takes time to discuss the situation with the instructor.

The mental tone of the classroom and laboratory is likewise important to a healthful environment. The student-instructor relations are friendly yet objective in nature. There is a continuous attempt to explore and clarify values. The student feels free to question the instructor's statements. Student progress is evaluated in terms of growth in understandings, appreciations, attitudes, and skills.

Counseling services. A student may find it difficult to determine his vocational goals because he may not comprehend clearly the personal traits which are required to succeed in a specific vocation or because he may have an erroneous conception of his own personal qualifications. The counseling services of a college are established to help solve such problems.

A student owes it to himself to become informed about available counseling services and to take advantage of the assistance offered. A counseling center provides services to students with educational, vocational, and personal-social-emotional problems. These services include admission counseling, orientation activities for new students, educational advising, vocational testing and advising, housing information, counseling on religious matters, social activities, health services, and other personal and social aid. There exists a close relationship among the counseling service, the student health service, and the physical education and other departments, since all are vitally concerned with health guidance.

Living quarters. Whether one lives in a fraternity or sorority house, a dormitory, a club, a rooming house, a room in a private house, or at home, one's living quarters affect his health and efficiency. For example, good lighting can decrease eye fatigue, headaches, nervousness, and irritability; bright, cheery surroundings have a definite psychological uplifting effect; proper heating and ventilation reduce the likelihood of contracting respiratory diseases, such as colds, sinusitis, and pneumonia; adequate space in living quarters prevents the spread of a number of communicable diseases; properly equipped and arranged quarters, with intelligent use of appliances, prevent many home accidents.

College or university authorities concerned with the housing of students are giving attention to the requirements for good housing, as well as the deficiencies leading to substandard housing. Standards for the quality of good housing are controlled by the campus public health officer or committee or by the local health department in the community.

Some aspects of an individual's living quarters are beyond his control. He can report unhealthy conditions or make suggestions for improvement. In most instances, if his suggestions or recommendations are not carried out, he can change his residence. But there are a number of factors that the student himself can control. It is with these factors of environmental sanitation that the following discussion is concerned.

The unit of measurement of the intensity of light is the foot-candle, which is the intensity of illumination on a perpendicular screen 1 foot away from a standard candle. Proper illumination for eye health and comfort can be attained by having sufficient intensity of light, 30 foot-candles, on the seeing task. The quantity of light is assured by having lamps of sufficient wattage to provide the proper intensity. The local electric-light company will send a representative to measure the light in one's living quarters. Light meters also can be obtained from the college or university maintenance division, from the campus public health officer, and from the sanitation division of the local health department.

Freedom from glare is a basic principle of proper illumination. All lamps should be provided with shades deep enough to cover the bulbs and lights should be properly placed so as to avoid glare. Semi-indirect lighting fixtures give a soft, glareless light which is well-diffused throughout the whole room. Light contrasts are avoided by having sufficient light in enough places throughout the room. Reading by a lamp that is the only source of light in the room is a frequent cause of eye fatigue because of the constant adjustment and readjustment necessary when the eyes glance from the printed page and back again. Approved study lamps have a large part of the light directed to the ceiling as well as on the study desk. Ceiling fixtures are designed for light to be reflected down from the ceiling rather than projecting directly down from the fixture. The combination of study lamps and ceiling fixtures assures proper distribution of light and eliminates dark and bright spots in the room. The color of the walls is important, too, for balanced lighting. Better reflective value and consequently more even distribution of light occur when (1) the ceilings are painted a dull white, cream, or ivory; (2) the walls are light pastel colors; and (3) the furniture is light-colored with a dull finish. The direction of light on the visual task must be correct. This is a factor quite controllable by the student. Floor lamps, table lamps, and study lamps of all types must be so arranged that the student is not facing the light. Light should come over the left shoulder for right-handed persons and over the right shoulder for left-handed persons to avoid shadows falling on the work.

The student has some control over heating and ventilation. Frequently, this is a matter of being aware of the situation. Artificial heat is necessary when the natural temperature is 68°F. or less. It is important that a temperature of 68 to 72° be maintained for comfort and general good health. Overheating is common in the winter season. Discomfort results from an operating temperature over 75°.

Proper ventilation with sufficient air exchange reduces bacterial concentration in the air and disperses body odors and odors from cooking or heat sources. An air exchange of 10 cubic feet per person per minute is an adequate standard [4]. This is obtained automatically in cold weather by normal leakage through doors, windows, ceilings, and walls. In other seasons, the student can make use of windows, transoms, fans, and air-cooling systems. This procedure merely requires good judgment.

Noise has a definite effect on personal efficiency, particularly on study and sleep. Noise is measured in terms of decibels. A decibel is a unit of measurement of sound similar to the foot-candle of light. It is the ratio of sound to the smallest distinguishable noise. Noise surveys have shown that the average noise level for homes varies from 22 to 45 decibels and should not exceed 50 decibels [4]. Much can be done in the construction of modern buildings to reduce noise. The student's recourse in noisy living quarters is to determine whether or not the noise is from a temporary source that can be stopped, to rearrange his study schedule to avoid noisy periods, or to move to a different location.

The student should realize that adequate space in sleeping rooms is necessary in controlling communicable disease. Three feet between cots is proper spacing. This spacing, with ceiling heights of 7 feet 8 inches to 8 feet, gives the necessary 50 square feet of floor area to prevent spread of communicable disease [4].

The student can do much to prevent accidents from electric shocks, burns, gas poisoning, and falls. He can see that all live conductors are placed in such a way as not to be exposed to contact. He can check to be sure metal enclosures of electrical appliances are well-grounded. He knows that wall switches are dangerous if touched by a person in a bathtub or shower. He can be careful with portable appliances to make sure that individuals are not permitted to come in contact with the appliance and a plumbing or gas pipe simultaneously. He must be careful with gas heaters, since carbon monoxide has caused many deaths. He understands that to prevent carbon monoxide poisoning from heaters it is necessary to have proper vents to flues. He also knows it is unwise to use an unvented heater in a bedroom when one is asleep or likely to fall asleep.

The functions of the healthful-environment aspect of the college health program are the most diversified of any of the administrative divisions. Because of this fact, only a few of them have been described; however, these serve as illustrations of the activities, facilities, and interpersonal relations constituting this important phase of the college health program. Furthermore, these examples point out the responsibilities of the college or university administration, the faculty, and the student, who together play a part in creating and maintaining a safe, healthful environment.

Physical education. Although physical education is usually administered in a separate department from health services or other divisions of the college health program, it, too, plays an important role in enabling the college student to live an active, satisfying, effective life. Physical education is concerned with the total development of the student through physical activities.

Purposes and objectives. Participation by the student in physical education activities under the guidance of well-prepared leaders contributes significantly to the student's health through the development of organic fitness and psychological strengths. It provides experience in democratic citizenship, skills, and appreciation for leisure-time pursuits. Such experiences are vital for women as well as for men. Every college woman's life is enriched through participation in physical education activities, particularly in dancing and in indoor and outdoor sports. The student achieves the following purposes and objectives through this division of the college health program [6, 11, 13, 15]:

1. The ability to see himself as he is through self-appraisal of his capacities and limitations.
2. An appreciation of, and responsibility for, a healthy body.
3. Skillful performance in a number of activities providing fitness in terms of strength, endurance, and reserve power.
4. Skills in physical activities to provide continuous recreation in later years.
5. An understanding of the importance and need for rest and relaxation.
6. Leadership ability, as well as appreciation for the talented performance of others.

7. Ability to participate cooperatively and effectively in group activities.
8. Emotional control and release of emotional strains and tensions.
9. Achievement of a normal condition by remedying defects correctable through physical activity.
10. An appreciation of physical activities as a participant and as a spectator.

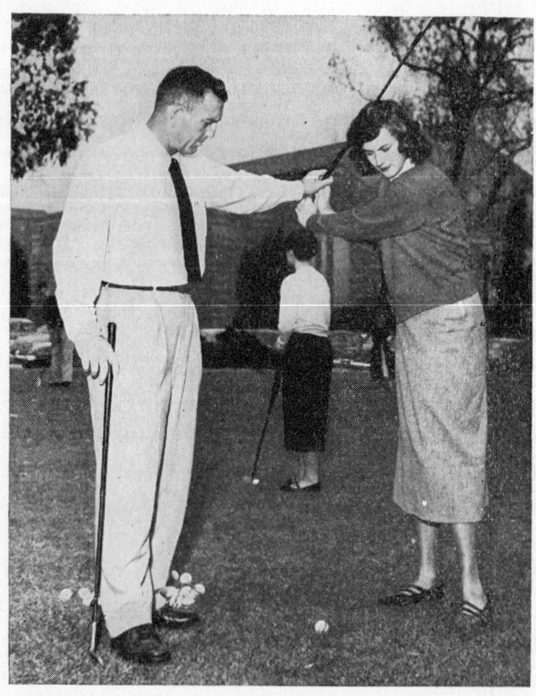

Fig. 3.5. Skills for men and women developed in carry-over physical education activities are valuable assets for continuing recreational activities in future years. (*Photo by Lee Hansen.*)

Functions of physical education. The physical education department carrying out the above objectives includes the following components: instructional courses in physical education on a required and/or elective basis, adaptive or corrective activities, a teacher-education program for physical education majors, recreational activities, and, in a number of institutions, intercollegiate athletics.

Guidance opportunities. A unique guidance function is performed in physical education. This occurs through the informal personal-social relationships between the faculty members and students due to (1) the nature of the activities, (2) the method of conducting the activities, and (3) the interest of well-qualified physical education instructors in the welfare of students. By means of this guidance function, physical education supplements and complements the other divisions of the college health program.

It is through the personal-social relationships with students that the physical education instructor is able to cooperate with the student health service in observing, screening, referring, and following up the student with a health problem. The adaptive or corrective program, supervised by health service and physical education personnel on an individual-need basis, serves as an important means of correcting remediable defects. This cooperative phase of the program also provides a medium for carrying out the classification of activities according to the findings of the student's medical examination. For example, the student who is appraised as "healthy" may participate in any or all physical education activities offered him. However, the student who has a serious defect by necessity is restricted to certain activities.

Physical education contributes to health education through health guidance in such student problems as conditioning, preventing infection, cleanliness, bathing, and adjusting to the opposite sex, to mention a few examples. The permissive, democratic atmosphere in a physical education class in which the instructor promotes personal security, self-reliance, and social acceptance among the students is in itself an example of the contribution to a healthful environment. Other examples include the continuous effort for safety and sanitation of fields, gymnasiums, and locker rooms, the safety precautions in conducting activities, and a morale factor permeating the total student body. This factor results from the participation in, and appreciation of, skilled performance in physical education, including intercollegiate athletics. Skills developed in carry-over sports are valuable assets for continuous recreational activities in future years.

College physical education offers a variety of activities that are carefully selected and organized to assist the student in his total personal and social development.

The contribution of community health resources. Community health resources supplement and support the college health program, and their activities are considered a part of the college environment. In turn, college health resources contribute to the community health program. This reciprocal relationship may be compared to a modern freeway with traffic flowing freely in both directions. A detailed consideration of community health activities is presented in Chapter 17. This chapter presents information pertaining to the available resources in the community. A study of these resources reveals the many possible contributions that can be made to the college health program.

The contribution of the college to the community health program. The college or university contributes in many ways to the community health program through its numerous resources. A few examples are cited. The faculty of the college, with its many specialists in a variety of fields, serves as a reservoir of resource personnel. A professor of sociology may be called upon to serve as a consultant to a community committee studying the types of people composing the community group. A psychologist may be asked to help in developing a public-opinion poll as a device to assist in determining health problems. A dean may be chairman of the community health council. A college health educator working with the public health educator may plan a mental health educational campaign.

The college or university today is a recognized research center. Community problems can be solved through the research of faculty members in such schools as medicine, public health, bacteriology, economics, and business administration, to mention but a few. The students, from the many fields represented in the college, contribute to the community health program by completing projects, surveys, and field experiences involving community health resources.

Many of the college personnel and students live in the community. They participate in the planned activities of the community health agencies, assuming their civic responsibilities as lay citizens.

When Are the Experiences and Services Available?

The experiences and services begin the first day the student becomes a bona fide member of the student body and extend to the last day he spends in the college environment. This period of time may terminate after receiving the first degree or after participation in advanced graduate studies leading to multiple degrees.

Each division or facility has its own schedule of hours, and it behooves the student to become acquainted with these schedules and to take full advantage of the experiences and services provided. However, the description of the types of experience and service shows clearly that healthful living in a college environment is not limited to an eight-hour day but must be considered on a round-the-clock basis.

Summary

The experiences and services comprising a college health program, including the supplementing and supporting activities of the community health resources, are considered in this chapter. The discussion is organized around the framework of why, who, how, what, where, and when.

Suggested Activities

1. Appraise your college health program. Work out a division of labor within your class to obtain answers to the following questions pertaining to your health program: What is its history? How was it developed? How is it organized? Who administers it, and how? How is it coordinated? What are its major divisions and activities? How are funds derived to support its activities? Whom does it serve? What part do students play in the program? How can students make additional contributions? What are present and future plans for improvement?

2. Invite the administrator responsible for the college health program to talk to your class about the health opportunities made possible through the program.

3. Interview the director of the student health service to determine the educational experiences and services available to students. Obtain information relative to the objectives, personnel, facilities, means of support, utilization of community resources, and extent of medical and hospital care provided.

4. Investigate the health education activities in your college or university. Determine the extent of health education courses and experiences offered through your college curriculum.

5. Report on the vocational opportunities offered in school health education. Obtain from your college health educator or send for the pamphlet "Health Education as a Profession" (American Association for Health, Physical Education, and Recreation, a department of the National Education Association, 1201 W. 16th St., N.W., Washington).

6. Report on the vocational opportunities in public health education. Contact your local public health educator or refer to "Educational Qualifications of Community Health Educators" (*American Journal of Public Health,* 38:843–850, June, 1948).

7. Obtain from the American Public Health Association (1790 Broadway, New York 19, N.Y.) information regarding other careers in the field of public health.

8. Determine the departments of the college or university responsible for maintaining and improving a healthful environment. What are the functions of each? How are these functions coordinated?

9. Explore the opportunities on campus for recreational activities which contribute to healthful living. Is there a college or university recreation association for students? What faculty leadership is provided? Are community resources utilized?

10. Report on the counseling service in your institution.

11. Obtain permission from the proper college or university authorities, request the assistance of an instructor, sanitarian, health officer, or representative from the local electric company, and conduct a lighting survey in your classroom, library, or other facility. Borrow a light meter to determine the intensity of light in various parts of the facility surveyed. For standards consult the pamphlet "American Standard Practice for School Lighting" (Illuminating Engineering Society, American Institute of Architects, Washington, 1948).

12. Outline the opportunities afforded you by your college health program in terms of activities, services, and protective functions.

13. Explore the community health resources contributing to the college health program. How much do they supplement and support the program? What resources are not utilized at present? Why? How can greater college and community coordination of effort be effected?

Suggested Readings

1. De Weese, A. O., "Health Education on the College Level," *Journal of School Health,* 21:206–209, June, 1951.

2. Dickinson, F. G., and E. L. Welker, "Second Survey of University and College Health Services: 1949–1950, Bureau of Medical Economic Research, *Bulletin* 88. Chicago: American Medical Association, 1952.

3. Diehl, H. S., and C. E. Shepard, *The Health of College Students: A Report to the American Youth Commission.* Washington: American Council on Education, 1939.

4. Ehlers, V. M., and E. W. Steel, *Municipal and Rural Sanitation,* 4th ed. New York: McGraw-Hill Book Company, Inc., 1950.

5. Joint Committee on Health Problems in Education of the National Education Association and American Medical Association, *Health Education.* Washington: National Education Association, 1948.

6. Kozman, Hilda, Rosalind Cassidy, and C. O. Jackson, *Methods in Physical Education.* Philadelphia: W. B. Saunders Company, 1952.

7. Marshall, H. L., "Changing Horizons in College Health Services," American Student Health Association, *Proceedings,* 29:7, 1949.

8. Moore, N. S., and C. D. Darling, *Student Health and the Changing Order.* Ithaca, N.Y.: Cornell University Press, 1951.

9. National Society for the Prevention of Blindness, "An Eye Health Program for Schools," *Publication* 141. New York, 1951.

10. Nelson, M. J., "The College Health Program," *Journal of School Health,* 21:298–300, November, 1951.

11. Oberteuffer, Delbert, *Physical Education.* New York: Harper & Brothers, 1951.

12. Oberteuffer, Delbert, *School Health Education.* New York: Harper & Brothers, 1954.

13. Physical Education Department, University of California, Los Angeles, *Group Process in Physical Education.* New York: Harper & Brothers, 1951.

14. Pond, M. Allen, "Housing and Health: Sanitary Aspects of the Dwelling," *American Journal of Public Health,* 39:456, April, 1949.

15. Report of the Third National Conference on Health in Colleges, *A Health Program for Colleges.* New York: National Tuberculosis Association, 1948.

PART TWO

Developing a Healthy Personality

4. Appraising Mental Health

Mental health is concerned with the individual's everyday living and today is recognized as an important facet of his total health status. It is a basic contributory factor in the maintenance of physical health as well as social effectiveness.

The increase in problems of mental health is due partly to the inability of the individual to understand himself and his fellow men and also to his failure to apply the fundamental principles of mental health in adjusting to present-day society with its speed, competition, pressure, strain, and anxiety. There is no doubt that these factors also are present in the college environment. This is reason enough to consider mental health, in its various aspects, as they pertain to the college student.

An appraisal of mental health involves a consideration of the following questions: (1) What is the meaning of mental health? (2) What are the recognizable characteristics of optimum mental health? (3) What does an examination reveal of the foundational factors underlying the development of the healthy personality, the emotionally mature individual?

The Meaning of Mental Health

Mental health is a normal state of well-being, a positive but relative quality of life. It is a condition which is characteristic of the average person who meets the demands of life on the basis of his own capacities and limitations [2]. As with the word "health," the term "mental health" connotes a quality of *wholeness* or *soundness*. Mental health is not mere absence of mental illness but is an active quality of the individual's daily living. Mental health governs how he feels about himself, how he feels about others, and how he is able to face the realities of life. It is rooted in his ability to balance feelings, desires, ambitions, ideals, and competencies. It is not some mysterious endowment bequeathed the individual entirely through heredity but is, to a great extent, the result of his own actions, his own adjustments to life situations. The emotionally mature person, described as a wholesome personality, is one who exemplifies sound mental health.

Mental health: a relative quality of life. The degree of mental health is relative, since no one has all the traits and characteristics of mental health all the time. The individual's condition, or state, of mental health is continually changing depending upon his own actions and the factors and forces acting upon him. In appraising his physical health, the individual recognizes that he may have minor deviations from normal or temporary symptoms of ill health, such as a headache. The same is true of mental health. The individual may have a bad day, may be depressed in spirits, or may unconsciously depend upon rationalization in adjusting to a particular situation. Also, he may deviate from normal in one particular, yet make his everyday adjustments. A person under such circumstances is not called abnormal; he is merely described as deviating in one special way. Since mental health is a matter of degree, one person may have a higher degree of mental health than some of his friends who are likewise considered normal.

Normality. What is meant by normal? It is important to understand the term "normality," since it is so frequently used to describe the condition of the mentally healthy individual. In one sense, normal is a synonym for "typical." This is a statistical use of the word, meaning with reference to an individual that he is average. The classic example sees the individual as average in height and weight for his age. One can obtain such averages by depositing a penny in the scale in front of the corner drugstore or by consulting the more accurate age, height, and weight tables which have been carefully devised by using statistical procedures.

A second concept refers to one's overt behavior judged by society's standards. For example, a normal behavior characteristic of the adolescent is "showing off." This is expected of the adolescent because it is natural at this developmental period. Therefore, it is considered normal behavior. This same characteristic in an adult would be considered abnormal, for it is not a mark of emotional maturity.

The third concept of normality pertains to the individual's health status. The individual is well, as opposed to being sick. One may say of a student that he is small in stature for his age, he does some queer things, but he is healthy. This means that he is an active, alert person with a good color and an interest in doing things. Important in this concept is that all normal people have problems to solve. It is when one becomes overpowered by his problems that his condition deviates from normal [12, 17].

Normality, although it is only a relative term, has considerable value in appraising one's mental health. The best single index of normality is a consideration of the total life situation of the individual. His total life situation would include (1) his behavior while making adjustments to his family group; (2) his own inner life, exemplified by his philosophy of life, his self-confidence, and his emotional stability; (3) his relations with friends, acquaintances, fellow students, and professors; and (4) his efficiency in work and study [7].

Mental ill health: a description. Mental ill health is deviation from the normal, the most important point being the degree rather than the kind of deviation [2]. The individual is *mentally ill* who does not make adequate adjustments in society, who is unable to face reality, who does not meet the demands placed upon him in social situations. The *psychoneurotic* individual deviates from normal in that he suffers from a partial separation from reality marked by eccentric behavior. He relies upon a number of escape mechanisms to meet the demands placed upon him. He uses defense mechanisms such as rationalization, projection, and the like, to a greater degree than the normal person, who only occasionally adjusts by means of such mechanisms.

A *psychotic* individual is one who is acutely ill. He is unable to meet his obligations to society. He cannot face reality. He is mentally ill to an even greater degree than the psychoneurotic. These conditions are discussed further in Chapter 5.

People who are making adequate life adjustments are continually striving for optimal mental health in relation to individual capacities and environmental influences. One of the fundamental considerations for the college student is that it is possible for the individual to change his present state of mental health and thereby improve his quality of living.

Mental health and wholeness. In Chapter 1 the concept of psychosomatic unity was developed. In a consideration of mental health, it is necessary to reaffirm the position that the individual is a complex being composed of mental, emotional, and physical traits which are interwoven and interdependent. The individual is considered as a whole rather than in separate parts consisting of mind and body.

Mental health means the efficient and harmonious working of the body as a unit with *all* parts interrelated and interdependent. This implies integration of the mind, the emotions, and the body. Mental health lies in the interrelationship between thinking, feeling, and action. The term "mental" refers to the above aspects of human behavior, each but a part of the total organism, which reacts as a whole to each situation. While the mental and physical factors mutually affect each other, they also are affected by many hereditary and environmental influences. All these influences lead to sound or unsound mental health.

Definition of mental health. Mental health is difficult to define, and no single definition is universally accepted. However, mental health is defined here as the ability of the individual to make personal and social adjustments, to face problems and make choices, to find satisfaction, success, and happiness in the accomplishment of everyday tasks, to work efficiently and to live effectively with others, to demonstrate socially considerate behavior, and to contribute to the betterment of society [5, 8, 10].

Basic terminology. The two key words in the above definition and in most definitions of mental health are "adjustment" and "happiness."

Adjustment. Adjustment is the product of the individual's experiences during the process of development. Each person brings to adjustment his unique personality, which includes his own assets and liabilities. An individual makes an adjustment when he attains a satisfactory relationship between himself and his environment and/or between his needs and his desires. In fact, life is a continuous process of adjustment. Achieving satisfactory adjustments leads to a *well-adjusted* personality, a mature person.

Inability to adjust to everyday situations brings about *maladjustment,* ranging from minor to severe conditions. Some adjustments are physical, such as responding to changing temperature. When one does not make adequate physical adjustments, he becomes ill. Some adjustments are social, such as responding to the social life of the college, for example, joining an interest group—a club, sorority, fraternity, and the like—or participating in the social activities provided by the college. When one fails to make satisfactory social adjustments, he loses his friends and his status in society.

Some adjustments are personal, in which one makes decisions in regard to his own needs and interests. For illustration, one decides between conflicting desires—to stay home and finish an assigned paper which is due for the next day's class or to go to a movie with a girl friend. Inadequate personal adjustments lead to tension and chronic worry. The terms "well-adjusted" and "mentally healthy" are used synonymously in this chapter to describe a person with good mental health.

Adjustment, then, means meeting the demands of a situation. Such action may call for compromises. It implies improving one's own abilities to keep up with a certain group if that is necessary for adjusting to that group. It also implies that one can contribute to the betterment of his own situation without absolute conformity. For example, one can persuade, demonstrate, or prove his point or his ideas in order to alter the demands of parents, friends, and even professors. An individual's adjustment is appraised on the basis of his whole life situation. Such an appraisal should consider the following: To what situation does the individual have to adjust? Examine the setting. In what ways does the individual make good adjustments? In what ways does he make poor adjustments? In other words, how does he adjust? Finally, is he improving in making adjustments [12]? These are questions one may ask himself as a means of self-appraisal.

Happiness. The well-adjusted individual enjoys life. His experiences are, for the most part, pleasant ones. Happiness is the by-product of resolving conflicts, of meeting goals successfully. It indicates that one enjoys human contacts, that he gets along well with people, that such associations enrich his life. On the other hand, chronic unhappiness is a symptom of maladjustment.

Criteria for optimum mental health. Specific characteristics of a well-adjusted mature individual serve as basic criteria of optimum mental health. These characteristics give insight into and an understanding of mental health. The following criteria are derived from the clinical experience, careful observation, and research studies of several mental health authorities [2, 7, 16, 18, 27].

The well-adjusted individual possesses:

1. *An understanding of himself as a personality.* He has some insight regarding his motives and desires, as well as his weaknesses and strong points. He attempts to evaluate his own behavior as objectively as possible. He is able to laugh at himself and his own mistakes.
2. *A sense of personal worth.* He feels worthwhile and important. He has self-respect. He makes use of his natural capacities. He is well-regarded by others. He feels secure in a group.
3. *Personal security.* He feels that he is wanted; he feels comfortable and safe.
4. *Self-confidence.* He has faith in his ability to succeed; he believes he will do reasonably well whatever he undertakes. He solves his problems largely by his own initiative and effort. He does not overestimate or underestimate his abilities. He feels able to deal with the demands of everyday life.

5. *Sound physical health.* He maintains a daily program of health practices promoting healthful living with regard to nutrition, excretion, sleep, rest and relaxation, physical activity, personal cleanliness, protection from disease and defects, etc. His mental health is proportionate to his physical health.

6. *Well-defined, realistic goals.* He establishes socially approved goals and makes reasonable progress toward attaining them. He has some understanding of his environment and of the forces with which he must deal. He plans ahead but does not fear the future. He develops a philosophy of life that gives meaning and purpose to his daily activities.

7. *Ability to get along with other people.* He has understanding of the motives and problems of other people. He respects the many differences he finds in people. He considers the interests of others, and he is able to give, as well as receive, love and affection.

8. *Emotional maturity.* He meets each situation as it arises. He welcomes new experiences and new ideas. He accepts his responsibilities. He takes life disappointments in his stride. He does not go to pieces as a result of his fears, worries, anger, or guilt feelings. He develops a wholesome attitude toward sex. He is capable of making a good heterosexual adjustment.

9. *Integration of personality.* He functions as an organized unit. He thinks clearly and constructively in solving his problems. His mind is adaptable and resilient, and he is able to make adjustments to constant changes and life situations. He is so organized as to control his body, mind, and emotions.

10. *Vocational abilities.* He experiences a reasonable degree of success in his vocational endeavors. He puts his best efforts into his chosen vocation and gets satisfaction out of doing so.

11. *Basic harmony.* He achieves a fundamental harmony with his environment. He feels a sense of responsibility to his neighbors and fellow men. He gets satisfaction from simple, everyday pleasures. He is able to modify his ambitions if they conflict seriously with the rights of others. He strives to improve the society in which he lives.

Mental health implies the satisfaction of human needs and interests and the fullest development of the personality. It also implies the adjustment of the individual to personal relationships and to the stresses and strains of a competitive society, thus precluding behavior disorders. The highest degree of mental health implies a maximum contribution to society over and above the greatest attainment of personal success [18].

Foundations of Mental Health

Mental health is based upon not one but many factors. The basic factors are (1) the total make-up of the individual as a biological organism—his interrelated physical, emotional, and mental traits; (2) the influences of the environment, including the society in which the individual finds himself; and (3) the interaction process between the individual and society—the experiences by which the individual influences other people and is influenced by them. This is the process by which individuals learn and develop into maturity. The individual, within his biological limits, develops into his eventual personality on the basis of his experiences.

The developing person is sometimes spoken of as the self, a unique personality. This personality is a composite of the biological self, the social self, and the self ideal. The biological self is determined by the hereditary endowment. The social self develops from the individual's interaction with his environment. The self ideal, superself, or psychological self is the individual's conscious or unconscious concept of his own behavior, including what he aims to be and do. The psychoanalysts would term these aspects of the self the "id," the "ego," and the "superego" [3]. These interrelated selves have a direct bearing upon the individual's mental health.

For the sake of simplicity in understanding the foundations of mental health, the basic factors have been broken down into common terms. Some of these major factors which are selected for discussion are (1) heredity, (2) some physical factors, (3) the fundamental social forces—the home and family, the school, the neighborhood, and the community.

Heredity. Heredity is the foundation force that provides the raw material, the potentialities of the individual, and sets the limits for his mental health. Heredity itself does not ensure mental health, although the exact role of heredity in mental health is not yet fully known. It is known that heredity accounts for the initial potentialities of the individual.

Hereditary traits are transmitted from parents to offspring by means of determiners of heredity called genes. A new life begins when the sperm cell from the father and the egg cell from the mother unite as a single cell, a fertilized egg. This cell grows and then divides into two cells. Cell division continues until a human body develops, consisting of millions of cells.

The individual's heredity is determined at the time the sperm and egg unite. The single cell contains twenty-four chromosomes from the egg cell and twenty-four from the sperm cell, making a total of forty-eight. These chromosomes are the rodlike living substances that contain the genes. When the cell begins to divide, the chromosomes line up along the center of the cell nucleus, and the chromosomes divide also, making forty-eight pairs. This means that there are two cells with the same sets of chromosomes and identical sets of genes. Every cell has forty-eight chromosomes except the germ or sex cells, which contain only twenty-four. Each cell has the same hereditary material, the genes, as the original fertilized egg. It is the genes, then, that provide the functional potentialities of the individual. The offspring has inherited potentialities pertaining to growth, appearance, intelligence, personality, and the like.

The genes are not contained in an environmental vacuum. They are influenced by both the internal and the external environments of the individual. Any trait or characteristic of the individual, therefore, including intelligence and personality, results from the interplay of both heredity and environment. Primarily it is capacity that is inherited, such as a capacity for thinking, feeling, and acting. How that capacity is utilized depends upon environmental influences.

The part heredity plays is clearer for physical than for mental traits. There is no doubt that one's physical features are inherited. As Scheinfeld [1] points out, "Making faces happens to be one of the most interesting jobs done by genes . . . your size and shape are pretty closely determined by your genes." Since each individual is different from all others, it is obvious that individuality results from the genes. Genes may combine in a great variety of ways and with only minor differences. The present problem is to discover how important these differences are with regard to specific functions. For example, it would be helpful to know which traits enable one individual to live more effectively than another.

Much remains to be learned concerning the inheritance of specific mental traits. Present evidence indicates that the mental potential or native intelligence is hereditarily determined and that the environment determines the extent to which this potential is realized. Studies on identical twins compared with fraternal twins show the importance of heredity. There is evidence that when an individual is well motivated and has ample opportunity, intelligence quotients can be slightly improved. It is also true that damage to the brain resulting from injuries or disease may lower mental capacity. Similarly, an unfavorable and culturally impoverished environment may limit the extent to which mental potential is developed and utilized.

There is no doubt that superior mental traits are found in those persons with superior hereditary endowment. Lorge [2] of Columbia University

[1] Amram Scheinfeld, *The New You and Heredity*, p. 87. Philadelphia: J. B. Lippincott Company, 1950.

[2] As cited by Scheinfeld, *ibid.*, p. 383.

states: "Superior intellectual ability is not a miracle. It is as natural as superiority in height or weight. Basically it is genetically constituted, but what the superior individual will do with his intellect will certainly be conditioned to a large degree by his environment and his education." Genetic studies also show a hereditary basis for special capacities such as musical, artistic, and mechanical ability.

Fortunately for mankind most persons are normal (that is, within a normal range), owing to the efficient workings of the mechanism of heredity. Hereditary defects are generally recessive, while normal traits are dominant. There are a few exceptions as in the rare disease, Huntington's chorea, caused by a single dominant gene. This disease results in complete degeneration, finally terminating in death. There is no known cure.

In most cases there is insufficient evidence of the precise role of hereditary factors in mental illness. Such evidence as there is indicates that most mental illnesses are not directly inheritable. It is apparent, however, that heredity may predispose a person to development of a particular type of mental illness, such as schizophrenia or manic-depressive psychosis, when he is placed under excessive stress. It is possible, too, that heredity plays a contributing role in psychopathic personalities and in the psychoneuroses, such as compulsive neuroses, anxiety neuroses, hypochondrias, and the like.

Heredity plays an important part in the production of many of the mentally defective or feeble-minded—idiots, imbeciles, and morons. It is often a factor in convulsive seizures. The term "epilepsy" (meaning "seizure") is applied to a chronic nervous disorder usually characterized by convulsions. Most authorities agree that epilepsy is not inherited directly, but that a tendency or susceptibility to epilepsy is inherited. This condition does not develop unless there is a weakness or defect in the brain or nervous system and, in addition, a stimulus, such as some accident or injury, an infectious disease, a metabolic disorder, or the like. Two factors are necessary, then, for epilepsy to assert itself: (1) a constitutional tendency or susceptibility, (2) an environmental stimulus.

Wallin [3] concludes that "defective heredity may furnish a fertile soil for the development of mental and nervous diseases, but that so far as minor personality maladjustments are concerned heredity supplies only a predisposing condition, just as do the stresses and strains that accompany the processes of maturation."

[3] J. E. Wallace Wallin, *Personality Maladjustments and Mental Hygiene*, 2d ed., p. 58. New York: McGraw-Hill Book Company, Inc., 1949.

Implications for the college student derived from the available data on heredity in mental health are as follows:

1. It is important for the individual to know his own limitations and potentialities.

2. Of even more vital concern is maximum or greater utilization of his potentialities. Good material has made many football coaches successful in the public eye. The greatest coaches from the viewpoint of the coaches themselves are those who have the ability to get the most out of their players, the material at hand. Improving mental health may be viewed as a parallel: almost everyone can further develop his potentialities, since few persons today are living up to capacity.

3. It is wise for the college student contemplating marriage to choose a mate of sound heredity and to know his own hereditary history as well as that of his mate.

4. Much research is needed to determine further the effect of heredity on mental abilities and specific traits.

5. Finally, the extent to which the individual's potentialities are developed depends upon the other foundation forces, particularly the environment and personal behavior. Heredity is but one factor in the development of personality.

Physical factors. The premise of the total individual functioning as an integrated unit is still upheld in this discussion of physical factors. However, a brief analysis of the physical factors involved in mental health is presented for the purpose of clarifying the foundations upon which personal and social adjustment rest. A major portion of the book is devoted to physical health and the reciprocal influence of the mental and physical aspects. Chapter 9, Maintaining a Healthy and Attractive Body, contains a more detailed account of the total physical aspects of effective living.

From the available data it is apparent that physical health factors make a significant contribution to mental health. The development of a wholesome, pleasing personality, resulting in a well-adjusted individual, is based partly on this foundation of physical health. An erect posture, a winning smile, color in the cheeks, and a feeling of exhilaration promote a sense of personal security and have a marked influence on other people. Strength, good looks, and robust health provide a social advantage in the development of personality characteristics.

A feeling of physical well-being makes possible intellectual alertness, enthusiasm, a good disposition, a desire to live, to achieve, and to be happy. Not all individuals in good physical health have good mental health; however, in most cases the better the physical health, the better also the mental health [2]. There is evidence that mental vitality, not intelligence, is improved by physical health. But the motivation and drive through which the individual applies his intelligence are increased, bringing about added intellectual efficiency.

One can remember without too much difficulty that his own mental health is poor when he is physically tired from hunger, overwork, or loss of sleep. Sick people, particularly the chronically ill, have a more difficult time making life adjustments. The malnourished are persons with whom it is difficult to get along. The data show that vitamin deficiencies lead to poor health and consequent personality difficulties. For example, vitamin B deficiencies result in restlessness, anxiety, and a quarrelsome attitude. In pernicious anemia, a deficiency of red corpuscles produces characteristic symptoms of apathy, irritability, depression, and anxiety. Persons suffering from serious physical defects tend to have similar problems of adjustment, though there are exceptions. On the other hand, the individual who follows a hygienic regimen pertaining to food, drink, elimination, bathing, physical activity, work, sleep, rest, relaxation, prevention of disease, and correction of defects is more likely to have good mental health. The effect of the physical factors is a contributory, foundational one to mental health.

From the mental health point of view, it is necessary to remember that the individual is a person in a body. Actually, the person and the body are one and the same. On the other hand, the body becomes an instrument of the self, the person. After heredity has provided the body form and set the limits as to what it can do, it is through the body that the interaction itself takes place. Contact with the environment is made through the actions of the body, and, in turn, the environment influences the body and the person in the body.

Social factors in mental health. The social factors pertain to the individual's environment, the society in which he lives, and the interaction process, his social functioning with other persons. Of special importance is his ability to make adjustments in social situations and with other people as he participates in everyday activities. These social forces have a foundational effect on the individual's mental health. The goal to be striven for is indicated in David Klein's [4] modernization of an old Latin adage, "A sound mind in a sound body in a sound society."

The environment in which the individual finds himself from birth influences him in a variety of ways. From his own particular environment

[4] David Klein, *The Psychology of Personal Adjustment,* p. 17. New York: Henry Holt and Company, Inc., 1944.

he gains his social heritage. The stimulation he receives, the knowledge he acquires, the skills he develops, the interests he utilizes, the attitudes he forms, the habits he establishes, the values and goals he develops are shaped by his environment. He enters this society which is already established; so he learns to adapt to it and acquire from it the content of his behavior.

From the very beginning of life, the individual is a part of society. He soon notices a few people, who in turn notice him. He uses his equipment—the sense organs, the muscles, and the nervous system—and begins to integrate what he sees with what he does. Interaction takes place when the infant, using his equipment, perceives and responds to others who are perceiving and responding to him in ways that are characteristic of the culture. By this medium the individual gradually changes himself. He learns, he develops a unique personality, and he participates in his society.

The home and family. The first experiences which develop the individual into the person he becomes take place in the home or family. Investigations have shown that young children learn to pattern their behavior after that of their parents. In most cases, both boys and girls are closer to the mother during the first ten years than to the father. The mother contributes to mental health by giving the child affection and security and by guiding his development efficiently and effectively. The child reflects the mother's fears and her ideas of right and wrong [7]. Reports of college students describing their mothers indicate that the mother contributes to mental health when she is gentle, agreeable, and even-tempered. Conversely, mothers tend to cause insecurity when they are nervous, tense, self-centered, and insecure. Mothers affect their children adversely when they are overprotective, reject the child emotionally, are domineering, are unreasonable or inconsistent in disciplinary practices, have favorites among their children, and are not well-adjusted themselves, with a resultant reflection of their frustrations in their children. The mother plays an important role in establishing ideals, attitudes, and practices which are of extreme significance in making adjustments.

The father as a provider generally has less contact with the children, though his role seems to take on greater importance as the children grow older. This is especially true if the father takes time to share his life with his family, if he shows interest in the development of his children, plays with them, works with them, shares their joys and troubles, is just in his discipline, and becomes an ideal in the eyes of his children.

Older children also influence the development of mental health in the family. Often older children, as in the case of parents, provide affection, security, and guidance for younger children, assisting them in establishing ideals and values. Negative influences result if older children dominate and create feelings of insecurity through constant friction. Sibling rivalry is a definite factor in emotional development.

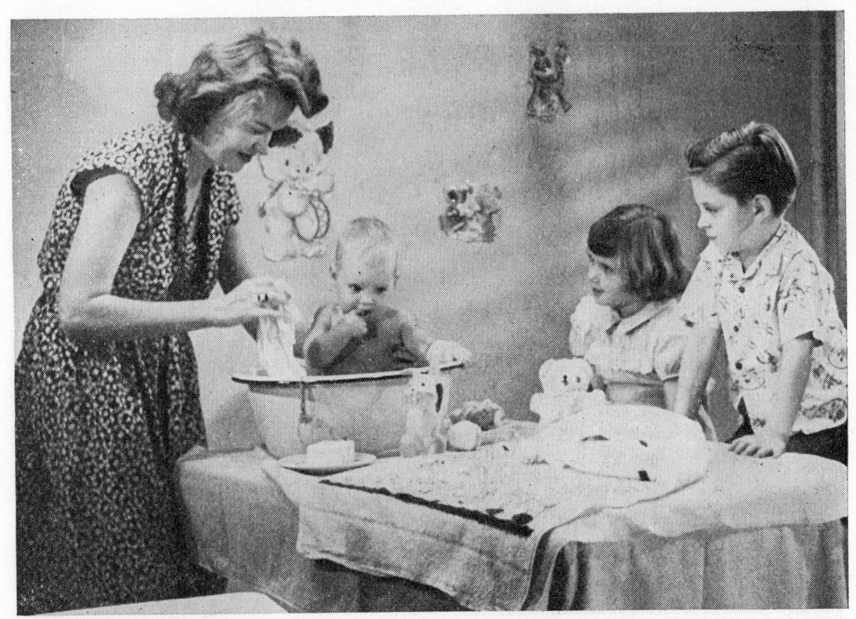

Fig. 4.1. The mother plays an important role in establishing ideals, attitudes, and practices which are of great significance in making adjustments. (*Arnold Eagle Photo, courtesy of Dr. Lester Beck.*)

Evidence from studies shows that broken homes produce a larger percentage of children with adjustment problems than do stable homes. However, not all broken homes result in maladjusted children. A home with one understanding parent is often superior to one in which there are two parents in constant conflict, creating an atmosphere of discord [16].

A good home is one in which there is: (1) genuine affection for each member; (2) a harmonious relationship between parents; (3) understanding on the part of the parents of the needs and interests of the children; (4) assistance on the part of the parents in helping children to realize their needs and interests; (5) consistent, firm discipline; (6) opportunity for children to participate in activities involving responsibilities, engage in play and recreation, and invite friends into the home.

In a study of the relationship between mental health and the family situation, the investigator [5] concludes that "the most important function of modern family life is psychological in nature. Family life meets certain basic human requirements more directly than is possible in any other area of life. In the family situation are provided the setting, the stimulation, and the guidance which determine, very largely, whether the child

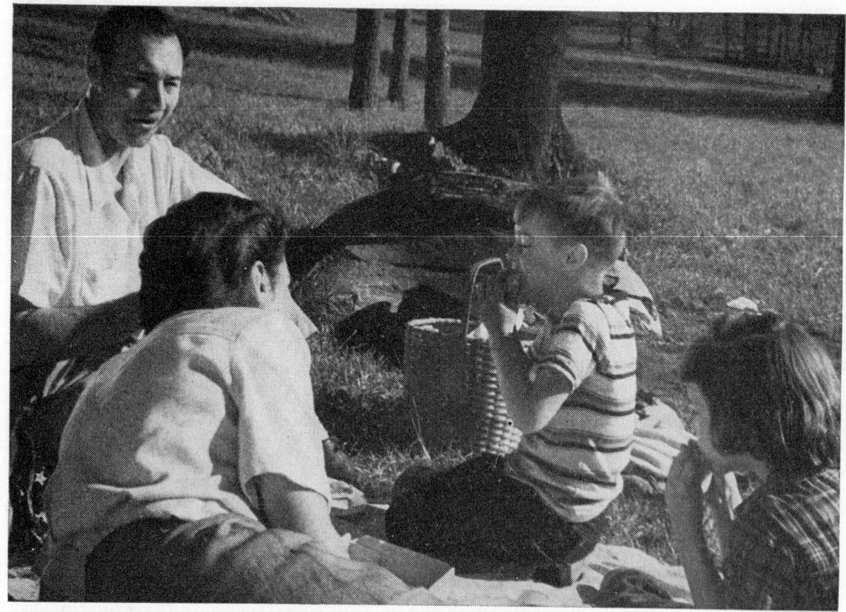

Fig. 4.2. Family life meets certain basic requirements more directly than do other areas of life. (*Courtesy of Dr. Lester Beck.*)

shall develop into a personally well-adjusted and socially useful individual."

The school and mental health. The school is the chief continuing and supplementing institution in which individuals develop sound mental health practices. The school is charged with providing experiences to develop the total individual through self-realization, human relationships, economic efficiency, and civic responsibilities. School experiences are designed to enhance growth and development, stimulate learning, and develop good behavior patterns. This calls for pupils participating in an enriched curriculum, under the guidance of well-adjusted teachers and

[5] Leland H. Stott, "Personality Development in Farm, Small Town, and City Children," University of Nebraska Agricultural Experiment Station, *Research Bulletin* 114, pp. 28–34, 1939.

administrators, in a wholesome environment. To achieve the purposes of the school, the experiences comprising the school curriculum are designed to meet the fundamental individual needs for (1) a feeling of personal worth; (2) social competence in winning acceptance from associates; (3) physical satisfactions necessary to the well-being of the body; (4) freedom to play and to accomplish purposeful tasks; and (5) developing interests and activities providing social values [6, 15].

The experiences in school, in addition to experiences in the home, determine, to a large degree, one's sense of personal worth. The result of schoolwork is not always positive from a mental health standpoint. Self-realization is achieved to the extent that successful adjustments are made and satisfactory progress results. On the other hand, if the school experiences cause many emotional stresses, do not provide affectional responses, and offer few chances for success, there is likelihood that the individual will adjust by using socially undesirable defense mechanisms. The pupil is expressing feelings of insecurity, anxiety, or frustration if his conduct in school takes the form of antisocial destructive behavior or if he shows withdrawal or regressive tendencies.

Social growth outside the family is developed to a great extent in school. The feeling of personal acceptance which one acquires lays the groundwork for socializing with others. The individual learns to respect the rights, feelings, and property of others in school. He learns to win the approval of his associates and to feel secure in the presence of others.

The school shares with the home in the development of social and cultural values. The attitudes and habits which become the attributes of mature adults are determined to a large measure through school experiences. The school exerts a dominant influence in the formation of attitudes and practices relating to customs, morals, politics, sex, marriage, and principles of living in general. These attitudes, whether positive or negative, are instrumental in determining the effectiveness of the behavior of the individual in society.

The school contributes to the development of sound mental health, assisting in preventing behavior disorders, when it provides the following:

1. Respect for the pupil as an individual.
2. Regard for the whole personality as an integrated unit.
3. An enriched curriculum of activities, cooperatively planned, meeting the needs and interests of pupils.
4. Extraclass activities, a part of the curriculum, such as dramatics, clubs, athletics, and recreational pursuits, for the development of broad interests of pupils.

5. Developmental tasks for each student, allowing some freedom in accomplishing the tasks.
6. Tasks adjusted to the level of development of each student.
7. Activities which develop habits of cooperation, an attitude of civic responsibility, and a creative approach to life.
8. Well-adjusted teachers and administrators.
9. Individual and group counseling.
10. A wholesome environment for pupils and school personnel.

In addition to the above preventive measures, the school attempts to identify children with problems and refer cases with behavior disorders to child guidance clinics. The school attempts to provide well-adjusted classroom teachers, specially prepared teachers in health education, family-life education and counseling, psychologists, and psychiatrists in child guidance centers. Also, the existing mental health resources of the community are utilized for carrying out this corrective health service program.

The Delaware public schools, working with the Delaware State Society for Mental Hygiene, have organized classes in human relations which in actuality are direct teachings in mental health. The objectives of this program are to assist in the growth and development of children by improving their ability to [6]

> . . . make decisions, accept responsibilities, learn from their own emotional mistakes, make and keep friends, bring their fears out into the open, carry on to the best of their ability when emotionally disturbed, accept themselves and depend less on artificial entertainment, face the past or the future without fear, face up to unpleasant fearful or distasteful events of the present, look at unknown future changes as interesting adventures to be faced.

The community and mental health. It is only within recent years that the community has been considered a foundational factor in mental health. The modern concept of mental health stresses more and more the importance of community life, as well as the practices engaged in by the individual and family. According to this modern concept, the mental health of the individual in a group is of concern to all members of that group. Likewise, the individual's mental health is related to his ability to fulfill his family responsibilities; to his efficiency in his chosen vocation; and to his acceptance of social responsibilities in his neighborhood and his community, which assist in bringing about changes in the

[6] H. Edmund Bullis, "A Positive Mental Health Program," *American Journal of Public Health*, 40:1114, September, 1950.

cultural pattern. "The community furnishes the framework and climate within which the family lives and develops; it must therefore provide a healthy atmosphere and a well-organized network for public and private community services of the highest possible quality." [7]

Also, the community provides supplementary services for mental health for all its people. When families fail to satisfy mental health needs,

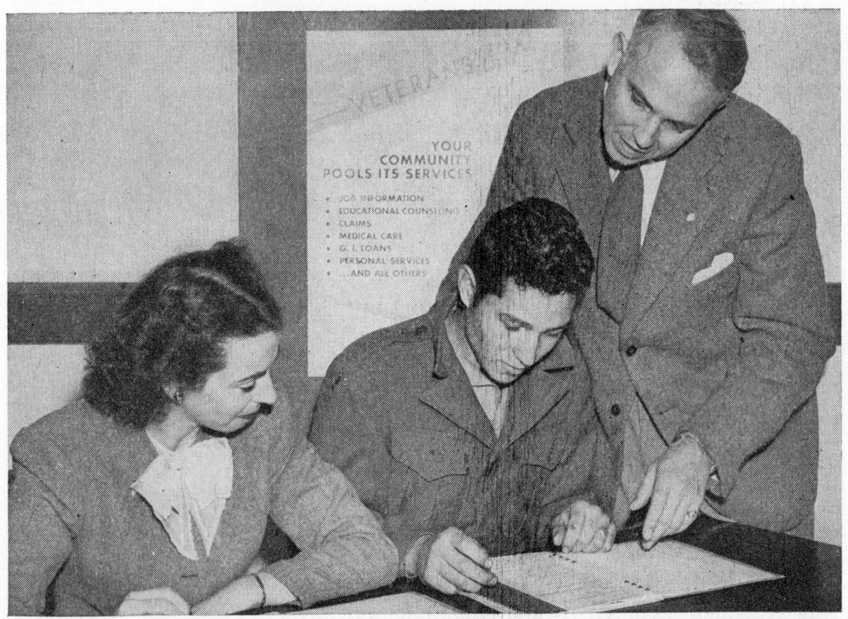

Fig. 4.3. The community provides services for the mental health of all its people. (Courtesy of *Dr. Lester Beck.*)

such as love and affection, a feeling of belonging, encouragement, and opportunities for group participation and for emotional release, then the communities must offer ways and means to supply these individual needs.

The mental health needs of the community have been determined by authorities through study of healthy people for the preventive approach and of the mentally ill for the treatment, or clinical, approach. The results of these studies indicate the mental health needs of the community to be (1) education of the general public to understand the forces and factors that maintain and improve mental health as well as impair it (this means educating the citizens of the community with regard to the

[7] Committee on Consultants on Community Reorganization, *A Consultant's Report: Reorganization of Community Services,* p. 9. New York: The Woman's Foundation, 1945.

basic principles of personal and social adjustment, such as how personality develops, the motivational drives, and how mental illness is related to the mismanagement of these drives); (2) a well-rounded recreational program conducted by well-qualified personnel with adequate equipment and facilities; (3) united efforts to strengthen the family, family groups making up the neighborhood, and communities, in order to hold together homes that might be broken up because of mental illness; (4) counseling services for people who are troubled by the cares and strains of everyday living; (5) early detection, diagnosis, and treatment of minor maladjustments; (6) treatment of those mentally ill who do not require hospitalization but are outpatients or ambulatory cases; (7) treatment for seriously disturbed or psychotic individuals who need hospitalization; and (8) procedures for the return of the mentally ill to useful citizenship [13, 14].

To meet these needs, criteria for community services have been summarized by a national group of community consultants: [8]

1. Educational facilities of standard quality for children and adults organized in accordance with individual needs, interests and capacities and closely related to the economic and social life of the community.
2. Family counseling and adjustment services and provisions for insuring the economic security of the family.
3. Services and care for children in their own homes and provisions whereby substitute homes or institutional care may be provided when necessary.
4. Mental hygiene clinics for children and adults.
5. Adequate children's court and detention facilities.
6. Provisions for the care of children of working mothers and adequate standards in child labor laws and full enforcement of such laws.
7. Recreation facilities and leadership for children, youth and adults.
8. Vocational guidance service for children and youth and counseling for adults.
9. Employment services for youth and adults.
10. Provision for adequate care, adjustment and recreation for the aged.
11. A community health program designed to provide both preventive care and treatment for adults and children of all ages and economic status, including hospitals and outpatient clinics.
12. Adequate and well-trained personnel in education, health, welfare and recreation.

The average citizen, including the college student, has a responsibility to understand and appreciate the principles of mental health and to

[8] *Ibid.*, pp. 15–16, 32.

accept his social obligation for the mental health of others. The latter may be accomplished by recognizing maladjustments in others and by accepting leadership in neighborhood and community activities for improving the community in order to make it a better place to live for his family and his neighbors.

Development of Mature Behavior

Each member of society assists in establishing and maintaining the social order by what he knows, thinks, feels, and does; also, each member responds to the social order that he has helped to establish. The aspects of behavior, such as interests, attitudes, and habits, that pertain to the individual's activity are significant because they exert a powerful influence on the individual's growth into maturity. A further examination is made of these selected aspects of behavior to determine their role in developing mental health.

Interests. In Chapter 2, it was pointed out that an interest implies the recognition of a need. It also may be stated that an interest refers to the special attention the individual pays as he is directed toward activity. The activity may relate to an object, an area, or persons within the environment. Such activity brings about pleasure and satisfaction, with consequent increased motivation. The value of interests lies in their significant effect upon the life of the individual. For example, interests that lead the individual to active participation rather than to a passive role are more desirable, since greater personal development results [1]. Also, interests in activities which stimulate the individual to create and discover bring about greater personal development than do the passive activities.

Many interests are temporary in nature. They change as people age and differ from person to person. Greater satisfaction comes from more enduring and lasting activities. The more enduring interests often lead to vocational choices as well as recreational pursuits. In addition, activities which can be shared with others bring about development to a greater degree than do those performed alone. Interests are preferred which develop personality through increased understandings, shaping wholesome attitudes and practices.

As the individual matures, his interests increase. The infant is interested primarily in food, sleep, and affection. The mature person seeks out the many activities within his environment. Some environments restrict while others broaden interests. Lehner classifies life activities as social, political, religious, educational, industrial, and recreational [6*a*]. Anderson proposes a different, more specific interest-classification system. He organizes life interests as follows: (1) manipulation and construction activities, illustrated by the child's interest in toys and the adolescent's construction of objects and machines; (2) sports and athletics, in which children, youth, and adults develop muscles, build up coordi-

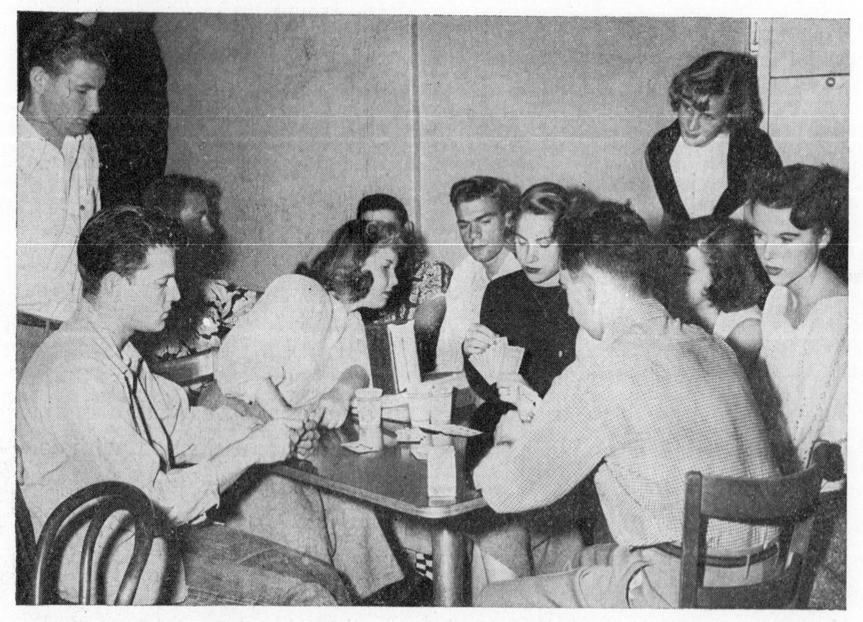

Fig. 4.4. Interests provide a means for releasing tensions. (*Photo by Stanley Troutman.*)

nations, and make personal and social adjustments; (3) outdoor life, exemplified by camping as practiced in the youth organizations, such as the Boy Scouts and Girl Scouts, exemplified for adults in hunting, fishing, and traveling; (4) clubs and social groups, such as ski clubs, service clubs, fraternities, sororities, and the like; (5) stories, reading, and literature interests, such as the child's interest in pictures and stories about objects and animals, the adolescent's interest in fiction, later on leading into religious and philosophical material and ranging from incidental appreciation to professional activity in reading and writing; (6) the comics or serial stories in newspapers and magazines; (7) motion pictures; (8) radio and television; (9) acting and the theater; (10) music; (11) dancing; (12) artistic activities; (13) hobbies; (14) religious endeavors [1].

Interests provide a means of releasing tensions, realizing new satisfactions, projecting one's inner life outward, seeing oneself in a new perspective, and obtaining needed companionship. Interests are vital to the development and maturity of the individual, as they enable him to acquire new attitudes, habits, and traits along with increased ability to make personal and social adjustments.

Attitudes. An attitude is defined as a "system of ideas with an emotional core or content."[9] Attitudes are tendencies to respond composed both of ideas and emotional factors. They are the result of many experiences involving points of view and feelings. They are the by-product of a situation rather than a response resulting from direct stimulation. For example, the late Franklin D. Roosevelt influenced many persons' attitudes through his speeches, not so much by what he said in his talks, as by the manner in which he presented his statements. Since attitudes are important in influencing behavior, they become a powerful force in the individual's development and his growth into maturity. A person develops negative attitudes, such as prejudice and bias, as well as positive attitudes, in the form of attachments and loyalties to individuals, objects, and ideals.

Home life shapes attitudes in the closely knit family association. The examples set by parents aid in attitude formation. Parental control, love, and affection and family social activities have a powerful effect on attitudes. Important, too, in attitude development are relationships with associates of the same and the opposite sex. The social life of the community exerts a potent influence on the development of attitudes. Advertising in the newspapers, magazines, over the radio, and on television is specifically directed toward shaping attitudes of children, youth, and adults. School experiences are planned by teachers, students, and parents with a primary purpose of modifying beliefs and attitudes.

On the national and international level, political-science attitudes play a major role. In a democracy, there is less attempt to control attitudes through the state. The process of attitude formation is based on the intelligence of each individual. It is an educational approach in which there is a free exchange of ideas. Decisions are arrived at through rational processes, after weighing the evidence on both sides of an issue. Individual self-directive behavior, leading to the optimum development of the individual, and civic participation in solving problems are the de-

[9] John E. Anderson, *The Psychology of Development and Personal Adjustment*, p. 283. New York: Henry Holt and Company, Inc., 1949.

sired results, not indoctrination by the state on preconceived principles directed by a selected few. The individual's critical evaluation, by the problem-solving method, of health information gained from various communication media—radio, television—is an illustration of the mature shaping of attitudes in a worthwhile manner.

Habits or practices. The individual is what he is because of his habits. The well-adjusted person has established a set of habits which permit him to perform his everyday tasks with ease and efficiency. Old habits tend to guide him unless he himself breaks the old and develops new ones. It is possible even at the college age to develop new habits, though it is much easier to develop good habits during early years.

Habits are a type of learned behavior so often repeated that the action becomes automatic, calling for little or no attention. "Habits are any response actions which may be initiated by a particular set of stimuli and terminated by a particular reaction." [10] Habits are not static; rather, they are in a constant state of change. For this reason, the development of wholesome practices for improved mental health is possible if the individual so desires, that is, if he exerts conscious control over his actions. New habits can be established by following these steps [2]:

1. Clearly state the purpose of the new habit.
2. Plan how this habit can be carried out.
3. Begin the new plan vigorously.
4. Do not permit any exceptions to the new habit, particularly at first.
5. Continue to perform the new habit.

Old habits may be broken by applying the same method; however, an old habit must be replaced by a new, improved habit so as to direct attention to another interest which will not permit one to indulge in the old habit. The mature, well-adjusted individual exerts conscious control of his emotional behavior by rational processes. By such action he is able to change old habits for new, improved ones and to develop habit patterns which aid in the development of sound mental health and more effective living.

Criteria for appraising mature behavior. The following criteria [11] serve as a guide and summary for the student in appraising his own behavior:

[10] H. W. Bernard, *Toward Better Personal Adjustment,* p. 87. New York: McGraw-Hill Book Company, Inc., 1951.

[11] Judson T. Landis and Mary G. Landis, *Building a Successful Marriage,* 2d ed. (copyright, 1953, by Prentice-Hall, Inc., New York), p. 111. Reprinted by permission of the publisher. Material in brackets added by present authors.

Criteria of Mature Behavior	*Criteria of Immature Behavior*
The mature person:	The immature person:
Is able to be objective [views his own interests, attitudes, and practices realistically]	Blames others for his failures
Is emotionally independent of parents	Is dependent upon parents
Makes decisions for himself [maintains practices that permit him to perform tasks with ease and efficiency]	Reverts to childish behavior
Acknowledges and takes responsibility for his mistakes	Refuses to accept his chronological age
Is heterosexual in his sex interests [utilizes a variety of interests]	Lets others make his decisions
Accepts his chronological age [welcomes new experiences and new ideas]	Is selfish
Is willing to wait for future pleasures	Is aggressive and domineering
Profits by his mistakes [takes life disappointments in stride]	Is quick to judge others
Accepts the moral codes	Defies social codes
Tries to understand others [appreciates the interests, attitudes, and practices of others]	Requires immediate satisfaction
Gets along with other people	Holds a fantasy conception of mate selection
Accepts the present and looks to the future	Sees sex as vulgar and dirty, or as the chief end and interest in life
Sees sex expression as a normal and satisfying phase of life	Shows lack of consideration for others
Is willing to use reason rather than fantasy in mate selection	Is self-centered
Can evaluate himself and his motives	

Summary

The preceding discussion has attempted to acquaint the student with the foundation factors in the development of sound mental health. A number of concepts involved in the meaning of the term were considered. A definition was presented. A set of criteria was outlined. Then the foundational forces of mental health—heredity, some physical factors, some social factors, such as the home, school, and community—were discussed. Finally, three aspects of behavior, namely, interests, attitudes, and habits, were appraised because of their significance in the development of the mature individual.

Suggested Activities

1. Formulate your own definition of mental health.

2. Indicate your family background by preparing a family tree. Start with your great-grandparents, and work to your immediate family. Note significant characteristics or achievements and defects or deficiencies of each person.

3. Appraise your hereditary background in relation to the development of your mental health. Refer to the section on Heredity.

4. Review the functions of the nervous system in a basic physiology or biology reference, or in references 1, 8, and 22. What part does neural activity play in mental health?

5. Evaluate your family home, using the criteria of a good home outlined in the section on The Home and the Family. Indicate what changes you would make when you establish your own home.

6. Write an anecdotal account of your grade school and high school experiences. Point out your pleasantest experiences, some embarrassing moments, and situations which have acted as definite learning experiences affecting your development.

7. Indicate several vocational possibilities you are considering. Give pros and cons for each.

8. Outline your participation in social activities. Do you like people? Do you make friends easily? What characteristics do you particularly like about your friends? Do you enjoy friends of both sexes? What do you believe are your social assets? Your liabilities?

9. State what values you have received from your favorite community. List some community activities which appeal to you for future participation.

10. Examine Lehner's classification of life activities in the section on Interests. Do you have some interests in each of his categories? If not, indicate which categories you need to think about in order to develop broader interests for the future.

11. Analyze your habit patterns. What old detrimental habits can you break? What new positive ones could you develop that would improve your personal and social adjustment?

12. Preview, show, and discuss audio-visual aids pertinent to mental health, such as the following: (*a*) *Heredity and Environment* (sound), McGraw-Hill Text-Film; (*b*) *Habit Patterns* (sound), McGraw-Hill Text-Film; (*c*) *Nation's Mental Health* (sound, 18 minutes), available from Text-Film Department, McGraw-Hill.

Suggested Readings

1. Anderson, John E., *The Psychology of Development and Personal Adjustment.* New York: Henry Holt and Company, Inc., 1949.

2. Bernard, H. W., *Toward Better Personal Adjustment.* New York: McGraw-Hill Book Company, Inc., 1951.

3. Cassidy, Rosalind, and Hilda Clute Kozman, *Counseling Girls in a Changing Society.* New York: McGraw-Hill Book Company, Inc., 1947.

4. Dysinger, Robert, "Mental Health in the United States," *Annals of the American Academy of Political and Social Science,* 286:1–174, March, 1953.

5. Joint Committee on Health Problems in Education of the National Education Association and American Medical Association, *Health Education.* Washington: National Education Association, 1948.

6. Katz, Barney, and George Lehner, *Mental Hygiene in Modern Living.* New York: The Ronald Press Company, 1953.

6*a*. Lehner, George F. J., *Explorations in Personal Adjustment: A Workbook.* New York: Prentice-Hall, Inc., 1949.

7. McKinney, Fred, *Psychology of Personal Adjustment.* New York: John Wiley & Sons, Inc., 1949.

8. Menninger, Karl A., *The Human Mind,* 3d ed. New York: Alfred A. Knopf, Inc., 1945.

9. Mid-century White House Conference on Children and Youth, *A Healthy Personality for Every Child: Fact Finding Report.* Raleigh, N.C.: Health Publications Institute, Inc., 1951.

10. Moore, Bernice M., and Robert L. Sutherland, *Family, Community, and Mental Health: Profiles of Community Action.* Austin, Tex.: The Hogg Foundation, 1950.

11. O'Kelley, Lawrence I., *Introduction to Psychopathology.* New York: Prentice-Hall, Inc., 1949.

12. Redl, Fritz, and William W. Wattenberg, *Mental Hygiene in Teaching.* New York: Harcourt, Brace and Company, Inc., 1951.

13. Ross, Mabel, "A Community Mental Health Program," *American Journal of Public Health,* 41:950–953, August, 1951.

14. Stevenson, George S., "When a Community Plans for Mental Health," *The Child,* 13:1–3, November, 1948. (Reprints available.)

15. Thorpe, Louis P., "Guiding Child and Adolescent Development in the Modern School," *Educational Bulletin* 16. Los Angeles: California Test Bureau, 1946.

16. Thorpe, Louis P., *The Psychology of Mental Health.* New York: The Ronald Press Company, 1950.

17. Vaughn, Wayland F., *Personal and Social Adjustment.* New York: The Odyssey Press, Inc., 1952.

18. Wallin, J. E. Wallace, *Personality Maladjustments and Mental Hygiene,* 2d ed. New York: McGraw-Hill Book Company, Inc., 1949.

Popular Readings

19. Barry, Herbert, Jr., *The Mind . . . "in Sickness and in Health. . . ."* Boston: John Hancock Mutual Life Insurance Company, 1951.

20. Beers, Clifford, *The Mind That Found Itself*, rev. ed. Garden City, N.Y.: Garden City Publishing Company, Inc., 1950.

21. Child Study Association of America, *What Makes a Good Home? The Beginnings of Emotional Health.* New York, 1951. (Pamphlet.)

22. Hughes, Margaret, *The People in Your Life.* New York: Alfred A. Knopf, Inc., 1951.

23. Menninger, W. C., *You and Psychiatry.* New York: Charles Scribner's Sons, 1947.

24. Preston, George H., *The Substance of Mental Health.* New York: Rinehart & Company, Inc., 1943.

25. Scheinfeld, Amram, *The New You and Heredity.* Philadelphia: J. B. Lippincott Company, 1950.

26. Slaughter, Frank, *The New Way to Mental and Physical Health.* New York: Grosset and Dunlap, Inc., 1947.

27. State Department of Mental Hygiene, State of California, *Mental Health Is 1, 2, 3.* New York: National Association for Mental Health, 1951. (Pamphlet.)

5. Making Life Adjustments

The meaning of mental health and its foundation factors have been explored in Chapter 4. The point was made that mental health is an asset to be achieved, as is true of physical health. In both cases, heredity plays its part. The important thing is to make the most of heredity by intelligent participation in life activities. This means making personal and social adjustments within the family, the neighborhood, the community, the college, and the widening environment of total society. Obviously, a basic aspect of mental health for the college student is knowing how to make appropriate personal and social adjustments and applying this knowledge in everyday life situations.

The discussion of personal and social adjustment is organized to assist the student in answering the following questions: (1) What are the adjustment problems facing the college student? (2) What are the characteristics of a well-adjusted personality? (3) How does one adjust to everyday situations? (4) What are the common adjustment mechanisms? (5) How do personality maladjustments develop? (6) What are the serious personality maladjustments, and how can they be prevented? (7) How does one develop and maintain maturity? (8) How does one make satisfactory sex adjustments? (9) Where or to whom can one turn for assistance in making life adjustments? (10) What constitutes a sound mental health program for college students?

Personality and Adjustment

Adjustment problems facing the college student. Of special importance in a discussion of the adjustment process applied to everyday living are the common mental health problems confronting the student in the college environment. Students are especially interested in the ways and means by which such problems may be solved and personal goals achieved. These problems have been stated in Chapter 2 in terms of the general mental health needs of college students and are more specifically outlined below. Recent studies [2, 6, 7] reveal the following common mental health problems facing students in the college environment:

1. Failure to relinquish home and family relationships.
2. Renouncement by students of parental and home situations.
3. Lack of motivation and self-direction (poorly defined goals, lack of personal drive and ability to accomplish tasks, disparity between goals and capacity to achieve them).
4. Lack of social adjustment (social inferiority or superiority, antisocial behavior).
5. Lack of emotional adjustment (emotional immaturity expressed in overstimulation, fears, anxieties, and the like).
6. Sexual relationships (maintaining standards and codes, inadequate sexual adjustments).
7. Scholastic difficulties (pressure of making grades).
8. Lack of economic adjustment (lack of opportunity to earn sufficient money, and unwise spending of funds).
9. Inability to adjust to housing and transportation conditions (lack of adjustment with large groups of individuals in dormitories, clubs, fraternities and sororities, and other housing groups, inability to withstand strains of commuting long distances with poor transportation facilities).
10. Poor health conditions.

The well-adjusted personality. The individual with the ability to make satisfactory adjustments to life situations is referred to as a well-adjusted personality. Personality is a difficult term to define because of its many connotations and because of the many things about it which are not yet known. However, in relationship to the well-adjusted individual, personality is defined as the whole person, including all his assets and liabilities, as he interacts within his environment. It is assumed that personality is a result of a combination of inheritance, environment, and behavior.

As a sum total of assets and liabilities, personality includes all one's traits—knowledge, attitudes, and skills. Personality is more than traits, however, for it involves the ways of making adjustment to life problems, too. Certainly it includes a person's thinking, speaking, feeling, and doing aspects of behavior. This concept is a biosocial viewpoint of personality according to which the individual is making personal adjustments and exhibiting social effectiveness. Such a view expresses the total pattern of behavior which the individual demonstrates in his family, his neighborhood, and society in general. It sees the whole individual as he is and as he changes from participation in all his life activities [17].

Characteristics of the well-adjusted personality. The well-adjusted personality is capable of making personal adjustments based on a sense of personal security and social adjustments based on feelings of social security. Such a person also attempts to strike a balance between personal and social adjustments. The well-adjusted individual, in terms of characteristics, is described in the following outline [2, 14, 15, 20]:

The well-adjusted individual:

1. Makes personal adjustments based on a sense of personal security.
   a. Knows himself.
   b. Works toward well-planned, attainable goals.
   c. Has a sense of his personal worth.
   d. Has gained personal freedom, regulation of his own life.
   e. Has a sense of belonging in his family.
   f. Shows an ability to get along with people in general.
   g. Participates in physical activities, such as individual, group, and team games and sports.
   h. Participates in work activities as a means of self-support; knows the value of money; engages in worthwhile work contributing to society.
2. Makes social adjustments based on feelings of social security.
   a. Recognizes and appreciates social standards and the rights of others.
   b. Exhibits social skills; likes and understands people, is considerate and diplomatic.
   c. Participates in college activities; engages in cooperative activities, as musical organizations, dramatics, clubs, committees, and the like.
   d. Participates in community activities; belongs to groups, such as the YMCA or YWCA, church groups, service clubs, professional groups; takes pride in commercial enterprises.
   e. Participates in social activities; associates with members of both sexes, enjoys mixed parties, dancing, and the company of boy and girl friends.
   f. Maintains friendly relations with his neighbors.
   g. Respects laws and regulations for protection of all citizens.

The process of adjustment. The individual establishes a satisfactory relationship with his environment when he meets his needs. The fulfillment of needs results in healthful, effective living. When needs are not met, the individual functions ineffectively and unsatisfactorily; in fact, he is uncomfortable. People's actions are an indication of their attempt to satisfy their needs. Thus some people are happy, successful citizens enjoying life, while others become troublemakers, alcoholics, or criminals—mentally disturbed persons.

Basic human needs. A need has been defined in Chapter 2, where the specific health needs of college students were presented. This definition pointed out that needs constitute "the demands, both internal and external, made upon an individual as he seeks to adjust to his environment." Katz and Lehner classify these demands into two basic human needs. They state that the motives for behavior stem from the person's attempt to satisfy these needs expressed as physical, or organic, and psychological, or ego, needs [15].

The physical need is the need to maintain physical health or well-being. This need refers to hunger, thirst, fatigue, lack of sleep, physical pain, excessive heat or cold and the like. These cause tensions in the individual that must be relieved. The tensions in turn motivate the individual to behave in such a manner as to meet these needs, by achieving a state of balance, or equilibrium. In such action the individual seeks comfort and pleasantness [15]. For example, a good meal satisfies his hunger. A cool drink quenches his thirst. A vacation with a chance to rest and sleep or a change of activity may relieve his fatigue and enable him to face more realistically his classwork or his job.

To maintain such well-being the individual functions on three different levels as follows: [1]

> 1. Automatically—certain healing and other processes maintain a condition of physical pleasantness. For example, the white corpuscles in the blood fight off infection. . . .
>
> 2. Unconsciously—the individual makes an effort to maintain his physical comfort . . . he unconsciously lifts his arms to cover his face when something is thrown at him. . . .
>
> 3. Consciously—the individual is quick to safeguard his physical well-being . . . he carefully selects what he eats in an effort to keep from becoming ill. . . .

The need to feel adequate and important serves as a motive for solving one's personal problems adequately and well. It constitutes the drive for making a success of whatever one undertakes. It is the reason for people seeking public recognition. Satisfying this need, too, is basic to good personality and sound mental health [15, 25].

When an individual's state of equilibrium has been disturbed by hunger, anger, rejection, love, and the like, he endeavors to respond by establishing a new state of equilibrium by securing food, resolving a conflict, gaining acceptance, mating, and the like. The individual acts in almost all life situations to meet his basic needs. This is a *field force* or *stress* concept of needs.

[1] Barney Katz and George Lehner, *Mental Hygiene in Modern Living*, pp. 16–17. New York: The Ronald Press Company, 1953.

Frustration. An individual is not always successful in satisfying all his needs in all situations. Generally speaking, the individual is motivated to meet his desires and demands. However, in attempting to satisfy his needs he meets a barrier or an obstacle causing frustration. Frustration, then, is the thwarting of desires or needs brought about by factors which interfere with normal and immediate adjustment of the individual. Frustration may be due to the individual himself, to life situations, or to society.

If frustrations are due to the individual himself, these are referred to as internal frustrations; they may be the result of defects, illness, injuries, or fears. If the frustrations are external, they may arise from various life situations involving finances, education, employment, and others. External frustrations also may be the result of society's control through the individual's contact with social mores or his interaction with social groups. For example, some groups do not approve of marriage outside their own group. An example pertaining to the college campus is the tradition in some colleges requiring freshmen to wear special costumes as a means of identity. Such restrictions may be frustrating to some individuals seeking to achieve their own personal goals.

The individual generally reacts to frustration or stress by attack, withdrawal, or compromise forms of behavior. These may be accompanied by emotional reinforcements, such as hostility, fear, and anxiety [5]. Reactions to stress frequently result in an act of hostility with emotional tension present. Expressions of hostility range from minor reactions, such as swearing, throwing away the golf club after a bad shot, or spreading gossip about a person, to such aggressive acts as fist fighting and even murder [15]. The more intense the frustration, the more intense the emotion. When frustration becomes a threat to the integrity of the ego, fear and anxiety are aroused. In such situations, the individual's reactive behavior utilizes more and more the defense mechanisms, many of which are socially disapproved. Each person has a frustration or stress tolerance. The ability to tolerate frustration depends upon the feelings of security and personal worth. When stress exceeds the individual's tolerance limit, he undergoes various degrees of personality disorganization. Adjustment depends on the individual's ability to withstand a strong frustrating situation or many mild barriers, such as disappointments in everyday life, without becoming disorganized.

In a consideration of frustration it is helpful to distinguish between satisfactions classed as (1) desires and (2) demands and to understand the behavior resulting from the blocking of each type of satisfaction. A *desire* is a need for a temporary satisfaction of a rather minor nature which the individual would like to have though he can well get along without it. A *demand,* however, is a basic need. If this need is not fulfilled, the resulting tension leads to maladjustment. When the demand is satisfied, the result is personal security and mental health. A schematic drawing of these results is presented in Figure 5.1.

Conflict. Frustration occurs when basic motives are thwarted. When basic motives oppose each other, the individual must make a choice be-

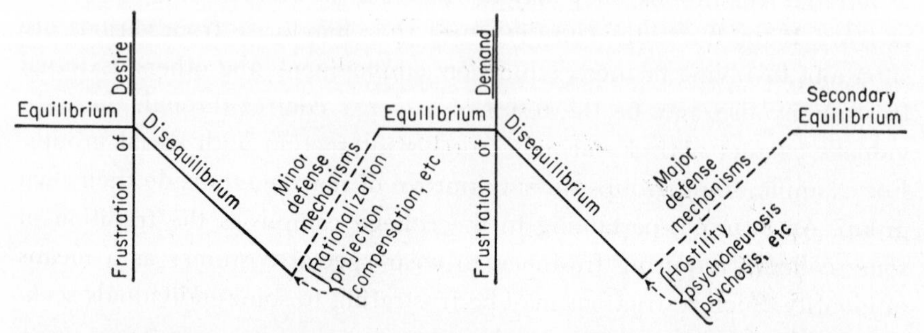

Fig. 5.1. Schematic representation of the results of frustration of desires and demands. (*Louis P. Thorpe, The Psychology of Mental Health, p. 57. New York: The Ronald Press Company, 1950.*)

tween motives in deciding upon a course of action. The state of tension occurring before the course of action is decided upon is called conflict.

All conflicts involve frustration. The stronger the motives, the more severe is the frustration. Time is a factor that often makes resolving a conflict difficult. In some circumstances, more than one motive might be achieved; however, the individual usually must act at once in only one direction. Most conflicts are easily resolved and result in only minor frustration. The choice of a life vocation often arouses a conflict in college students. A more frequently occurring conflict, however, concerns the satisfaction of the sexual desire. Should one marry before finishing college, engage in premarital sexual intercourse, practice masturbation, or suppress the sexual desire by participating in socially accepted activities?

Conflicts may be conscious or unconscious in nature. The majority of conflicts resulting in disordered behavior are unconscious and therefore beyond the individual's awareness. Such conflicts are associated with feelings of insecurity, feelings of guilt, or contradictory tendencies, such as love and hate of the same person. At this point, it is important to note that every person, including the well-adjusted individual, has frustrations and conflicts. Even in Paradise or Shangri-la conflicts or frustrations occur when human beings are present. However, the well-adjusted individual lives with these disturbances without experiencing serious symptoms of maladjustment.

All behavior involves conflict to a certain degree. Almost every situation tends to call for a variety of responses which cannot all be made at once. In many cases, first one, then another of these responses becomes dominant so that adjustments are made easily. When the degree of conflict is intense, the responses may produce hesitancy, tension, vacillation, or complete blocking. These responses indicate a more intense degree of conflict [12].

The sequence in adjustment. With respect to integration, all living organisms show a tendency to select patterns of adjustment which involve the least possible conflict [12]. This concept of behavior provides a basis for understanding the sequence of the process of adjustment. In learning to adjust to life situations the following sequence occurs:

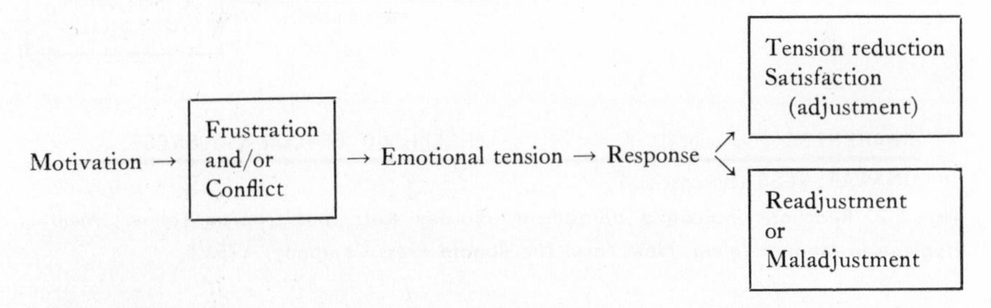

Principles of personality adjustment. The basic principles of human behavior become guide lines in meeting everyday problem situations. These principles, resulting from the adjustment sequence, are summarized briefly.

Every individual within his field or context has fundamental physical, or organic, and psychological, or ego, needs to be met. Needs motivate behavior. They must be satisfied or removed; otherwise tensions leading to maladjustments take place. Generally, needs are not easily satisfied because of the conditions within the field or context or in the mind which block their direct satisfaction. Therefore, frustration and conflict exist naturally and normally. To overcome frustration and conflict, the individual varies his behavior, selecting that which is most integrating and unifying. This behavior is based on influences from the total field of his past development and reflects his total self. His modified behavior resolves the frustration and conflict. In solving the problem, adjustment takes place, resulting in personal security and mental health [5, 12, 20]. Reactions indicating adjustment are shown in Figure 5.2.

A summary of the ways the individual makes life adjustments includes the following: [2]

1. Uses his abilities and capacities with satisfaction and enthusiasm.
2. Does his share in worthwhile group activities.
3. Gets along well with people, whether or not they are his superiors.

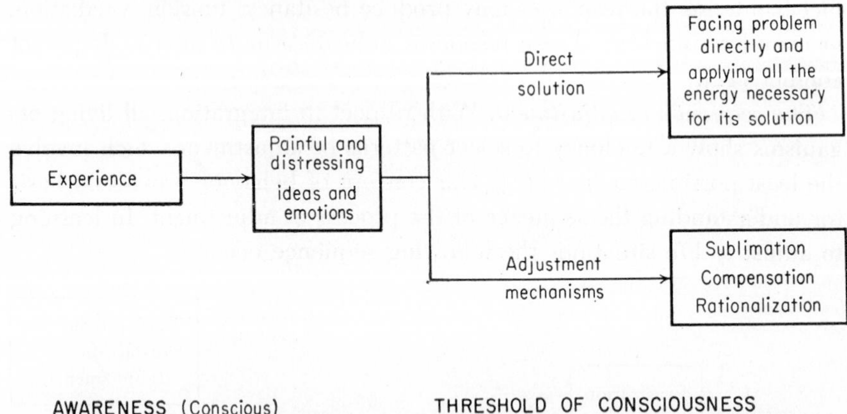

Fig. 5.2. Reactions indicating adjustment. (*Barney Katz and George Lehner, Mental Hygiene in Modern Living. New York: The Ronald Press Company, 1953.*)

4. Meets situations involving stress with constructive ideas and the will to succeed.
5. Tries to solve difficult problems or complete difficult tasks in spite of obstacles that may face him.
6. Does not permit daydreaming or wishful thinking to take the place of genuine accomplishment.
7. Is tolerant and understanding of the needs and desires of associates.
8. Gives as well as receives assistance and favors.

These principles of adjustment can be illustrated by a description of the actions of a college coed. Katherine Jamison was a college sophomore. Although not a beautiful girl, she was careful of her appearance and was considered attractive. Her budget for clothes was limited. She did not complain but selected with care what she was able to purchase so that she always looked nice.

She liked to play tennis and badminton and to swim, bowl, and skate

[2] *Ibid.*, p. 62.

and enjoyed other activities. As a consequence she had a good appetite and slept well. She ate a balanced diet and avoided stuffing herself. The doctor told her at her last medical examination that she was in fine physical condition. However, he warned her about doing too much and becoming overfatigued. She heeded his advice and added an hour's sleep to her daily schedule.

Katherine was a good student. She was not brilliant. However, by organizing her work and daily activities, she found adequate time for study. She listened attentively in class, kept up in her assignments, and received satisfactory grades.

Her mother and father loved her very much and gave her a feeling of security at home. Yet they urged her to attend college away from home. While she was in high school, they had given her freedom and expected her to assume responsibilities in the household. This was true even when she came home from college on visits. Her parents insisted that she make her own decisions. They would help her find out both sides of the question: the rest was up to her. She got along well with her older brother and sister despite the fact that they teased her continually. She soon learned to "dish it out" too.

Katherine realized her faults as well as her good points. She had discussed her faults with her mother, who showed her that her fine qualities far outweighed her shortcomings. She was well liked in her neighborhood. At one time she helped a neighbor whose daughter was seriously hurt in an accident.

Katherine was popular with college men. They liked to date her. She was good company, danced well, and was a fluent conversationalist but also a good listener. She could have a good time without wanting to go to places her date could not afford.

Since she liked people, she became interested in student-body activities. She ran for sophomore representative to the student executive committee but was defeated. In her campaign she made many new friends and had several interesting experiences. Although she was disappointed by her defeat, she decided it was good experience and she would try for office again after she became better known.

Katherine was a well-adjusted girl from a good home that provided her personal security. She was a healthy, normal coed. She liked to do things. As a result she had many accomplishments which gave her personal satisfaction. She had a number of good friends, both men and women. She liked people, and they liked her. She not only desired recognition in socially accepted ways but wanted to contribute to the welfare of her group and her college. She generally was successful in what she undertook, yet could adjust when she was unsuccessful.

Behavior Adjustments

Adjustment mechanisms. The individual develops a number of techniques to overcome frustration and conflict during the process of adjusting. These adjustment mechanisms are devices used to reduce tension by achieving an indirect satisfaction of a need. These are very common practices in everyday life and are not harmful unless used to excess. Some are defensive mechanisms similar to the body's lines of defense against infection and are socially desirable, while others lead to socially undesirable adjustments. A number of the common adjustment mechanisms are described in the following paragraphs:

1. *Regression* is a return to a former, somewhat primitive, and rather childish type of reaction. Examples of regressive reactions are furnished by the tennis star who throws his racket against the net when he receives an adverse decision or by the college student who leaves school and returns home because life is simpler there.
2. *Identification* is hero worship, identifying oneself with people or institutions that represent ideal qualities. Collecting autographs of famous people is an example.
3. *Projection* is the denial of one's own weakness by shifting a problem or the blame for a situation to other persons. An executive discharging a subordinate to cover up his own mistakes furnishes an example of this adjustive mechanism.
4. *Rationalization* is finding reasons for actions or conditions to justify them in the eyes of other persons and ourselves. For example, an individual buys a new car on the excuse that the tires of his old car are worn smooth. Actually, he needs new tires, not a new car.
5. *Transference* is an attachment to a person having a similar attitude to one's own. For illustration, if a person to whom one is introduced resembles a friend, one tends to be attracted to this new person.
6. *Repression* is a tension-producing mechanism. It is a process of selective forgetting in which the individual unconsciously tries to forget those aspects of his past or present behavior which may cause pain or discomfort. He fights to hold his desires down or pretends they do not exist. He feels one way and acts another. An illustration of repression is given by the marine who has undergone many unpleasant experiences and seen many horrible sights on the battle front but who represses his thoughts of these events, refusing to review them for himself voluntarily. It is a mechanism in which an individual represses feelings of horror, shame, guilt, or humiliation.

7. *Compensation* is a means of achieving satisfactions in a roundabout way. It may be the exaggeration of a desirable trait to reduce a feeling of inferiority resulting from an undesirable trait. Handicapped individuals who have achieved greatness illustrate this characteristic.

8. *Sublimation* is giving a desire a means of expression which will be useful and acceptable to society, overcoming frustration by striving for success in other situations. An illustration is provided by the college student who sublimates his sexual urges by substituting socially accepted activities, such as athletics, dances, parties, and the like, for premarital intercourse.

9. *Substitution* is a variety of the compensation technique. The individual reduces tension by changing from a frustrated activity to one that is more easily accomplished. An illustration would be substituting athletics for academic achievement, or vice versa.

10. *Egocentrism* is an exaggerated attempt to increase the importance of the self. Such behavior may range from temper tantrums to swimming the English Channel in order to gain publicity and public attention.

11. *Sympathism* is a technique by which the individual, to avoid facing a problem or an obstacle, tries to gain attention and receive expressions of concern over his difficulties. An example is the college student who fails a course and then seeks the sympathy of others to explain the failure, which in his mind was due to unfair treatment given him by the instructor.

12. *Dissociation* is a device by which the individual can satisfy motives which are contradictory, which would lead to conflict if allowed to operate simultaneously. Our present-day attempt to lead a normal existence under chaotic world conditions is an example of mild dissociation.

13. *Negativism* is persistent opposition to efforts made to aid or improve the individual. This device is common in children but occurs in adults as well. The patient who refuses to follow his doctor's orders or the advice of his family illustrates this mechanism.

14. *Fantasy* consists in unreal activities that have meaning and existence only for and within oneself. It is an indication, directly or indirectly, of the problems one is faced by, and its primary goal is escape from reality. Imagining oneself to be a chorus girl, a movie actress, a football star, or the owner of a lucrative business are examples.

Attitude of society toward adjustment mechanisms. Behavior mechanisms may be classified as follows according to their relative degree of social acceptance: [3]

1. Socially approved adjustment mechanisms: compensation, rationalization, substituted activities.

[3] L. P. Thorpe and B. Katz, *The Psychology of Abnormal Behavior,* p. 69. New York: The Ronald Press Company, 1948.

2. Socially tolerated adjustment mechanisms: identification, projection, egocentrism.

3. Socially criticized adjustment mechanisms: sympathism, regression, dissociation.

4. Socially disapproved adjustment mechanisms: repression, negativism, fantasy (daydreaming).

Psychosomatic conditions. In some individuals, when there is inadequate release of tension caused by excessive stress, functional bodily disorders, called psychosomatic disorders, develop. Psychosomatic disorders are bodily symptoms of ill health closely related to psychological factors. The symptoms are due to severe emotional stress and are commonly called tension symptoms. Emotional disturbances may affect any organ in the body and thus produce pain and discomfort.

Psychosomatic symptoms include chronic fatigue, aches and pains, digestive disorders, disturbances of eliminative functions, genito-urinary disorders, and cardiovascular dysfunctions. The most common specific symptoms include headache, neckache, backache, palpitation of the heart, pain in the region of the heart, tightness in the chest, tightness in the throat, choking sensations, loss of appetite, vomiting, indigestion, constipation, diarrhea, frequent urination, tiredness, weakness, and dizziness. Several common illnesses notably bronchial asthma, migraine, ulcers, and colitis are primarily psychosomatic in origin.[4]

Psychosomatic disorders may be corrected when the individual understands how the condition occurs and after he realizes the importance of seeking guidance from a clinical psychologist and psychiatrist. Generally, such competent assistance is necessary in order to eliminate the causes of the emotional stress.

Personality Maladjustments

Personality maladjustments result from the inability of the individual to meet his life needs. Variations in adjustment seem to differ primarily in degree rather than in kind [25]. Some of the minor personality maladjustments, such as inferiority feelings, feelings of insecurity, and nervous states, have been discussed. These minor deviations are characterized by feelings and tensions, for the most part are not serious, and are often only temporary in nature, with a return to well-adjusted behavior a real possibility. However, if not corrected, they may lead to greater degrees of maladjustment and serious mental disorders. Such maladjust-

[4] Katz and Lehner, *op. cit.*, p. 136.

ments also may result from disease, accidents, heredity, shock, intoxication, endocrine dysfunction, or continuous presence within the environment of frustration, conflict, and threats to security. These disorders are characterized by definite observable symptoms indicating the presence of emotional tension, with resultant loss of personal efficiency.

The major personality maladjustments are not of great concern to college students owing to the low incidence within this select group. However, an understanding of these disorders is important from a preventive aspect in later life and from the point of view of the total mental health problem in the general population.

Those suffering from the major mental disorders are classified as the psychoneurotics, the psychotics, and the psychopathic personalities and the mental defectives.

Psychoneurosis. Psychoneurosis, or neurosis, refers to the condition of a mentally ill person, commonly called a neurotic. The two terms psychoneurosis and neurosis are now used synonymously, although psychoneurosis is more widely employed to avoid confusion with medical terms relating to neurological conditions [25]. A psychoneurosis is a partial separation from reality marked by eccentric behavior. It is a behavior disorder due to emotional tension resulting from frustrations, conflicts, repressions, or marked insecurity. The psychoneurotic individual finds it difficult to meet his needs, his social obligations, and the demands of daily living, as his efficiency is limited by his emotional state. However, he still maintains some adjustive capacity within the limits of his social structure. It is estimated that 5 to 25 per cent of the population in the United States suffers from psychoneurotic disorders [25].

Psychoneuroses can be prevented by parents who understand and assist their children in solving their problems, particularly those related to fears, dislikes, and aversions. Treatment and correction of the psychoneuroses can be administered and achieved by psychotherapy, such as interview therapy and psychoanalysis.

The psychoneuroses are classified into five forms as follows: (1) hysteria; (2) psychasthenia; (3) neurasthenia; (4) anxiety; (5) hypochondriasis [5, 25]. Hypochondriasis is described as an example. For further details and description of each type, see references 5, 11, 24, 25, and 27.

Hypochondriasis. Hypochondriasis is a condition in which the individual exhibits great concern regarding his health. He is overanxious about his bodily organs and their functions, particularly those affected by emotional conditions as well as by organic disease. Heart disease, kidney disease, and ulcers are commonly feared. The hypochondriac's symptoms and suffering are greatly overestimated by himself. By an exaggeration of his condition, the individual gains sympathy and attention, which bring a feeling of security. The hypochondriac is often a health faddist looking for special diets or remedies which will improve or restore health.

Psychoses. The psychoses are serious mental disorders. They are commonly referred to in lay terms as insanity. A psychotic person is one who is not able to face reality and therefore is unable to meet his obligations to society. His whole personality is affected. His behavior may be such that he injures himself or other persons. The majority of psychotic persons are acutely ill and are committed to mental hospitals.

The behavior of some mentally ill individuals combines the symptoms of both psychoneurosis and psychosis. In some cases there can be no clear line of demarcation. Usually, however, a differentiation can be made, as the psychotic reactions are more severe, affect a greater part of the personality, and are more dangerous to the individual as well as to other persons [5, 24].

The psychoses are classified into reaction types as follows: (1) organic; (2) toxic; (3) functional.

The organic type. An organic psychosis is a major disorder of personality due to some physical or structural condition. All persons in this group are afflicted with brain disease or brain injury. The brain injury is for the most part responsible for the failure of the individual to adjust to his environment. Examples of conditions in this category include (1) senile psychosis (softening of the brain and hardening of the arteries) and (2) paresis, caused by advanced syphilis.

The toxic type. This type of psychosis displays two symptoms: (1) a disorganization of time, of place, and of the individual's own personality; and (2) hallucinations ranging from mild to extreme, producing great anxiety. Examples of the type include alcoholic psychosis and psychoses from drugs. Alcohol has a toxic effect on the central nervous system which is demonstrated by the emotional responses, the functional activities, and an effect on the nervous tissue. Alcoholic persons have some unmet need or hidden mental conflict which alcohol temporarily satisfies. While intoxicated, a person is actually mentally ill, and his behavior during this time is psychotic. However, because of the rapid recovery from this condition in some cases, the individual is not usually thought of as a psychotic case. It is the chronic drinker who suffers from hallucinations, delirium tremens, and loss of memory. Drug addicts, such as those who use morphine, find that the intellectual faculties are affected much more than the physical condition. The action of alcohol and drugs may eventually result in some form of brain injury.

The functional psychoses. In this class of psychosis the brain appears normal, but a malfunctional condition exists within the individual. Two common examples of the functional type are schizophrenia and manic-depressive psychosis. For further information and description of other psychoses, see references 5, 11, 24, 25, and 26.

SCHIZOPHRENIA (DEMENTIA PRAECOX). This is the most common and the most important severe mental disease, especially from a social standpoint. Approximately 53 to 65 per cent of all cases in state mental hospitals are schizophrenic cases, and for every one in a mental hospital there is probably one in a less disturbed condition cared for by relatives in private homes [11]. A great many criminals, prostitutes, and hobos are suffering from schizophrenia [25]. While the well-adjusted individual is an integrated unit, the schizophrenic person is one who lacks integration between thinking and feeling. The result is a complete withdrawal from human relationships. Such persons commonly are referred to as shut-in personalities. They show in their disorganization of personality a loss of interest in former activities. Also, they exhibit preoccupation and fantasy about sex, religion, money, or bodily functions, finding an illogical or unreal solution for their overemphasized problems. Hallucinations often support their illogical beliefs. Delusional experiences frequently occur about health, strength, or power. Frequently there is loss of feeling for others, in fact complete disregard for social living exhibited in a breakdown of habits of cleanliness and thoughtfulness.

MANIC-DEPRESSIVE PSYCHOSIS. In this type of mental illness the individual is disturbed in the way he feels about life and his experiences. His feelings are intensified and overemphasized to the point where his judgment and behavior are affected. Depression or elation becomes set, lasting as long as months or years. Although the name of the illness refers to alternating moods, there are cases in which only one mood appears; such conditions are called "manic-depressive manic" or "manic-depressive depressed." In the majority of cases there is a period of excitement and overactivity followed suddenly by a period of depression. The opposite order is seen less frequently. The period of depression usually lasts longer than the excited state. In most cases, chronic manic-depressive patients spend the last years of their lives in hospitals in a worried, despondent, unhappy state.

Sources of Assistance in Making Life Adjustments

Personality maladjustments of either minor or serious nature are not a disgrace. They can happen to anyone, and they do occur more often than is realized. Most deviations are temporary and cause no permanent damage if discovered early. In most instances, such conditions develop gradually, sending out warnings in advance. The majority of persons with adjustment problems can be helped to lead happy, normal, useful lives. The important fact is that mental illness demands prompt care just as does physical illness. To know where to turn for assistance when one needs help for himself, a member of his family, or a friend is the first step in making necessary adjustments.

When the student is confronted with a minor problem while at college, he can immediately contact the counseling center, the student health service, or a member of his family. It is more than likely that the counseling center will have a clinical psychologist trained and experienced in counseling techniques and skilled in handling personal-social-emotional problems. The counselor will refer serious conditions needing medical attention to a qualified psychiatrist. If the student prefers to talk with his own physician or the college physician at the student health service, this medical adviser can provide necessary assistance. When the problem is a serious one, the physician is an excellent person to recommend a qualified psychiatrist. A psychiatrist is a medical doctor with specialized training in the prevention and treatment of emotional disturbances and mental diseases. He has had experience in a mental hospital or a mental hygiene clinic.

If as a citizen in the community an individual is faced with such a problem, the logical person to consult is the family physician. Again, the physician will recommend a reputable clinical psychologist or psychiatrist if one is necessary.

The student or the citizen who does not have a family physician can consult the local mental hygiene clinic or mental hygiene association, the local public health department, or the state department of mental hygiene.

Beware of the quack or charlatan, the advertising self-appointed specialist. Psychological cultists are prevalent everywhere, preying on the uninformed public.

Maturity and Adjustment

The individual develops from relatively unorganized behavior to organized and structured behavior. He is motivated toward goals or purposes within his environment. From the environment or within himself, barriers or rival motives arise causing frustration and conflict. Conflict brings a necessity for choice between two different lines of action. A shifting back and forth may occur before a decision is made between the two existing tensions. The individual uses various adjustment mechanisms to resolve his conflicts. As a rule, he will use the socially desirable defensive mechanisms. As his behavior becomes more and more patterned, he achieves new goals and develops the capacity to work for remote goals. He gains self-control and self-management. He develops interests and wholesome attitudes and habits. He achieves a wholeness or balance of emotions and desires. Through his actions he gains in effectiveness and becomes a mature individual.

A discussion of maturity and adjustment calls for a review of the development of interests, attitudes, and habits (see Chapter 4, pages 77 to 82). Also, a consideration of the development and control of emotions is pertinent to this topic.

Development and control of emotions. It has been pointed out that, when the individual is under stress, he undergoes feelings of tension and excitement called emotions. Emotions are characteristic of the early stages of adjustment. They tend to decrease as the individual acquires the ability to satisfy his needs. Emotion is characterized as a "stirred-up" state. A condition may result in which the individual becomes so excited in an emergency situation that he is unable to act; conversely, he may be stimulated and keyed up to rise to new heights in his particular activity. Emotions may give him the most satisfying feelings or bring about trouble and disaster. Fear, anger, love, and jealousy are typical emotions.

Fear. Fear is an emotion that is often present when frustration and conflict occur. It is characterized by dread or expectation of harm. Fear is in reality an internal state of readiness to avoid or run away from whatever threatens. Typical minor fears are lack of confidence and fear of the dark. Such fears often are passed on verbally from generation to generation. Fear of the dark is conditioned either from actual experience or from stories which have been heard in childhood. Anxiety is a type of fear resulting from the unknown or unpredictable. It usually arises from conflict and frustration. Experience and education aid in reducing this type of fear, as motives become more easily directed and satisfied.

Worry. Worry is a form of anxiety. It may express itself in a variety of ways, for example, insomnia, a vague feeling of restlessness, indigestion, hyperacidity, overconscientiousness, or obsessions or compulsions which vary from minor disturbances to more severe ones.

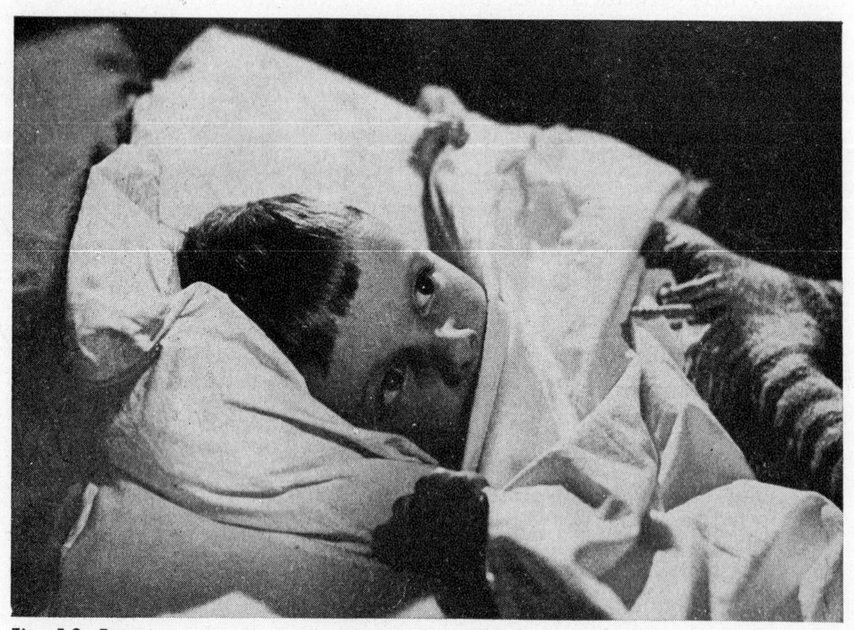

Fig. 5.3. Fear is an emotion characterized by dread or expectation of harm. (*Courtesy of McGraw-Hill Text-Films.*)

An anonymous writer has developed a worry table indicating what people generally worry about in our times.

	Per Cent
Things that never happen	40
Things over and past that couldn't be changed by all the worry in the world	30
Petty worries	10
Needless health worries	12
Real legitimate worries	8

Worry may be a symptom of mental conflict or of insecurity. In such cases, the feelings must be relieved, or the worry persists. Worry can be relieved by adjustment to the problem at hand, by a direct attack, or by formulating a definite plan to solve a problem. Talking or writing about his fears, worries, and anxieties often relieves the individual from the resulting disturbing factors. This aids him in regaining his equilibrium. Attaining experience, improving skills, and developing interests assist the individual in adjusting to these emotionalized reactions.

Inferiority feeling. An inferiority feeling is an emotional state of mind. The person believes he is a failure or is different from others in phys-

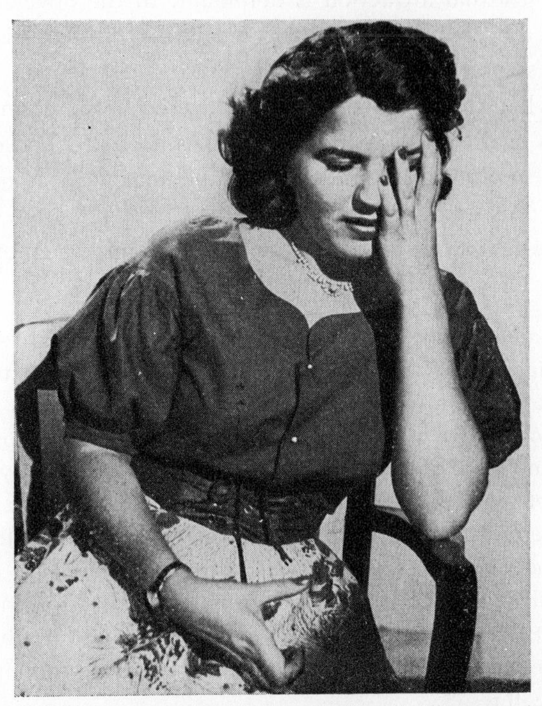

Fig. 5.4. An inferiority feeling is an emotional state of mind. (*Courtesy of Dr. Lester Beck.*)

ical, mental, or social standards. Often a feeling of inferiority differs from an actual inferior state measured by objective standards. In many instances an inferiority feeling is due to frustration in one's social setting. Such feelings are best adjusted by understanding oneself, by observing that most persons have similar feelings, by achieving success, by admitting inferiority in one field and transferring to another field where success can be achieved. Self-confidence is the opposite of fear, anxiety, and worry. The self-confident person faces his fears because he has made adjustments in personal and social relationships. He has gained success where he naturally excels and has extended his efforts into other areas, achieving new goals.

Love. Love is an emotion relating to an attachment and affection for other persons and objects. In normal development, love begins with self-love, spreads to an affection for parents, then to affection for persons of the same sex, and finally to an affection for the opposite sex. This development may be interrupted by circumstances at any stage along the way. Some individuals never progress beyond the stage of interest in which homosexual attraction is dominant. In the development of the love emotion a cycle prevails. First comes idealism, then disillusionment. Out of these stages there is a gradual development of true values. Many individuals when their love ideals are shattered never permit themselves to engage in further social interaction of this type. These persons do not progress to the heterosexual stage and marriage. A more detailed discussion of this emotion is presented in Chapter 6.

Guide lines for controlling emotions. In controlling emotions the following guide lines will help [1, 14, 20, 23]:

1. Strive to understand fears, anxieties, and worries. Information relative to the emotion and to the cause of the emotional response is often helpful. If one knows the situation bringing about the response exhibited and what the adequate response should be, behavior can be redirected. As previously suggested, some of the disturbing elements can be eliminated by meeting the emotions objectively, by talking about the fears and anxieties or writing about them. With the disturbing elements eliminated, the individual often has a new perspective and sees new ways to face these feelings.
2. Realize that emotions are stirred by the emotional responses of others. If one understands the fact that it is a first reaction to exhibit emotion in response to the emotions of others, this tendency may be restrained and emotional control will result.
3. Keep emotions isolated or in context with a situation, not allowing them to affect general behavioral responses. Emotional control keeps emotions segregated and concerned only with their original stimulus. Thus if a specific fear arises because of a disturbing event, it is not permitted to become a major problem and cause general inferiority feelings.
4. Do not worry over past mistakes. Approach new situations with confidence. Emotional adjustment comes through profiting from mistakes or failures, with a "comeback" in new situations. Brooding over past mistakes and defects only permits poor past behavior to influence present and future conduct. The well-adjusted individual has the ability to "come back," for he lives in the present and the future, not the past.
5. Use direct positive action in controlling emotions. Get at the basis of the conflict immediately. Determine what caused the real trouble. See your instruc-

tor, your boss, your father or mother. Talk the situation through, rather than withdawing and worrying over the affair.

6. Become reassured after the removal of emotional conditions. When the basic condition is understood and a plan of action has been formulated to remedy the situation, self-reassurance or reassurance by a friend gives added confidence and a greater chance of success.

7. Observe friends who meet emotional stress with calm and collected behavior. They can help one to meet similar conditions.

8. Maturity involves improvement in controlling emotions. Emotional reactions accompany stages in the process of adjustment. As individuals mature, experience and skill are gained in progressing from emergency reactions to skilled behavior.

9. Energy and enthusiasm are positive aspects of emotions and must be retained to make life adjustments.

Emotional maturity is reached when the individual develops a sound set of values, self-confidence, a sense of personal worth, and a sense of humor. Emotions may be helpful to the individual [10] when they:

1. Provide a stirred-up state that brings out reserves of energy.
2. Cause expressive changes, such as joy and tender feelings.
3. Free inhibitions, permitting ideas to be acted upon which otherwise might be stultified.

Emotions may be detrimental [10] when they:

1. Cause irrational action.
2. Impair motor skill.
3. Block mental processes.
4. Restrict the range of desirable activity and experience.
5. Impair health.

Adjustment to the Sex Drive

Sexual adjustment—an example of attaining maturity. Sexual adjustment is part of the individual's total development into maturity. The maturation of the sex organs, sex characteristics, and sex drives directs the individual along the pathway of development to adult attitudes and maturity. Sexual maturity helps to bring out what is best, most generous, and most constructive in the individual's life.

Sex is a basic drive upon which both race preservation and personal happiness depend. As a drive properly controlled, it becomes a powerful force aiding personal and social adjustment. From a positive point of view, it leads the young away from dependence on their parents toward finding independence and the responsibility of loving, supporting, and caring for a family. In this respect, sex is a powerful, constant stimulus toward mature attitudes. If sexuality does not evolve properly, the whole process of growth and development is influenced negatively. Too much repression of sex tends to impair freedom and ease of functioning to the extent that mating and sexual satisfaction are not attained. On the other hand, too much sexual freedom can interfere with normal adjustments in love and mating functions to the degree that sexuality remains on an infantile level, as a desire for play and personal pleasure only. Disturbances in sexual development can lead to personal and social maladjustments.

The sex drive is a natural aspect of life which needs to be both understood and controlled. It should be considered squarely and frankly as a meaningful and respectable part of life. The goal of the sex drive is biological sexual maturity—the capacity to love, mate, reproduce, and care for the young. However, sex has more than reproductive functions; it is a factor in a happy family life, which is a partnership with a sharing of interests and ideas, mutual acceptance of responsibilities, self-realization, and love.

In our culture, a person matures sexually years before he can establish a home and, according to social standards, give expression to his sexual impulses and desires. For his own good and for the good of society the individual is expected to conform to the conventions within the culture. This means that the sex drive must be controlled if sex is to become a positive force in the development of the personality. The requirement for self-control is not unreasonable when one remembers that any great power or drive has to be controlled or its creative force becomes a destructive menace, as illustrated by atomic power. The value of the drive depends upon how well its potentialities are understood and how skillfully it can be managed [30].

According to Kraines and Thetford,[5] self-control implies these elements:

1. Understanding one's impulses, both as to their function and normalcy and also as to their potentiality for good or harm.

2. Conscious setting up of values or goals which one wishes to attain both as a person with particular desires and drives and as a member of society with definite obligations and responsibilities.

3. The willingness and the requisite will power to postpone, and, if need be, renunciate immediate gratification for future satisfactions.

[5] S. H. Kraines and E. S. Thetford, *Managing Your Mind*, pp. 199–200. New York: The Macmillan Company, 1944.

Self-control motivated from within the individual is more effective than that resulting from outside forces. This implies that the student has the right to know as much as possible about his own sexuality if he is to exercise control and if he is to make his own sexual adjustment in relation to the demands of society. He needs to know what is expected of him and why. He needs to become familiar with ways and means of exercising control. Briefly, he needs to understand (1) the structure and function of reproduction (see Chapter 7, pages 153 to 159), (2) the emotional factors basic to developing mature sexual attitudes regarding loving and mating (see Chapters 6 to 8), and (3) the basic problems related to the sex drive.

Understanding sexual behavior. The premise has been established that an understanding of the basic problems relating to the sex drive is fundamental to developing self-control and self-direction. The aspects selected for discussion here because of their pertinence to the adjustment of the college student are the following: (1) nocturnal emissions; (2) masturbation; (3) homosexuality; (4) petting; (5) premarital sexual relations.

Nocturnal emissions. Nocturnal emissions, or "wet dreams," are the result of psychic stimulation during sleep and are considered a normal reaction in the male. Little attention has been given to the fact that similar orgasm during sleep is not uncommon in the female, particularly in the older and sexually more experienced female. This does not involve ejaculation as is the case in the male. Kinsey reports that 99 per cent of the males who go to college experience nocturnal emissions at some time in their lives [16]. The single males at the college level derive about one-sixth of their total sexual outlets from this source. Some individuals report a feeling of tiredness or weakness after a nocturnal emission. Generally, there is no serious aftereffect.

Masturbation. The term "masturbation" refers to the attainment of sexual gratification by the deliberate self-stimulation of the genital organs. The Kinsey study indicates that 92 per cent of American males and 96 per cent of college male students ultimately practice masturbation [16]. Other studies show masturbation to be common among females, though to a lesser extent than for males. At the college level, Kinsey reports that masturbation is the chief source of sexual outlet up to the time of marriage. Since masturbation is considered a common practice, it is not classed as a sexual abnormality except when an adult uses this means of sexual gratification in preference to heterosexual intercourse in marriage. It is, however, an undesirable sexual outlet, which belongs to a phase of development that can be outgrown by attaining complete sexual maturity and utilizing other, more socially accepted means of sexual adjustment [16].

Through the years masturbation has been blamed as the cause of ills ranging from pimples to insanity, including loss of manliness, feeblemindedness, genital cancer, and many other such conditions. There is agreement today among educators, clinical psychologists, psychiatrists, and many medical practitioners that the effects of masturbation are not fundamentally different from the physical effects of any other sexual activity. However, many mental disturbances occur from masturbation as the result of conflicts, such as feelings of guilt, inferiority feelings, fear of social disgrace, or worry about condemnation of such activity. There is no objective evidence that the manual act itself has a definite detrimental effect on physical or mental health or sexual virility [9]. However, other harmful effects may result from masturbation. The relationship between masturbation and sociosexual adjustments still remains to be determined. In some cases, masturbation may be so sexually satisfying that the individual does not desire to engage in sexual relations during marriage. This condition is considered a deviation from normal living [25]. A youth's attention may be focused on masturbation to the extent that he neglects his interests in school, recreational activities, and associations with the opposite sex.

Homosexuality. Homosexuality is a condition in which erotic interest is felt or sex relations are experienced between members of the same sex. Usually, homosexual acts include manipulation of the genital organs—interfemoral coitus, for example—to achieve sexual gratification. The three well-known theories as to the cause of homosexuality are (1) that it is due to an inherited tendency, (2) that it is a result of conditioning or maladjustment, such as unsatisfactory social relations with members of the opposite sex, and (3) that it is due to a sex-hormone imbalance. The causes are complex and difficult to ascertain; it is probable that any or all of these may be involved as multiple factors.

Kinsey's findings show that 37 per cent of the total male population has had at least some overt homosexual experience, while 4 per cent of the white males are exclusively homosexual throughout their lives [16]. Homosexual experience is less frequent among women than among men. Nineteen per cent of the females reported such experience [17]. Kinsey advocates the use of a three-point scale of heterosexual, bisexual (heterosexual and homosexual), and homosexual. He emphasizes how misleading is the tendency to consider an individual homosexual if he is known to have had a single experience with another individual of his own sex. Many persons in the population have had such experiences and then have developed normal heterosexual adjustments in later life [16].

Homosexuality is not confined to one or two lower social levels but occurs in varying degrees at every social level and among persons in every occupation and of most ages.

Petting. "Petting," the modern term for a practice that always has existed, is sexual expression through physical contact ranging from kissing and fondling to direct sexual stimulation stopping short of sexual intercourse. It may be classified as (1) the sincere expression of genuine love and affection and (2) a means of deliberate sexual stimulation through exploration and excitation of the other person, at the same time inviting gratification in return. Petting of the first sort is an important phase of the true art of love. It is a part of the technique of arousal, love play, which brings about the mutual relationship and feelings preliminary to the sexual act. It is preparation for mating.

Petting of the second type is a general experience of youth, ranging from "light" to "heavy." Light petting is described as stroking of the hair, the face, or the arms and hands. Heavy petting includes caressing or fondling of the body of either or both participants; usually, this includes the caressing or fondling of the breasts and genital organs of the girl.

The problem of petting is to keep it within bounds. Without self-control, owing to its progressive nature, it will lead to sexual relations or some other sexual outlet. If one decides to pet, some decisions should be made immediately. How far shall one go? Is it worth the resultant tensions? Pleasure to one person may mean a series of unfortunate consequences for another. For example, the dangers of pregnancy, abortion, and venereal infection may be involved even if *some* degree of self-control is used. On the other hand, some authorities maintain that petting guarded by self-control serves as an educative experience and is a step from immaturity to the full maturity of the heterosexual stage, serving as an outlet for energies and desires, as well as a stimulator of desire [3]. It is well to remember that the principles of fair play are involved, that petting affects not only oneself but the partner as well. The girl, who normally is slower in responding to such stimulation, may easily arouse the passions of her companion. She places him in a highly emotional state without realizing what she has done.

Since each case is different, no specific rules can be stated. It is important, however, to know what petting is, what type or kind is involved, where it leads, and the consequences. Then one may decide for himself whether or not to practice in a particular situation.

Premarital sexual relations. If there is any problem that must be faced squarely by the college student, it is that concerning premarital sexual relations. It is important to consider the issues involved and then to arrive at one's own decision, weighing the satisfactions against the natural risks. The decision may rest on the personalities and the emotional constitutions involved and the social situation in which the couple find themselves. This decision, however, should be based on critical thinking, not emotional rationalization.

Promiscuity is one of the most important social problems with which society must cope. Waggner [6] illustrates this point when he says: "Many of the revelations of recent sex studies are symptoms of an ailing society. But let us not confuse the ailment with the desired state of health, or change the temperature scales on the thermometer to make the fever normal."

The case for premarital sexual relations can be summarized briefly. Some authorities believe that such relations temporarily solve the problem of sexual desire and relieve tensions built up by this desire. They provide temporary physical pleasure. In some cases where there is strong sexual drive, they may prevent personality strains and possible distortions. However, in the majority of cases premarital relations create more problems than they solve.

The reasons for abstinence are good ones. Society sanctions sexual relations as a vital part of the art of love, an expression of deepest affection, in the marital partnership. It considers sex as a sacred thing. No scientific studies to date, only the rationalization of young people, give evidence that premarital sexual experience makes for better adjustment in marriage.

The House of Delegates of the American Medical Association, the British Social Hygiene Association, the American Social Hygiene Association, and others have collected data which prove that continence and chastity are not harmful to health.

The risks involved in premarital sexual relations always must be considered. One cannot ignore the possibility of the woman becoming pregnant. Even with the increased knowledge of birth control, medical authorities agree that there is no perfect contraceptive. Particularly is this true under the usual hurried, inconvenient circumstances of premarital

[6] Walter H. Waggner, "Must We Change Our Sex Standards? A Symposium," *The Reader's Digest,* 32:1–6, June, 1948.

relations. If the woman becomes pregnant, the question arises whether she will have the baby or submit to an illegal, induced abortion. The first choice is tragic for more than one person. Illegitimacy is a condition that no rational person would intentionally bring upon another human being. On the other hand, abortion is one of the greatest risks to life and health, with terrific psychological as well as physiological effects. There also is mental anguish for the woman who has had sexual experience and merely thinks she has become pregnant. Worry may upset the menstrual cycle, causing her period to be late or even missed. In this condition, it is easy for her to rationalize herself into using drugs, nostrums, which will not necessarily induce an abortion but will often cause severe illness. She may even become the prey of an abortionist who will perform an operation even though she is not pregnant. It is a good health practice to see a physician and have an examination for pregnancy regardless of one's marital status.

Premarital relations may lead to venereal disease. Two factors are important in regard to venereal diseases: (1) they rank high among the reportable communicable diseases; (2) it is difficult and, in some cases, impossible to tell from outward appearances whether or not venereal disease is present. It is true that the incidence of venereal disease is low among college students as compared with the general population. However, some college students do have contacts with prostitutes and "pickups" which increase the danger of such infection.

It is well to remember that mental conflicts, particularly worry, guilt, and fear, affect the peace of mind of both parties, especially the woman's. Emotional reactions often result even if pregnancy, illegitimacy, and venereal disease are avoided. Premarital intercourse, with its worries and fears, may result in an attitude about intercourse which prevents the establishing of normal sexual relationships in marriage.

The problem for young people becomes extremely difficult if they are unable to marry when they are ready to marry. Guilt complexes may result from indulging in premarital sex relations when couples are by necessity postponing marriage, though many couples who are not able to marry refuse to practice premarital sexual intercourse.

Many authorities in the field of marital relations, such as Dr. James Bender, Director of the National Institute of Human Relations, Norman E. Himes, noted author, and Paul Popenoe, General Director, American Institute of Family Relations, believe in early marriage as one practical solution to the problem. If the couple have found true love, are fit to marry, and have carefully considered the responsibilities involved, it is better that they should marry. Early marriage, from eighteen to twenty-five, is far superior to promiscuity and delinquency. In many instances, an early marriage would necessitate financial assistance from both sets of parents, if they are in a position to help. Financial assistance by parents is merely a return to the early days of America, when a newly married couple were given a few acres of land, a team and a wagon, a house, and the like, to give them a start. Both the scholastic and the marital records made by young veteran student families are proof of the soundness of the early-marriage concept.

Satisfactory sexual adjustments. Heterosexual adjustments, through social contacts and experiences with members of the opposite sex, indicate maturity of development from childhood experiences to adulthood. This development does not occur without many conflicts and frustrations. Hurlock suggests that two environmental conditions are essential for successful adjustments: (1) an environment in which there is a sufficient number of members of the opposite sex of appropriate age, intellectual status, and personality adjustment to give the individual an opportunity to select congenial companions and to have pleasurable social contacts with them; (2) an encouraging, sympathetic, and helpful attitude on the part of parents and other adults [13].

The fundamental attitude leading to maturity is shown in the ability to enjoy giving more than receiving and an interest in, and love for, the marriage partner, for children, friends, a profession, and hobbies. By properly developing self-discipline, the student is able to achieve self-development, personal maturity, and adjustment. Such maturity makes it possible for him to attain his highest goal—that of contributing to the betterment of society.

Formulating a Personal Program for Mental Health: A Summary

Undoubtedly, the college student has been following some type of mental health program for a number of years. It may have been sound or unsound, according to modern principles. It may have been planned intelligently or followed haphazardly. The chances are better than even that the program has been a good one because the college student has attained various goals and made many successful adjustments, resulting in a high degree of maturity. However, many desires, wishes, and goals are yet to be satisfied. A four-point personal program for mental health is suggested to enable the student to continue making successful life adjustments and to ensure improved personal and social relationships. This program consists of the following:

1. An understanding of mental health—its basic factors and forces, including the personal and social adjustment process.
2. The study and appraisal of mental health principles.
3. The application of mental health principles to life experiences.
4. Planning and replanning a course of action for happier, healthier living.

Developing an understanding of mental health. A fundamental assumption of this chapter is that the college student is capable of understanding the basic factors involved in the personal and social adjustment process. The student is aware that mental health is not a mysterious process but is the result of his everyday living in the home, in school, on the job, or in other community activities. He knows that he can do something about shaping his own thinking, feeling, and doing to live more effectively. He realizes that heredity has set limitations for him. He understands his environment with its particular mores and its stresses. He learns what his capacities are. He is aware of his assets and liabilities. He is assured that he has many unique abilities upon which he can capitalize. Also, he knows that most persons in our society are not utilizing their maximum capacities.

Insight into the adjustment process further enables the student to understand that it is natural for many of his goals to be attained with little or no difficulty. On the other hand, many goals are difficult of achievement, with frustration and conflict present as desires and wants are blocked. He realizes that some of these are blocked temporarily, while other barriers are permanent. In either case, new adjustments or readjustments are required. It is apparent to the student that the majority of his problems can be solved successfully by appropriate behavior, utilizing wholesome, purposeful experiences. He recognizes that he uses several of the mental or defense mechanisms occasionally for achieving adjustments. However, he is aware that he does use them. He makes sure they are not used excessively or to the extent that they become habitual forms of behavior. They do not inhibit his ability to face reality in making adjustments. For example, when a life problem occurs, he faces it realistically and applies all his attention and energy in working out a solution.

As the student gains a clearer understanding of mental health, he has greater opportunities to apply its principles in his everyday living in home, college, and community activities.

Study and appraisal of mental health principles. Some fundamental principles of mental health are reviewed and presented in the form of *guide lines* for effective living. These can be studied and considered by the student for incorporation into his own mental health program. The following specific suggestions or guides have been derived from a number of authorities in the field of mental health [2, 15, 20, 25, 26, 27]:

1. Have a practical plan for achieving a successful life centered in work, play, love, and faith. Develop your philosophy of life. Have several major attainable goals, and enjoy working toward them.
2. Keep yourself in good physical condition through a balanced program of physical activity, rest, wholesome diet, proper elimination, and personal cleanliness.
3. Gain confidence through making sure of some small successes and a few major ones.
4. Face your troubles, worries, and fears. Do what you can about them; then direct your efforts to more pleasant things. Gradually, do the thing you fear. Time and experience aid in the solution of problems. Remember that time heals.
5. Find desirable ways to express your disturbing emotions, rather than repressing them. Attempt to determine why you go off at a tangent. Know yourself. Control your emotions.
6. Feel the importance of dedication to a significant cause which is greater than yourself. This dedication may be to your family, your girl or boy friend, or your chosen vocation.
7. Adopt a wholesome attitude toward sex. "Love, but love wisely." Remember that sex functions when in keeping with the standards and mores of society are a source of rewarding satisfactions contributing to personality development.
8. Cultivate a variety of active interests. Special interests, such as sports and hobbies, are examples.
9. Cultivate a sense of humor. Admit your own mistakes, and be able to laugh at yourself for some of your "boners."
10. Accept criticism impersonally, and profit by it. Avoid brooding over past mistakes. Turn the next opportunity into a successful accomplishment.
11. Enjoy a social life with both sexes. Acquire a few close friends and companions with whom you can share your successes and problems.
12. Maintain a sensible independence. Gain independence from parents, but maintain your love and respect for them.
13. Accept responsibility with a willing spirit when given a job to do.
14. Find moments in each day to relax completely. Find serenity; avoid strain. Cultivate periods of contemplation, meditation, and appreciation as well as active participation.

15. Get along with others. Learn to live in your environment, getting along with yourself, your family, your neighbors, and your community.

16. Do the best you can. Do not try to reach all your goals at once. Do not try to do better than your best. Be satisfied with making some progress if it is the best you can do.

After carefully reading and thinking through the above precepts for sound personal and social adjustment, the student can check his own situation by using the principles as a check list (see Suggested Activities).

Planning and replanning a program for happier, healthier living. Meeting health needs and interests implies that the student takes time to think through and chart his desired course of action and life activities. This means deciding what he wants to accomplish in life, in what values he believes, what principles he is going to follow, and what course of action will enable him to attain his goals.

The student who plans his own program feels more secure in himself. He knows what he wants, where he is going, and how he is going to get there. Temporary blocks do not discourage him, because he is able to replan in view of new situations, modifying his goals if necessary to meet the changing situations, but making successful adjustments. His goals are in harmony with his needs and interests. They are not too remote, nor are they above or below his capacities. He substitutes planning for worrying. He is achieving an integrated, purposeful life.

The student's program based on his own needs and interests is a well-balanced program in terms of life activities. The student's goals formulated in relation to the major areas of life activities should include social, political, religious, educational, industrial, and recreational aims [19]. It is the responsibility of every mature individual to participate in activities in each of the above areas—in some areas more than in others, but a balanced program, which is what he strives for, should include a real interest in each.

Application of the principles of mental health. While an understanding of the principles of mental health is important to better personal and social adjustment, actually it is only a beginning step toward improvement. It is only when the principles become guides to action that real achievement occurs. It is paramount that the principles give intelligent direction to the student's own life activities. Only the student himself can shape his life the way he wants to live it. Only he can make life adjustments to find the happiness he seeks. It is well to remember Henry Drummond's remarks regarding the pursuit of happiness: "Half the world is on the wrong scent in the pursuit of happiness. They think it consists in having and getting and in being served by others, but it consists in giving and in serving others." To follow the precepts of mental health takes persistence and fortitude, but applying these principles to everyday living can bring about happier, healthier, more effective living.

Suggested Activities

1. Appraise yourself on the basis of the qualities and skills outlined in the section on Characteristics of the Well-adjusted Personality. What are your strengths and weaknesses as a result of your appraisal? What can you do about your inadequacies?

2. How do you usually react when your immediate goals are blocked and frustration and conflict are present? Describe your reactions.

3. Do you have any important problems that seem unsolvable? What have you done to solve them in the past? What alternate courses of action might you take?

4. What types of adjustment mechanism do you frequently use during frustration or conflict? What socially desirable behavior might you substitute for these?

5. What are your pet worries? How well-founded are they? Analyze them, and suggest ways of relieving them.

6. Describe aspects of your behavior that you believe exhibit immaturity. Outline suggestions for improving your present status.

7. If you have now or should have a personal adjustment problem, whom would you seek for assistance? Whom would you recommend to a relative or friend for a minor personality disturbance? For a major personality maladjustment?

8. Refer to the guide lines for effective living in the section on Study and Appraisal of Mental Health Principles. Preface each statement with the phrase "Do you." How does your present program compare with the above principles? How many of the sixteen statements are your strong points? How many are weak ones? In what categories do your strengths and weaknesses fall? Compare your analysis with the appraisal you made in item 1. Do your strengths and weaknesses check?

9. With your appraisals from items 1 and 7, formulate your personal mental health program.

10. Preview, show, and discuss audio-visual aids to making life adjustments, such as the following: (*a*) *Control Your Emotions* (sound, 12 minutes), Coronet Films, 1950; (*b*) *Emotional Health* (sound, 20 minutes), McGraw-Hill Text-Film, 1947; (*c*) *Breakdown* (sound, 41 minutes), available from Text-Film Department, McGraw-Hill; (*d*) *Feelings of Depression* (sound, 32 minutes), available from Text-Film Department, McGraw-Hill.

Suggested Readings

1. Anderson, J. E., *The Psychology of Development and Personal Adjustment.* New York: Henry Holt and Company, Inc., 1949.

2. Bernard, H. W., *Toward Better Personal Adjustment.* New York: McGraw-Hill Book Company, Inc., 1951.

3. Bowman, Henry A., *Marriage for Moderns,* 3d ed. New York: McGraw-Hill Book Company, Inc., 1954.

4. Carrol, Herbert A., *Mental Hygiene.* New York: Prentice-Hall, Inc., 1951.

5. Coleman, James C., *Abnormal Psychology and Modern Life.* Chicago: Scott, Foresman & Company, 1950.

6. Crow, Lester D., and Alice Crow, *Mental Hygiene,* 2d ed. New York: McGraw-Hill Book Company, Inc., 1951.

7. Diehl, H. S., and C. E. Shepard, *The Health of College Students: A Report to the American Youth Commission.* Washington: American Council on Education, 1939.

8. Fenton, Norman, *Mental Hygiene in School Practice.* Stanford, Calif.: Stanford University Press, 1943.

9. Fishbein, Morris, and Ernest W. Burgess, *Successful Marriage.* New York: Doubleday & Company, Inc., 1949.

10. Fry, Clements C., *Mental Health in College.* New York: Commonwealth Fund, Division of Publication, 1952.

11. Hartwell, S. W., *Practical Psychiatry and Mental Hygiene.* New York: McGraw-Hill Book Company, Inc., 1947.

12. Hunt, J. McVickers, *Personality and the Behavior Disorders,* Vols. I, II. New York: The Ronald Press Company, 1944.

13. Hurlock, Elizabeth B., *Adolescent Development.* New York: McGraw-Hill Book Company, Inc., 1949.

14. Josey, Charles C., *Psychology and Successful Living.* New York: Charles Scribner's Sons, 1948.

15. Katz, Barney, and George Lehner, *Mental Hygiene in Modern Living.* New York: The Ronald Press Company, 1953.

16. Kinsey, Alfred C., Wardell B. Pomeroy, and Clyde E. Martin, *Sexual Behavior in the Human Male.* Philadelphia: W. B. Saunders Company, 1948.

17. Kinsey, Alfred C., Wardell B. Pomeroy, Clyde E. Martin, and Paul H. Gebhard, *Sexual Behavior in the Human Female.* Philadelphia: W. B. Saunders Company, 1953.

18. Kluckhohn, C., and H. Murray, *Personality in Nature, Society and Culture.* Cambridge, Mass.: Harvard University Press, 1948.

19. Lehner, George F. J., *Explorations in Personal Adjustment.* New York: Prentice-Hall, Inc., 1949.

20. McKinney, Fred, *Psychology of Personal Adjustment.* New York: John Wiley & Sons, Inc., 1949.

21. O'Kelley, Lawrence I., *Introduction to Psychopathology.* New York: Prentice-Hall, Inc., 1949.

22. Redl, Fritz, and William W. Wattenberg, *Mental Hygiene in Teaching.* New York: Harcourt, Brace and Company, Inc., 1951.

23. Saul, Leon J., *Emotional Maturity.* Philadelphia: J. B. Lippincott Company, 1947.

24. Shaeffer, L. F., *Psychology of Adjustment.* Boston: Houghton Mifflin Company, 1936.

25. Thorpe, Louis P., *The Psychology of Mental Health.* New York: The Ronald Press Company, 1950.

26. Vaughn, Wayland F., *Personal and Social Adjustment.* New York: The Odyssey Press, Inc., 1952.

27. Wallin, J. E. Wallace, *Personality Maladjustments and Mental Hygiene,* 2d ed. New York: McGraw-Hill Book Company, Inc., 1949.

Popular Readings

28. *Brief Principles of Mental Hygiene.* Minneapolis, Minn.: The Minnesota Mental Hygiene Society. (Pamphlet.)

29. Doyle, Kathleen, "When Mental Illness Strikes Your Family," *Public Affairs Pamphlet* 172. New York: Public Affairs Committee, 1951.

30. Kraines, S. H., and E. S. Thetford, *Managing Your Mind.* New York: The Macmillan Company, 1944.

31. Menninger, W. C., *There Is Something You Can Do about Mental Health.* New York: The National Association for Mental Health, 1951. (Pamphlet.)

32. Pratt, Dallas, and Jack Neher, "Mental Health Is a Family Affair," *Public Affairs Pamphlet* 155. New York: Public Affairs Committee, 1949.

33. Polatin, Phillip, and Ellen Philtine, *The Well-adjusted Personality.* Philadelphia: J. B. Lippincott Company, 1952.

34. Strecker, E. A., and K. E. Appell, *Discovering Ourselves,* 2d ed. New York: The Macmillan Company, 1951.

PART THREE

Preparing for Effective Family Living

6. Choosing a Life Partner

Preparation for marriage and parenthood is a continuous process from birth to adulthood. It involves many profound changes in the development of the individual. The college student has undergone most of these developmental changes and has become, or is rapidly becoming, an emotionally mature person. He is ready to make his own decisions in attaining his goals. Choosing a life partner, an essential part of preparation for marriage and parenthood, is one of the common goals of students.

The individual seeks a life partner from within his field of eligible persons. In so doing, whether consciously or unconsciously, he attempts to choose a person who he believes will assist him in satisfying his physical and psychological needs. These needs have been discussed in Chapter 5.

It is especially desirable to have numerous contacts with others before choosing a suitable partner. This affords an opportunity for a testing of personalities involving emotional and intellectual appraisals which helps each member separately and both together in proving or disproving their mutual suitability. Many individuals do not use mature judgment in selecting a mate. As a college president once said: "You wouldn't pick a horse out by moonlight, but you choose a life partner that way." The discussion in this chapter is organized to aid the student in answering some pertinent questions pertaining to choosing wisely a husband or wife. These questions are as follows: (1) How does one gain mutual understanding of the opposite sex? (2) How does dating aid in selecting a life partner? (3) What are desirable qualities to look for in a lifetime partner? (4) What is love? (5) How does one know when love comes along? (6) What appraisals should be made when a couple is in love? (7) How important is the courtship and engagement period in preparation for marriage and parenthood?

Mutual Understanding between the Sexes

One of the common problems for both youths and adults is getting along with the opposite sex. It is well to remember that learning to get along with people begins at home. The same qualities that enable one to adjust in the home make it easy to adapt socially. Some examples of these social qualities are acting naturally, having something interesting to talk about, being interested enough in others to be a good listener, encouraging others to talk about their interests, expressing appreciation for kindnesses, showing consideration for others, understanding the behavior of others, and being friendly. The effect one has on others, that is, how he makes them feel toward him, is a significant factor in one's ability to get along well with them. In many instances, this involves subjugating one's own interests in order to express a genuine interest in, and concern for, his friends. A major factor involved is understanding the variations which exist between men and women. There are fundamental differences between the sexes apparent in terms of body build, functions, and behavior. Regardless of these differences, the sexes are complementary to each other.

Studies do not confirm the concept that women are the weaker sex [21]. Actually, women are ahead of men in most phases of growth and development. Puberty occurs in girls two years earlier than boys. Girls are approaching physical maturity at the age of twelve or thirteen, as evidenced by their developing feminine figures. This earlier development also is apparent in the social transition stage. Girls tend to possess a social drive in which sex urges are more general and more easily satisfied than is true of boys. Some of these satisfactions, both physical and psychological, are contacts with the same sex. Slumber parties, tea parties, fashion shows are illustrations of activities based on this interest. Girls do become interested in boys at this time. For this reason, the girl faces social problems, including boy-girl relationships, before she has the same amount of preparation as boys in mental development, education, and experience. It is characteristic at this point for one girl to become interested in boys while her very best friend of the same chronological age has not developed this interest. Often friendships between girls are broken off because of this difference.

Boys, on the average, show their rapid growth between the ages of fifteen and twenty. They possess a sex drive directly concerned with the primary sex organs. As indicated in the previous chapter, the sex drive is satisfied by means of orgasms through nocturnal emissions, masturbation, and, to a lesser degree, other sexual experience. At this time the adolescent boy is greatly concerned with his vocational or professional choice. Much of his thinking is directed toward his vocational future. The girl, too, may have to make good on a job; however, this usually is a temporary situation until marriage. During the teens, romances have more serious implications for girls than for boys. On the other hand, a boy gives less serious thought to his "love affairs." In the later years of high school and early years of college many girls find male classmates too young to be important to them socially.

Metabolism studies show that the male is more powerful and active physically, while the female adapts to the rapid changes called for by menstruation, childbirth, nursing, and menopause. It is general knowledge that man exceeds in muscular strength. Men adjust to extremes in physical exercise better than women, that is, to a variety of activities at high and low activity levels. Women adjust to temperature changes more readily than do men. Women are said to be 2° cooler than men; at least the thermometer must be raised 2° higher before women "glow." Therefore, men perspire more quickly. Women, on the other hand, withstand cold better, usually because of the insulating tissue below their skins and their more adaptable metabolic adjustment [21].

Men require more food calories than do women. A very active man weighing 154 pounds needs 4500 calories a day, while a woman of 123 pounds similarly engaged requires 3000. This accounts for the complaint that "men are always hungry." The fact that women, in general, eat less than men, yet still gain weight, is a discouraging problem for many women.

Women have more sickness, with less serious results. Men have less sickness, with more serious consequences. Women are more likely to admit illness and to see a doctor sooner. Women seem to have better resistance to disease and defects. Men are more likely to suffer a breakdown by reason of the strain involved in their more strenuous activities. Statistics show that women have a greater life expectancy than men at all ages. In addition, their gains in longevity are greater. The life expectancy of white females at birth in 1900 was three years more than that of white males. By 1948 life expectancy for white females had increased to more than five years greater [7].

A general social problem exists in the sex ratio, which has changed from a more or less even distribution of males and females to a shortage of prospective husbands in most parts of the United States. This is particularly true in comparing mating groups, the older males compared with younger females. The average difference in age between husband and wife is approximately three years. Distribution of marriageable males further complicates the problem, since the ratio of men to women is not distributed equally over the country. In the farming and industrial sections there is an excess of men, while in large cities and centers of population an excess of women exists.

There is conflicting evidence as to differences in personality traits between sexes. Differences exist because of their varied functions and pursuits. But individuals differ from group patterns, whether male or female. All women are not this way and all men that way. Women demonstrate their emotions more readily than men. Menstruation, childbearing, and menopause are associated with more marked emotional high and low peaks.

Biologically speaking, the male has greater freedom of action simply because sexual freedom does not affect his life to the same extent as in the case of the female. Woman does not seek sexual experience as does man. She seeks love, which is a fulfillment of her motherhood urge. Woman's primary interest in man centers in her being courted, pursued, captured, loved, and protected. Man may be bent on many feminine conquests, but only one wife. The wife is the one he loves and protects and also the one for whom he works. Along with more freedom for the man goes the greater responsibility for support and protection of his family. This is a paramount feature in the man's role as a family member.

Although differences between the sexes do exist, neither is superior or inferior. They differ by nature in structure and function. Each is dependent upon the other in accordance with their differences. In this sense, the sexes complement each other. Mutual understanding and cooperation are required for happy associations and for complete functioning as integrated personalities.

Dating

Dating may help to provide the necessary experience for understanding and adjusting to the opposite sex. Dating assists the individual in (1) making friends and keeping them; (2) mixing socially; (3) having a good time; (4) producing objectivity in judging members of the opposite sex; (5) serving as a basis for courtship; (6) learning to control or helping one to learn to control emotions and urges; and (7) making possible the choice of a life partner.

Dating may be an end in itself, or it may be rated in terms of a possible marriage. However, much of the emphasis during dating is upon present satisfactions rather than future needs.

A comparison of the values in dating and in marriage shows a sharp contrast. This comparison can be illustrated by a consideration of desirable qualities. The desirable qualities in dating are more superficial, while those desirable in a lifetime partner are necessarily deeper and more enduring.

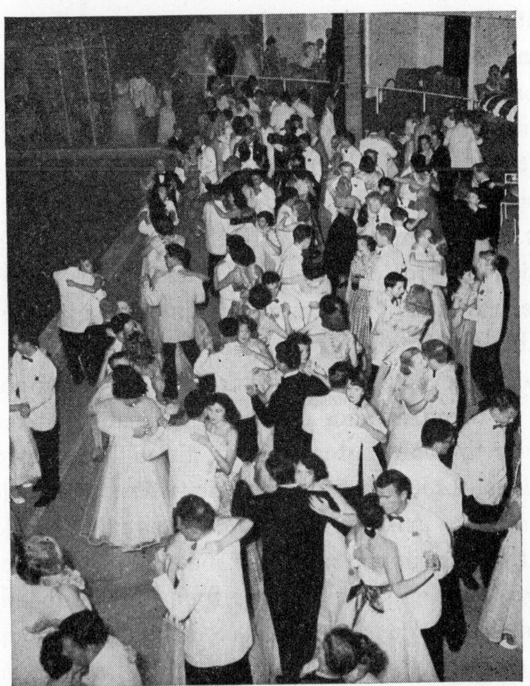

Fig. 6.1. Dating may help to provide the necessary experience for understanding and adjusting to the opposite sex. (*Photo by Stanley Troutman.*)

Bowman,[1] in a study of desirable qualities listed by Stephens College students, found the following:

Desirable Qualities in a Date	*Desirable Qualities in a Husband*
Ability to dance	Companionship
Ability to carry on a conversation	Ability to provide
Good manners	Understanding of wife
Consideration	Love
Pleasing personality	Ambition in vocation
	Intelligence

"Attractive appearance" could be added to the dating list, while, from a man's point of view, "good homemaker" would rate very high under desirable qualities in a wife.

[1] Henry Bowman, *Marriage for Moderns*, 3d ed., p. 162. New York: McGraw-Hill Book Company, Inc., 1954.

Although the contrast in qualities desirable in dates and spouses exists, there is also a positive relationship between the two lists. It is apparent that the desirable qualities of a date may develop into the more substantial qualities of a life partner. The experience of dating can be useful in determining whether or not the couple are companionable. The discovery of common goals helps to determine whether or not the man and woman may become compatible marriage partners.

Dating, with its inherent values, is worthy of intelligent planning. The college student may well consider the following questions: Does he have opportunities for making friends with the opposite sex? Is the circle of friends sufficient to provide wide acquaintanceship before marriage? Is he able to keep friends? Is he using his dates to appraise the desirable and undesirable characteristics of the opposite sex?

Circulation is a keynote for making friends. One does not meet people while sitting at home. Studies on dating indicate that dates are made most frequently through mutual friends, through contacts in school, at church functions, through recreational activities, at vacation areas, and at work. Planning for making friends should take into consideration those places where there are opportunities for meeting members of the opposite sex. In college these opportunities are found at get-together dances or parties, informal gatherings of a variety of kinds, in groups before and after classes, at the student union or the student social center, in clubs, at athletic contests, on trips in which a number of students participate, at the library, and in classes.

Since dating is the exploration period before selecting a life partner, it is the period when the individual can "play the field" to advantage. Marriage studies have shown that young adults with many friends tend to have a greater chance for marital success than those with a very limited number of friends. There are instances when a mate has been selected at an early age with the exploration stage omitted and a most successful marriage has resulted. However, this is not generally true. A number of friends provide a greater opportunity for selecting one who has the desirable qualities of a lifetime partner. Also, there exists a basis for favorable comparison and contrast if one has made a selection from a number of companions.

In the process of selection, keeping friends is as important as finding new friends. Friends appreciate loyalty, dependability, and common sense, combined with an interest in the friend as a person different or unique, especially in respect to his hopes and his ambitions. Friends like a variety of interesting activities. Boys appreciate girls who are considerate of their financial status on a date. Friends frequently are lost because of such factors as continual bragging about one's own accomplishments, frequent references to good times on past dates, the "handing out of a line," and "gold digging." Also to be considered are the individuals who immediately become too serious, who attempt right away to turn their friendship into a love affair.

Going Steady

There are advantages and disadvantages in going steady. If both partners have gone through the "playing the field" period, going steady is merely a natural step toward choosing a life partner. If, on the other hand, one or both parties are swept into going steady too soon, this experience may seriously interfere with making the right choice of a life mate. The decision to go steady is one of those innumerable ones which the individuals involved must make for themselves. It is important to weigh the evidence on both sides in the light of the case at hand, using critical thinking, not merely following temporary emotional desires.

The advantages and disadvantages of going steady, as listed by authorities in the marriage field, are as follows [8, 17]:

Advantages	*Disadvantages*
Makes it easier to gain invitations	May mean choice of mate before maturity, before best judgment is reached
Is a sure way to get to popular social affairs	Limits the choice of a life partner by eliminating chances for playing the field
Provides personal security, particularly to insecure persons	Fosters jealousy
Is a symbol of personal achievement	Becomes a habit and is difficult to break off
Enables a couple to get to know each other well	Breaking up often causes serious emotional disturbances
Signifies a couple is in love	Rarely lasts into marriage, thus postponing the exploration period to the time when one should have made the choice of a mate
Is cheaper and easier than exploring the field	Limits social experiences with different types of women and men
Is a preliminary to becoming engaged and being married	

During the dating or friendship period, with time and favorable conditioning, the feeling of appreciation and affection for one another may logically grow and develop into love. Studies indicate that one in six or seven love affairs leads to the altar, that is, that change is the common

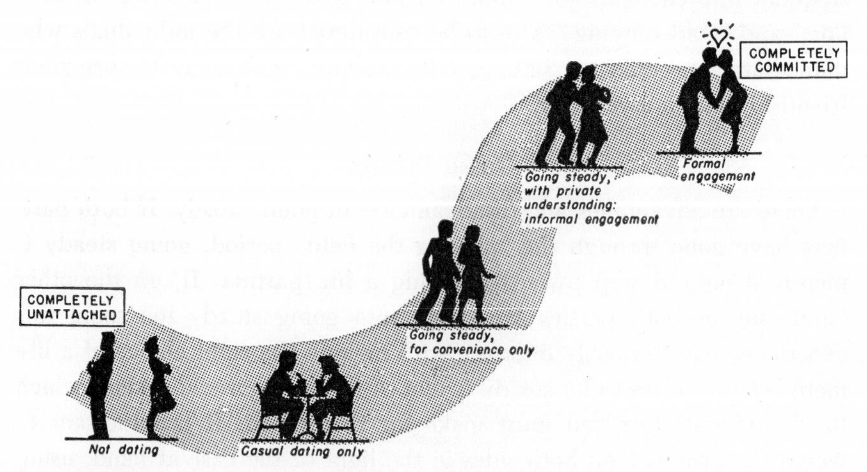

Fig. 6.2. Stages of involvement. (*Evelyn M. Duvall and Reuben Hill, When You Marry, rev. ed., 1953. Boston: D. C. Heath and Company, 1953.*)

practice during this exploratory period. Growing out of dating and several love affairs comes the ability to love and be loved.

Love, a Prerequisite for Happy Marriage

What is love? Do we know when love comes along? Does love last? These are sixty-four dollar questions; yet they are ones for which answers are needed in preparation for family responsibilities.

What is love? The poet Shelley gave a definition of love when he described it as "that profound and complicated sentiment which . . . is the universal thirst for a communion not merely of the senses, but of our whole nature, intellectual, imaginative and sensitive."

Love is a basic need or drive from childhood to old age. With love one grows and develops naturally and happily. Without it the individual may become frustrated and unhappy. The affectional responses begin in childhood. Children must receive love in order to give it. If the child is accepted and his individuality respected, he learns to love and be loved. If he is neglected, excluded, or repulsed, he attempts to defend himself, protecting his ego, but remains unsatisfied. Satisfaction may come later through affection from friends and sweethearts. William C. Menninger,[2] noted psychiatrist of the Menninger Foundation, in an interview said: "I think the best thing parents can do is to teach their children how to love." Individuals influence those about them to love when they have developed their own capacity and express their love to others.

Love is more than possessiveness. It is not making another person over into one's own image. It is not dependency, nor is it self-sacrifice, though love usually requires sacrifice. Investigators have established that one must qualify for love by loving himself if he expects to love others. Robert H. Felix,[3] Director of the National Institute of Mental Health in Washington, D.C., defines self-love in this way: "One has a feeling of dignity, a feeling of belonging, a feeling of worthwhileness, a feeling of adequacy —yet a healthy sense of humility."

Erich Fromm [4] says: "To love a person implies caring for and feeling responsible for his life, not only for his physical existence but for the growth and development of all his human powers."

Romantic love. Romantic love is the total pattern of love behavior characterized by thrill and excitement. It is but one ingredient of mature love. However, it is most important in the selection of a life partner and in assisting in evaluating each person's strengths and weaknesses.

Other elements in the romantic complex which are frequently played up in popular music and the movies are the following: [5]

Romantic love is the only valid basis for marriage. Love is a mysterious attraction of two people for each other.

One stumbles into love when the right person comes along.

There is a "one and only" right person for everybody. Finding this person insures lasting happiness.

Mature love. Mature love is that type which leads to a happy and satisfying marriage. It is what holds a family together. It is the love a wife has for her husband despite his coming home irritable and cross from a hard day at the office. Or it is the husband's love for his wife even though she prepares a poor meal. It is the couple's love for each other that persists when the money saved for a new home is applied on the

[2] Reported by Howard Whitman, "Science Discovers Real Love," *This Week Magazine,* June 4, 1950, p. 5.

[3] *Ibid.,* p. 20.

[4] *Ibid.,* p. 4.

[5] Meyer F. Nimkoff, *Marriage and the Family,* p. 375. Boston: Houghton Mifflin Company, 1947.

young son's emergency operation. Mature love includes romantic love but is of a more permanent and enduring character. It provides security and personal worth for both partners. Mature love is total love based on the realities of everyday family living [6].

Does one know when love comes along? There are still many people who believe in "love at first sight." Landis [6] found: "When 735 college students were asked whether they believed in 'falling in love at first sight,' 34 per cent of the men and 50 per cent of the women said they did not; but 39 per cent of the men and 34 per cent of the women said they did. The rest were undecided."

Love probably begins as a reaction to good looks, good clothes, popularity, physical attraction. It may arise out of an inner feeling, for example, at a dance or sitting close to someone in an automobile. This is the natural sex attraction of men and women. However, this physical attraction is merely the starting point in love; it is not love itself. Love encompasses additional qualities of personal attachment over and above the sexual drive. As has been stated previously, it is manifested in one's whole personality, his ways, qualities, patterns of thought and action, tenderness, devotion, sympathy, and understanding. Such love is no longer blind; rather, it is conscious and free. Love is developed by two people's discovery of mutual interests and goals, their companionship and congeniality based on similar personality traits or complementary ones.

Distinguishing between infatuation and love aids in answering the question, "Do we know when love comes along?" Infatuation may come suddenly, but love takes time. Infatuation can be based on one or two traits (usually including sex appeal), whereas love is based on many traits. In infatuation the person is "in love with love," whereas in love the person is in love with another person. In infatuation the other person is thought of as a separate entity and employed for self-gratification. In real love there is a feeling of identity with the other person. Infatuation produces feelings of insecurity and wishful thinking, whereas love produces a sense of security. In infatuation one suffers loss of ambition, appetite, etc., whereas in love he works and plans to please the other person. The physical element is much more important in infatuation than in love. Infatuation may change quickly, but love lasts [4].

[6] Unpublished study by Judson Landis, reported in Judson T. and Mary G. Landis, *Building a Successful Marriage*, 2d ed. (copyright, 1953, by Prentice-Hall, Inc., New York), pp. 45–46. Reprinted by permission of the publisher.

Adams and Packard [7] present some conditions that are usually present before love can develop:

The two persons have had experiences together that have caused each to react favorably to the other.

Each has found present in the other qualities, standards and ideals which they admire.

Their sexual feelings have been so favorably conditioned, without their realizing it, that they find great pleasure just in each other's presence.

Each one in some way fulfills some of the needs that are of importance to the other, such as desire for social approval, or, with a man, mastery.

Does love last? The enduring kind of love comes to the fore when romance wears off. Daily attention and sympathetic understanding are needed for love to grow and become permanent. This daily process of loving, successfully practiced by both man and woman, is the answer to the question, Does love last? Such love calls for a real partnership, with both partners working at the job continuously. One person alone cannot make it succeed. Partners conscious of and practicing attitudes of thoughtfulness, tolerance, and cooperativeness develop the companionship which makes love last. Good insurance comes through avoiding nagging, faultfinding, greediness, selfishness, the attitudes of boredom, uncooperativeness, and inconsiderate actions. The partnership then is based on satisfying companionship, exemplified in the motto, A family that plays together stays together. Indeed, lovers must be true friends to make love last, believing that it takes more than romantic love to guarantee a successful marriage, but that no marriage can be a happy association without love. Love lasts when it is mature love—when it expresses concern for the partner's happiness and well-being, when there is a "we" feeling, when it is realistic, when it grows with time [8].

Courtship

Courtship is the period during which partners find out about each other. It is at this time that the couple should stop to appraise themselves, and each other, to determine whether or not their match presents elements that show they are headed for successful marriage. It is a time to look ahead intelligently, forgetting momentarily the emotional aspects, to try to determine whether or not marriage will survive after the prenuptial ardor and interest have worn off.

[7] Clifford R. Adams and Vance O. Packard, *How To Pick a Mate,* p. 50. New York: E. P. Dutton & Co., Inc., 1946.

Appraising the prospective life partner. Perhaps more than any other point, the couple should keep in mind that love leading to successful marriage takes time to mature and develop. Such love grows best out of a happy courtship, with intelligent planning and genuine companionship.

Although the suggestions of authorities can prove of significant value in assisting a couple to know whether or not love has come along, one must remember that research studies and evaluation devices are indicators only, not mathematical equations which accurately measure the love status. Nevertheless, these appraisals serve as guide lines for young couples seeking clarification of their own situation.

Personal characteristics of a life partner. What are the personal characteristics one should consider in choosing a life partner? Terman [8] in his study of 792 married couples found that the following ten background characteristics are most predictive of marital happiness:

1. Superior happiness of parents.
2. Childhood happiness.
3. Lack of conflict with mother.
4. Home discipline that was firm, not harsh.
5. Strong attachment to mother.
6. Strong attachment to father.
7. Lack of conflict with father.
8. Parental frankness about matters of sex.
9. Infrequency and mildness of childhood punishment.
10. Premarital attitude toward sex that was free from disgust or aversion.

Of minor significance to marital happiness are these factors:

1. Age at marriage.
2. The amount of schooling.
3. The length of premarital acquaintance or engagement.
4. The amount of adolescent petting.

Race, religion, and social and economic status, although important, did not outrank the first ten above.

Personality factors are of the greatest significance on both the positive and the negative side in choosing a life partner. Terman's study [9] showed that one of the greatest dangers to marriage "is the all around unhappy temperament of one or both of the spouses."

The findings of the Burgess and Cottrell study on prediction of success

[8] Lewis M. Terman, *Psychological Factors in Marital Happiness,* p. 372. New York: McGraw-Hill Book Company, Inc., 1938.

[9] *Ibid.,* p. 101.

or failure in marriage for the most part substantiate Terman's data. The following are illustrative conclusions from the study: (1) prediction before marriage of marital adjustment is feasible; (2) problems of sexual adjustment in marriage, with the majority of couples, appear to be the result not so much of biological factors as of psychological characteristics and of cultural conditioning of attitudes toward sex. The outstanding factors in marital adjustment seem to be those of affection, temperamental compatibility, and social adaptability [5].

Since personality factors are so important to marital success, lovers should find out how the prospective life partner reacts under emotional stresses or strains. *To be* the right person is more important in a successful marriage than it is *to find* the right person. Lovers can make it a point to discover how the prospective mate reacts to disappointments, to slights, to reverses. Does he or she have the ability to control emotions? If not, does the partner complement or counterbalance the other in emotional control?

The factor of physical attraction definitely is present if love exists. This factor is not to be forgotten in the evaluation process, for it is a vital element. This attraction ranges from the day-by-day stages of developing love to the ecstasy of sexual relations. Sexual adjustment is primarily a matter of knowledge of sex functions and of mental attitudes, environmental influences, and time. This has been discussed more fully in Chapter 5.

Appraisal devices. Eckert suggests three tests in appraising the prospective life partner.[10] Since it takes time for love to grow, the first test is the *test of time.* People do not *fall* into love, they *grow* into love. Infatuation may appear during or after the first meeting and then develop into love. To prove that love is more than physical attraction, the second test is the *test of separation.* Do you feel the same about a person after being away from him for days, weeks, or months? The third test is the *test of companionship.* Do you have a lot in common when you are together? How much do you really enjoy a person while participating in everyday activities? The three tests of *time, separation,* and *companionship* can be used as an appraisal device in making intelligent decisions relative to "true love."

Edson[11] has developed a set of standards (which may also serve as an appraisal device) for choosing a home partner. The partner should be:

[10] Ralph G. Eckert, "So You Think It's Love," *Public Affairs Pamphlet* 161, pp. 4–6. New York: Public Affairs Committee, 1950.

[11] Newell W. Edson, *Choosing a Home Partner.* New York: American Social Hygiene Association, 1951. (Pamphlet.)

First, a partner closest to your ideal—a practical ideal.
Second, a partner of sterling character.
Third, a partner who perennially interests you in thought, speech, and action.
Fourth, a partner in whom you have confidence—genuine respect.
Fifth, a partner you can live with and who can live with you.
Sixth, a partner with a harmony of tastes, standards, and conduct with no serious clashes.
Seventh, a partner in good health.
Eighth, a partner of skills—skills of hand, of head, of heart.
Ninth, a partner worthy to be the parent of your children.
Tenth, a partner who brings out your best—"your best bet."

The Engagement Period

The engagement period is a natural outgrowth of dating and courtship experiences. It is the declaration of the partners that a mutual understanding has been reached. In most cases, there is a public announcement stating their intention to marry, thus presenting to their friends notice of their serious purpose. The declaration gives the couple new status in that they are recognized as future life partners.

There is much more to the engagement than the joyful, proud announcement. It is a time for the couple to get to know each other in a more private and intimate fashion. It is a time for loving and being loved. The extent or degree of physical intimacy is a question the couple must face squarely. To be considered is the fact that conditions, though more intimate than before, are not the same as during marriage. The environment is different, and the feelings of stability and permanence are closer, yet they are not cemented as in marriage. Social approval is not the same as during marriage. Evidence from marital studies does not show that premarital sex experience enhances marital adjustment. The question of premarital sexual relations has been discussed in greater detail in Chapter 5. All these factors indicate that the wise course to pursue is that in which full intimacy is postponed until after marriage.

The late Professor Frank W. Hoffer,[12] an authority on courtship and marriage, told students at the University of Virginia:

> Intimacy involves an integrating of personalities; a passionate interest in the other's ideas, hopes and aspirations; interchange of thought; respect for the other's dignity and worth. While in popular thought the physical relation is assumed to possess the greatest degree of intimacy and while this in one sense may be true, I wish to stress that the ultimate in intimacy may occur in a

[12] Whitman, *op. cit.*, p. 5.

congenial conversation, looking at a sunset together, partaking of a meal. The sense of intimacy does not arise from mere physical contact. It is mental rather than physical.

The strongest bonds to hold the new relationship together are love and affection unselfishly expressed.

Another important aspect of the engagement period is the mutual planning for the coming marriage. This is the time to double-check the choice of the partner, before the life partnership begins. It offers a chance to predict by a closer and more tender relationship future marital adjustment. Questions which lead to marital adjustment may well be raised and answered to the satisfaction of both parties; for example, when can the marriage take place? This problem for young people becomes extremely difficult if they are unable to marry when they are ready to marry. As indicated, guilt complexes may result from indulging in premarital sex relations. Many couples not able to marry at once refuse to practice premarital sexual intercourse, and the natural result in this case, if the situation is prolonged, is the production of stresses or strains which are bound to affect personalities. It has been stated previously that a number of authorities in the field of marital relations believe in early marriage as one practical solution to this problem. If the partners have found love, are fit to marry, and have considered carefully the responsibilities involved, it is better that they marry early and not prolong the engagement over a period of years.

Other questions related to becoming better acquainted and making definite plans for the marriage may be answered if both parties complete a marriage prediction schedule (see references 5 and 5*a*).

Health Status

One's health status in terms of physical and mental fitness is an important factor to be considered in the preparation for marriage and family living. No one has perfect health; therefore, one cannot expect such a degree of health from his life partner. However, it is good premarital planning to ascertain one's health status and that of his prospective mate.

Health is a factor often influencing the choice of a life partner. Many men and women are not attracted to those who do not appear healthy. In other instances, a known defect or disease condition does not influence selection, and marriage takes place. When this occurs, both partners must understand the condition and accept it in order to prevent serious disturbances during marriage. Physical appearance does not tell the complete story of one's health status. Defects and disease are at times not apparent during courtship, especially in the brief, whirlwind variety.

Only on the advice of a physician should one marry if he is afflicted by such serious conditions as acute rheumatic fever, high blood pressure, tuberculosis of the lungs, or acute or chronic kidney disease. It is important also to know that both persons are free from venereal disease.

From the standpoint of eugenics (improvement of the race), each person has the right to know if his prospective mate comes from sound hereditary stock. This can be a protective measure to prevent the transmission of a hereditary defect to one's offspring and to avoid the tragedy of abnormal offspring. Persons with conditions such as epilepsy, dementia praecox (schizophrenia), or manic-depressive psychosis, described in Chapter 5, should not marry unless advised by competent medical counsel. In addition, one must consider whether or not he is a possible carrier of a defective trait though he does not have the disease himself. Also, one has the right to ask his partner whether or not his or her grandparents, parents, brothers, and sisters were normal. This is important. Progressive deafness, deaf-mutism, hemophilia (the dread bleeding disease), cleft palate and harelip, stub fingers, and brittle bones are such hereditary handicaps. Further reference is made to Chapter 4, in the section on Heredity, and to references 4, 7, 9, and 20.

Health examinations before marriage. Health status is best determined through complete physical and psychological examinations. Such examinations (1) attempt to establish the state of general health. (2) test the blood for syphilis and for the presence or absence of the Rh factor, (3) detect anatomical defects that might affect sexual adjustment and child-bearing functions, (4) provide an opportunity for intimate personal counseling, and (5) assist in the inquiry into the family background. Some medical examinations are complete health examinations and cover all the above items. Others are limited in scope, including only a physical examination and blood tests. Usually, one's family physician is the best person to provide the *complete* health examination. Also, local health centers are assuming such responsibilities as a part of their maternal and child health or health education functions. These services from the health center, the local tax-supported public health agency, are free and of high quality. Many colleges, likewise, provide the above services as a part of their college health program through the student health service, as indicated in Chapter 3.

Where examinations are not complete health examinations but are limited to physical inspections, the student or citizen of the community may be forced by necessity to consult several sources before his health status can be appraised adequately. In addition to the physical examination in a doctor's office or a health center, useful information can be secured from the college counseling center, the marital counselor, the community family service agency, family institutes, and the like.

Thirty-nine states in the United States in 1951 had laws requiring premarital examinations [7]. The state-required examinations for the most part include a superficial physical examination and a blood test for syphilis. Hence the prospective couple attempting to determine their fitness to marry need to go further than the law dictates.

The couple are wise to plan the examination with the family physician or with a urologist or gynecologist far enough in advance of their marriage in order to fulfill the suggestions and requirements outlined by the health adviser. Sufficient time must be allotted during the examination to allow for frank discussion of personal questions. This is an excellent opportunity to receive authoritative advice relative to planned parenthood, fertility, and the like, for those who desire such information. The advice and counsel of medical and family-life education authorities are extremely important in determining fitness to marry.

Summary

Choosing a life partner and participating in a wholesome courtship are basic factors in preparation for marriage and parenthood. In all the studies by sociologists, psychologists, and marital counselors the prime factor in choosing a life partner seems to be "to find a socialized, stabilized individual with a happy temperament—a healthy personality, an emotionally mature individual." The couple must be emotionally companionable, sexually normal, and eugenically sound to produce children. Both parties need to be able to appraise their own strengths and weaknesses and make adjustments accordingly.

Successful family life depends upon the selection of the right person for a life partner. But even more important is the ability of each partner to make life adjustments so as to *be* the right person and thus ensure healthful living in the family.

Suggested Activities

1. Analyze your friendship status. Do you make friends easily? Do you keep your friends? Do you have one or two very close friends in whom you can confide?

2. Hold a round-table or panel discussion on the advantages and disadvantages of going steady.

3. Make a list of the qualities you desire in a mate. How does your present girl or boy friend rate in regard to these qualities?

4. Compare your list of qualities with Newell Edson's standards on page 134. Does your girl or boy friend rate favorably?

5. If you think you are in love, complete Dr. Clifford Adams's evaluation schedule, "Are You Really in Love?" (see reference 2). How do you score? How does your girl or boy friend score?

6. For a further check on your love affair refer to Paul Popenoe, *Marriage Before and After,* for the "Does He Love You?" test, or send for pamphlet reprint (American Institute of Family Relations, 607 S. Hill St., Los Angeles).

7. Study your family tree. From the hereditary standpoint, are you fit to marry? How about your girl or boy friend?

8. Studies indicate the great importance of personality factors in a successful marriage. If you are seriously contemplating marriage, make a list of your positive, wholesome personality characteristics or traits. Ask your prospective partner to do the same. Do you both possess sufficient personality factors to help ensure a successful marriage? Do you complement each other? Do you think this partnership should not result in marriage?

9. If you intend to marry your present choice of a life partner, fill out the Burgess "Marriage Prediction Schedule" (see reference 5*a*). Score yourself and your prospective partner. Should you or should you not marry?

10. If you are having difficulty in finding or keeping girl or boy friends, as the case may be, consult one or more of the following: a marriage counselor, a physician, a marriage counseling agency (see list of agencies in reference 12), or a close, reliable friend.

11. Preview, show, and discuss the following audio-visual aids: (*a*) *How Do You Know It's Love?* (sound, 12 minutes), Coronet Films; (*b*) *Are You Ready for Marriage?* (sound, 16 minutes), Coronet Films, 1950; (*c*) *Choosing for Happiness* (sound, 14 minutes), McGraw-Hill Text-Film, 1950; (*d*) *This Charming Couple* (sound, 19 minutes), McGraw-Hill Text-Film.

Suggested Readings

1. Adams, Clifford R., *Preparing for Marriage.* New York: E. P. Dutton & Co., Inc., 1951.

2. Adams, Clifford R., and Vance O. Packard, *How to Pick a Mate.* New York: E. P. Dutton & Co., Inc., 1946.

3. Becker, Howard, and Reuben Hill, *Family Marriage and Parenthood.* Boston: D. C. Heath and Company, 1948.

4. Bowman, Henry, *Marriage for Moderns,* 3d ed. New York: McGraw-Hill Book Company, Inc., 1954.

5. Burgess, Ernest W., and Leonard S. Cottrell, *Predicting Success or Failure in Marriage.* New York: Prentice-Hall, Inc., 1939.

5*a*. Burgess, E. W., "The Marriage Prediction Schedule" from E. W. Burgess and H. J. Locke, *The Family*, pp. 760–771. New York: American Book Company, 1945.

6. Cavan, Ruth S., *The American Family.* New York: The Thomas Y. Crowell Company, 1953.

7. Dublin, Louis I., and Mortimer Spiegelman, *The Facts of Life from Birth to Death.* New York: The Macmillan Company, 1951.

8. Duvall, Evelyn M., and Reuben Hill, *When You Marry.* Boston: D. C. Heath and Company, 1953.

9. Fishbein, Morris, and Ernest W. Burgess, *Successful Marriage.* New York: Doubleday & Company, Inc., 1949.

10. Foster, Robert, *Marriage and Family Relationships*, rev. ed. New York: The Macmillan Company, 1950.

11. Groves, Ernest R., Edna L. Skinner, and Sadie J. Swenson, *The Family and Its Relationships*, rev. ed. Philadelphia: J. B. Lippincott Company, 1948.

12. Landis, Judson T., and Mary G. Landis, *Building a Successful Marriage.* New York: Prentice-Hall, Inc., 1953.

13. Landis, Judson T., and Mary G. Landis, *Readings in Marriage and the Family.* New York: Prentice-Hall, Inc., 1952.

14. Levy, John, and Ruth Munroe, *The Happy Family*, rev. ed. New York: Alfred A. Knopf, Inc., 1952.

15. Moore, Bernice M., and Dorothy M. Leahy, *You and Your Family*, rev. ed. Boston: D. C. Heath and Company, 1953.

Popular Readings

16. Eckert, Ralph G., "So You Think It's Love," *Public Affairs Pamphlet* 161. New York: Public Affairs Committee, 1950.

17. Himes, Norman E., *Your Marriage*, rev. ed. New York: Rinehart & Company, Inc., 1940.

18. Mead, Margaret, *Male and Female.* New York: William Morrow & Company, Inc., 1949.

19. Popenoe, Paul, *Marriage Before and After.* New York: Funk & Wagnalls Company, 1943.

20. Scheinfeld, Amram, *The New You and Heredity.* Philadelphia: J. B. Lippincott, 1951.

21. Scheinfeld, Amram, *Women and Men.* New York: Harcourt, Brace and Company, Inc., 1944.

7. Planning for Marriage

Marriage is a primary concern of a majority of the individuals in our society. Of all the persons in this country who reach the age of fifty years, approximately 90 per cent are or have been married. All who attain marital status are expected to accept definite responsibilities. It is evident that adequate preparation for these responsibilities is needed.

Relatively few college students are married. Nearly all, however, are looking forward to the day when they will marry. The ideal adjustment pattern for most individuals includes a successful marriage, a happy home life, and well-adjusted children of their own. Young adults can be making plans for a successful marriage and for establishing their own family. Some of the questions to be answered during this planning period are, What are the common pitfalls to avoid in planning a marriage ceremony? What are some of the adjustments to be made after the marriage ceremony? What can be done prior to marriage to assure successful achievement of adjustments? What basic information should one have about the physiology of marriage? What are some of the problems associated with unsatisfactory marriage?

Marriage should have the best efforts of both partners who unite for life in what can be a deeply satisfying and worthwhile relationship. The likelihood of successful marriage is greater if the partners enter the relationship with an awareness of its significance and the adjustments required to assure its success.

Significance of Marriage

Marriage is not the same today as it was in the past. Social institutions such as marriage must be flexible to the extent that they can be adapted to the changing needs of the individuals involved. Marriage is unsatisfactory if it becomes so root-bound that it fails to satisfy the reasons for which it exists. Fortunately, it does not show signs of becoming obsolete, as some have suggested. Monogamous marriage has contributions to make which cannot be duplicated by any other relationship.

MacIver [1] describes the family as "a group defined by a sex relationship sufficiently precise and enduring to provide for the procreation and upbringing of children." The marriage relationship established and accepted for this purpose has withstood the challenge of time. However, this definition is not adequate to cover the type of marriage relationship required to satisfy the needs of man and wife in our present-day democratic society.

Each of the marriage partners desires happiness. This happiness is most likely to be achieved if the marriage is successful. The marriage does more than provide for children. Affection, security, sympathy, understanding, and companionship needs are satisfied through marriage. The sex drive cannot be satisfied adequately in any other way because of the psychological concomitants of marriage.

There can be little doubt regarding the importance of marriage if one notes the attention focused on this relationship. People talk about it, religion sanctifies it, magazines and books record what writers are thinking about it, lawmakers attempt to regulate it, and countless numbers of men and women continually attempt to make it successful.

Legal aspects. Unfortunately, the legal aspects of marriage vary widely from state to state. Lawmakers are not in full agreement in their attempts to provide regulations offering maximum opportunities for successful marriages. The established regulations, in most instances, have a bearing on the health of the individuals involved. It is important to be aware of the reason for the controls which are established. If the importance of the protective regulations were more widely understood, it is likely that a common set of laws might be accepted in all the states.

Premarital physical examinations. Regulations concerning premarital health examinations for the prevention of venereal diseases are accepted in some states and rejected in others. All except eight states require certificates showing freedom from venereal infection before individuals are permitted to marry [17]. Some persons discover through the premarital examination that they have contracted a venereal disease. As a result of this discovery, they are able to have the disease treated by a physician. The discovery is beneficial to the individual because it enables him to escape the secondary effects of an untreated venereal disease. The marriage partner is protected by the elimination of a disease which might be transmitted during sexual relations. The fetus is protected from infection during pregnancy, and its chance for normal birth is increased.

[1] Robert W. MacIver, *Society: A Textbook of Sociology,* p. 196. New York: Rinehart & Company, Inc., 1937.

In addition, other members of society profit because a potential source of infection is discovered and eliminated.

Premarital health examinations contribute to successful marriage, especially if the examination includes a more thorough appraisal than the test for venereal disease (see Chapter 6 for additional information regarding premarital examinations).

Waiting period. Many states require a waiting period between the date of application for a license and the date of the marriage ceremony. This waiting period is required because marriages resulting from a spur-of-the-moment decision are not likely to be successful. A three-day waiting period is not a hardship to persons who have planned adequately for their marriage, and the delay prevents many from undertaking marriages which have little chance of success. Dublin indicates that in the United States the number of marriages is 1 to 3 per cent below the number of marriage licenses which are issued [17]. It is fortunate indeed when individuals find themselves to be incompatible before they marry and are able to avoid a mistake which can cause much unhappiness.

Prohibited marriages. Nearly all the states prohibit marriage to certain groups of individuals. An examination of the restrictions indicates that health is an important factor in determining the limitations. Some states prohibit the marriage of individuals with advanced tuberculosis. Insanity and feeblemindedness, to a varying degree, are barriers in all states. The basic reason for establishing these controls is the inability of such individuals to fulfill social obligations. In addition, the possibility of producing abnormal children is of major significance in determining restrictions.

The hereditary factor is the basis for controls over the marriage of close blood relations. Inbreeding results in the combination of genes which produce defective conditions such as hemophilia (in which the blood fails to clot properly) and a hereditary form of deafness. An example of the danger of such inbreeding is the family of four sons and two daughters who developed a hereditary form of deafness, which neither parent developed but which was present in the families of both parents; the parents were first cousins [13]. Limitations on the marriage of blood relations are in force in all states. The degree of relationship of persons forbidden to marry differs considerably from state to state. The soundness of some of the restrictions is questioned by some authorities. Amram Scheinfeld [20] indicates that inbreeding can produce superior children. However, at the present time, Scheinfeld would agree with the ban on cousin marriages unless it is known that the family is free of serious defects which are hereditary.

Getting Married

The actual marriage ceremony takes only a few minutes. Planning for the event may extend over a period of days, weeks, or months. This planning period provides many happy memories for the couple after the wedding ceremony. The beginning of the new family unit is deserving of much consideration. Another phase of the family cycle is entered. This beginning is worthy of more than a spur-of-the-moment occasion.

Social approval. Marriage is more than a relationship between a bride and groom. Society also is concerned with a partnership which begins a new family group with all its opportunities and responsibilities. Social custom decrees the nature of the ceremony. The desires of the couple and also the approval of the social group are considered when the plans are made. The type of ceremony—the church wedding, the home wedding, the simple, planned ceremony before the justice of the peace, the elopement, or the secret marriage—is an important element in beginning the marriage favorably. When a couple are making plans for their wedding, it is recommended that they take time to consider the pros and cons regarding the different types of wedding ceremony.

Secret weddings. The secret wedding, not announced until a much later date, may give rise to unfavorable speculation on the part of associates of the couple. Parents are displeased because they are not informed of the plans or the event. Marriage is commenced behind a screen of secrecy which makes the normal adjustments more difficult. Little can be said in favor of this type of wedding.

Elopements. Elopements are, in many instances, the result of a desire to escape. The opposition of parents, the high cost of elaborate weddings, and publicity are cited frequently as reasons why couples elope. Pregnancy is another possible reason.

In the case of an elopement, friends may be offended because they are not permitted to enjoy the occasion with the bride and groom. Parents may feel that their children are unfair. All in all, the marriage partnership begins under rather unfavorable circumstances. Popenoe in a study of 738 elopements concludes that marital adjustments made by couples who have eloped are less satisfactory than adjustments made by couples married in the home or church in a planned ceremony [19].

Planned ceremonies. The well-planned wedding ceremony is more likely to be followed by a satisfactory marriage. This type of ceremony indicates that the couple has taken time to prepare for the occasion, that each is acquainted with the strong and weak traits of his proposed life partner, and that both are aware of the step they are taking. The marriage thus is the result of a decision based on sound thinking and not on the fancy of the moment. Some of the hazards associated with "picking a mate by moonlight" are avoided.

Planned ceremonies, however, also may have pitfalls. An elaborate wedding which leaves the bride and groom emotionally and physically exhausted launches the marriage under unfavorable conditions. The elaborate wedding may cost so much that the honeymoon and the early weeks of married life are complicated by financial difficulties. The couple is fortunate if the parents of the bride or the groom are able to pay for the wedding ceremony. Emotional, physical, and financial limitations are factors to consider as plans for the wedding ceremony are being made.

The extent to which the church is involved in the wedding ceremony is dependent largely upon the religious beliefs of the bride and groom. It is wise for the couple to consider the importance of the church in relation to the wedding ceremony in the light of future relationships with the church. The late Noel Keys, family-life counselor at the University of California, in his talks with students stressed the fact that three out of four American couples choose to have a religious service instead of a civil ceremony. Marriages begun under the auspices of a minister, priest, or rabbi are much less frequently ended by divorce.

It is important for the well-being of an individual that he plan wisely for marriage and provide a wedding occasion which is recalled with pleasure many times during the years of married life.

The honeymoon. In many ways the honeymoon is part of the process of getting married. The legal requirements of the marriage are satisfied by the wedding ceremony. The honeymoon, however, plays an important role in the transition from the status of an engaged to that of a married person. An expensive ship is launched with care; likewise, it is advantageous to launch carefully a life partnership of husband and wife.

The honeymoon provides the first opportunity for the partners to be with each other intimately and continuously with the approval of society. These early days of marriage may establish the pattern of relationship between man and wife. It is advisable to avoid the common mistakes which are made when a honeymoon is planned haphazardly.

The honeymoon is a time for activities which the partners mutually enjoy. In addition to providing for social activities, ample time should be allowed for rest and relaxation. For a few days the newlyweds simply enjoy the companionship of one another. Soon, however, it becomes expedient to plan activities which help in passing the time pleasantly. On the other hand, it is a mistake to plan too many things and to be so busy going places that little time is allowed for enjoying each other's company.

The cost of the honeymoon is dependent upon finances. Like the wedding itself, the honeymoon is not supposed to use up money needed by the couple to establish the home in which they begin their married life.

The honeymoon above all other factors requires privacy. This is an occasion which calls for the newlyweds to be by themselves. The third person, relative or friend, is not only unnecessary but may jeopardize the partnership. This is a time for sharing with no one but the new mate. Intrusion upon this privacy by an outsider can do little good, and it may cause much difficulty.

For the first time these partners are completely on their own. They make their own decisions. The apron strings are severed. The success of the new partnership is dependent upon the ability of the partners to adjust during the honeymoon as well as in the other stages of marriage.

Adjusting in Marriage

In Utopia all marriages are completely successful. Both husband and wife derive a maximum of happiness from their partnership, which in all cases is terminated only by death. It is apparent that this happy state of affairs does not always exist in our society. Many marriages are terminated by divorce. Many other marriages provide little in the way of satisfaction. Therefore, it is advisable to be aware of the adjustments to be made to assure success in marriage.

In spite of the fact that approximately one marriage in four is not successful and a divorce results, it is a rare person who does not believe that "this is for life" when the marriage vows are exchanged. There is, deep within both bride and groom, the hope that their marriage is to be a truly happy and successful lifelong partnership.

From the time the individual first begins life in this world to the time for establishing a marriage partnership, forces are at work preparing him for this experience. The actual process of getting married is only a point on his life line. He is not transformed suddenly by a ceremony which in the eyes of other persons makes him a member of a marriage partnership. He does change, but the change seldom is extreme. The changes are only phases of his attempt to adjust to a new and different relationship and usually are comparatively slow in occurring.

The problems associated with making the necessary adjustments vary from one marriage to another. For some couples most adjustments do not involve problems, because a solution is forthcoming for each new experience. Individuals who readily adapt to such circumstances are mature persons. They are able to call upon the unlimited resources of an adequate personality and a wealth of individual experiences.

Areas of adjustment. Judson Landis suggests seven areas of adjustment in a study on the time required by couples to attain a mutually satisfying adjustment in marriage [8]. His list includes mutual friends, in-law relationships, spending family income, social activities, religion, children, and sex relations. In the following consideration of adjustment, one additional area is presented, involving the personality adjustment of one person to another over and above the personality factors implied in the other areas.

Getting along with one another. It is advisable to begin marriage with the understanding that some conflict or difference of opinion is normal and natural. The marriage in which husband and wife are in perfect agreement at all times, on all matters, and under all circumstances is nonexistent. The task confronting the partners is to resolve differences of opinion in a mutually satisfactory manner. The desirable solution of differences enables each person to retain his own individuality and self-respect. It is in this area of adjustment that the aspects of adjustment discussed in detail in Chapter 5 should be carefully considered.

A statement by Foster [2] indicates the importance of personality factors in achieving adjustment: "The majority of problems in husband-wife relationships are, basically, personality problems, essentially conflict situations between a husband and wife or other family member, and most so-called money, sex, social, or other types of problems are only symptomatic of the underlying problem."

A mature, married individual respects the personality of his mate. He knows and understands those things which set the mate apart as an individual. Decisions are reached by mutual agreement. Undoubtedly, one person exerts more influence in decisions relating to situations about which he is better informed. Even so, decisions need the backing of both persons if follow-up action is to be mutually satisfactory.

One should not be so engrossed in the big things as to forget the everyday "little things." Remembering the birthday and anniversary and failing to remember the 360-odd additional days is an example of inadequately directed attention. The words and actions which make a person feel wanted each day are the basis for a mutually satisfying relationship in marriage.

[2] Robert Geib Foster, *Marriage and Family Relationships*, p. 124. New York: The Macmillan Company, 1950.

The exchange of wedding vows implies that a mate is accepted for what he is. The person who weds with tongue in cheek and plans to reform his mate following the wedding ceremony should avoid taking on such a task. Efforts should be directed toward finding a mate who does

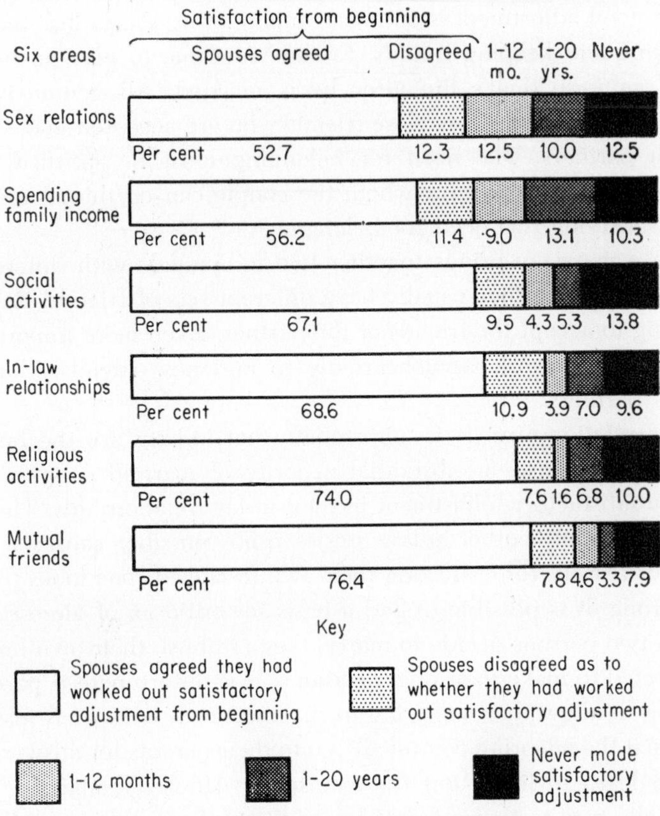

Fig. 7.1. Percentages of 409 couples reporting various periods of time after marriage required to achieve adjustment in six areas. (*Judson T. Landis, "Length of Time Required for Adjustment in Marriage," American Sociological Review, p. 668, December, 1946.*)

not need reforming. A mate should be chosen wisely and accepted for what he is. It is helpful to remember that all individuals have their limitations and that perfection cannot be expected in a mate.

A sense of humor does much to relieve tensions which so easily become obstacles to success in marriage. Life is pleasant if one looks for the fun offered in everyday living.

A final point to be considered in getting along with one another is the need for reducing sources of annoyances, on the one hand, and seeking areas of agreement and mutual pleasure, on the other. This is accomplished by exploiting to the fullest those things enjoyed by both persons and by continually attempting to discover new sources of pleasure and satisfaction for all members of the family group.

Mutual friends. In Chapter 5 it is pointed out that an individual who makes a good adjustment is one who, among other things, has the facility for making and keeping friends. Friends continue to play an important part in an individual's life after he is married. All genuinely happy couples have at least a few close friends who are accepted and respected by both partners. The need for belonging must be satisfied. Mutual friends, with whom and for whom the couple can do things, are important in satisfying this need for belonging.

When a marriage brings together two individuals with differences in social background, they usually have different sets of friends. Each must be willing to accept the friends of the partner. Even more important, the partners should work wholeheartedly to find new friends who accept them as partners.

In-law relationships. It is unfortunate that in-laws are the butt of so many jokes, because a substantial majority of married couples make a mutually satisfactory adjustment in their in-law relationships. The steady bombardment of mother-in-law stories quite possibly causes a few to search for reasons for criticizing their own in-laws. If one looks for something wrong, it is possible to find a basis for criticism of almost anyone.

When two persons decide to marry, they establish their own home and are expected to make their own decisions. It is unfortunate if parents are unwilling to allow their offspring to run their own lives. It is just as unfortunate if the offspring continually go to their parents for answers which they can learn to figure out for themselves. However, married persons occasionally turn to their parents for advice and assistance without jeopardizing their independence.

Factors such as a housing shortage, men being called into service, or a desire on the part of in-laws to help young married couples get a start are responsible for some couples living with parents or other in-laws. In addition, many young married couples find it necessary to have one or more of their in-laws living in their newly established home. Despite the fact that it is best for the newlyweds to have a home of their own, many couples make a satisfactory adjustment while living with in-laws.

Tact, intelligence, and the realization that the new relationship comes first can resolve most difficulties which arise in relationships with in-laws if all persons concerned attempt honestly to cooperate.

Spending family income. Few people are financially able to purchase everything they desire. Most families are confronted with the problem of determining how limited finances are to be expended to satisfy their needs. Budgeting, credit buying, insurance, and getting one's money's worth are phases of this problem to be considered by the members of the family group.

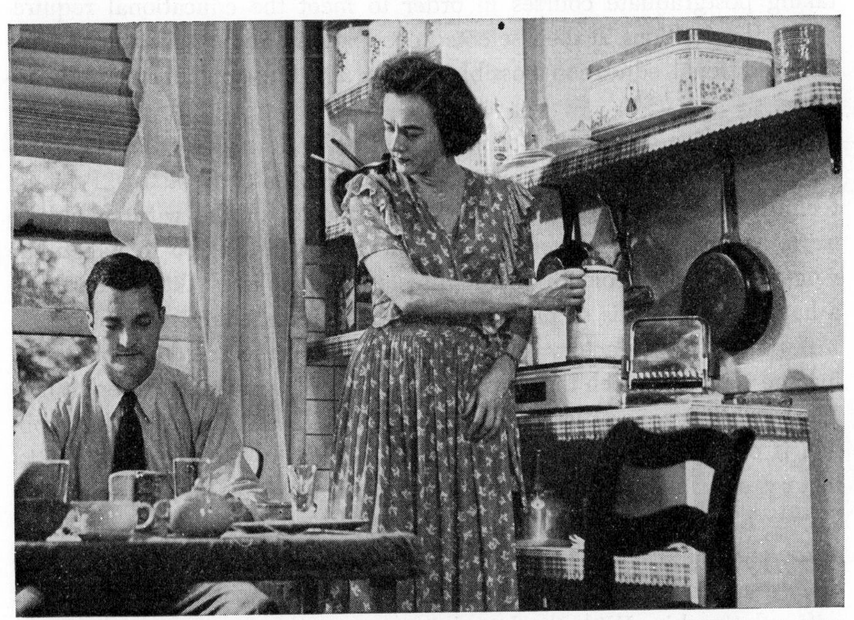

Fig. 7.2. Married students have adjustment problems due to cramped living quarters. (*From "Who's Boss," McGraw-Hill Text-Film, McGraw-Hill Book Company, Inc.*)

Among the items requiring attention is a plan for providing health service for the family. In addition to providing for medical care, the family members decide on the health products to be purchased. They should have a basis for evaluating both products and services to be assured of the most adequate protection in return for what they have to spend. This is discussed in more detail in Chapter 12.

In addition to spending the family income, the man and wife may have to consider the matter of supplementing this income by having both partners at work outside the home. Should the woman seek employment or remain at home and devote all her efforts to maintaining a home for her family? This question confronts many couples in our society today. As in other areas of adjustment, there is no one stock answer to the question. If the marriage of two ideally suited partners can be commenced sooner by having the wife work for a period of time, perhaps it is advisable to reach some agreement concerning a period of work for her. For some couples, this is better than postponing the marriage. During the years following World War II, many wives worked to supplement the GI education allowances and permit their husbands to continue their schooling. Many college graduates are confronted with the necessity for taking postgraduate courses in order to meet the educational requirements for positions in their selected occupations. Some wives have made this additional education possible by working to supplement family income.

The decision on whether or not the wife should seek employment outside the home is based on a long-term consideration of all factors. Personal feelings regarding temporary work or a career for the wife should be expressed by both partners before marriage. The degree to which the woman's absence from the home affects the couple's ability to establish a happy home life is of primary importance in reaching a decision.

A basis for satisfactory adjustment regarding the spending of family income is one in which the partners cooperatively plan their expenditures. The need for cooperative planning is indicated by the fact that this problem is one which requires more time in which to reach mutually satisfactory adjustment than does any other area except sex relations (see Figure 7.1).

Social activities. The use of leisure time presents many possibilities for discontent and as many opportunities for enrichment of the husband-wife relationship. With the breadwinner in many families working less hours than in the past, there are more hours for leisure. Planning for leisure time deserves the serious consideration of all members of the family group. The happily married couple discovers activities which are enjoyed mutually. The pleasure derived from this companionship is one of the essential factors in making the marriage a happy one. These same partners discover that each person has some activity or activities in which he participates with individuals outside the family group. It is worthwhile for the husband to play golf, go fishing or hunting, or enjoy the comradeship of other men in a service organization. Likewise, the wife profits from her association with other women in a bridge club, a knitting or sewing group, a service organization, a tennis or golfing group, on community projects, or in some other activity.

It is sometimes necessary, and in most instances well worth the effort, for both partners to learn and to take part in some new activities which can be enjoyed together. Many leisure hours are passed in company with other married couples. For this reason it is important for married persons to develop skills in activities which are participated in with other couples.

With many forces operating to draw members of the family away from the home for their leisure-time activities, it is advisable to plan for activities which are enjoyed by the whole family. Group activities within the home and outside the home are recommended. The pleasure derived from well-planned family activities helps to develop happier and more secure individuals and families.

Religion. The basic point to stress in regard to religion and marital adjustment is the need for a common interest and a respect for the partner's beliefs. It is expedient to consider carefully the possibilities of differences arising from religious preferences and practices. It is advisable to reach decisions prior to marriage regarding situations which require agreement.

The extent to which religion enters into marriage can be noted by the previously stated fact that three-fourths of the marriages in this country begin with a religious ceremony. Individuals seek the sanction of the church even though the civil ceremony suffices for legal purposes.

Problems arise in relation to church attendance by the partners and by their children. If one of the partners does not attend church, is this accepted by the other? Does the individual who fails to attend church accept the fact that Sunday is set aside for church attendance by his or her mate? Which church are the children to attend if the parents are of different faiths? Such problems must be met squarely. Possible disagreements should be anticipated and a solution agreed upon before the marriage vows are exchanged. Decisions should not be delayed until tensions are created by unresolved problems. Two individuals whose religious convictions are definitely in opposition may find it advisable to refrain from becoming man and wife.

There is no single answer to the problem of religious adjustment for married persons. Each couple has its own peculiar problems to solve. The solutions are more likely to be satisfactory if they are based upon respect for one's partner and for his basic beliefs.

Children. On the basis of the sociological definition of the family given earlier in this chapter, one can see that children, their procreation and upbringing, are a foundation of marriage in our society. Most parents agree that their children provide many of the happiest and most satisfying experiences of their lifetime. These same parents indicate that children are the center of many problems which create tensions between man and wife.

Associated with procreation are such problems as the following: Shall we have children? When shall we have children? How many children shall we have? Most couples desire children of their own. If this feeling is not mutual, the individuals have been unwise in their selection of a mate. Complicating the desire to have children are such factors as lack of sufficient income to provide for children, inadequacy of housing facilities, and physical inability to have children.

Couples who have children find it expedient to agree on the way in which the children are handled. Disagreements between parents, resulting in an inconsistency in parent-child relations, are difficult for the parent and for the child. Fortunately, the modern parent has many resources upon which to depend for valuable assistance when the need arises.

The following chapter provides more detailed information concerning parent-child relationships and indicates valid sources of information for parents.

Sex relations. Landis reports that fewer couples achieve mutually satisfactory adjustments in sex relations than is the case in any of the other adjustment areas. He also reports that adjustments in sex relations and in spending family income require a longer period of time than do adjustments in any of the other areas [8].

An improved understanding of the physiology and psychology of sexual relations in marriage is helpful to many married couples. Likewise, every effort should be made to establish favorable attitudes concerning sex relations. Emotional blocks resulting from poor attitudes make the adjustments in marriage extremely difficult, if not impossible, for some. Sexual relations between well-adjusted marriage partners serve as a strong unifying force to make the marriage relationship a richer and more satisfying experience. Such persons appreciate sex relations as more than a mere physical relationship.

Rice lists procreation, self-expression, and security as three purposes of sex [4]. An understanding of these purposes eliminates many of the obstacles to successful adjustment. The procreative function needs little elaboration at this point except to indicate that too few persons understand and appreciate the intricate pattern involved in the beginning of a new human life.

It is a misfortune indeed not to appreciate fully the deep inner quality of intimate association in normal sexual relations. The physical satisfaction is in reality insignificant in comparison with the deep emotional compensation which comes from the love expressed by two persons who not only accept but desire sexual relations as a necessary and valuable component of family living.

The everlasting quest for security permeates the thoughts of mankind. This quest is aided immeasurably when sexual relations between husband and wife are such that the bond between them is strengthened. The feeling that "He is mine and I am his" provides security for the mates as they face their responsibilities within and outside the family. Parents who feel secure, who love one another and can depend upon this love, transmit a feeling of security to their children.

Physiology of Marriage

The misinformation in relation to the reproductive function of human beings is extensive and, to say the least, unfortunate. Accurate information concerning reproduction is important in determining whether happiness in marriage is achieved. Those who know little and recognize their inadequacy will seek accurate information; but people who believe they have all the answers are unlikely to search further.

Anatomically the male and female reproductive systems are complementary. This enables the sperm and the egg to unite to begin a new life within the mother. Structurally, in all but a small minority of cases, sexual relations between male and female are free of complications. On the other hand, because of attitudes toward sexual response, some individuals have difficulty when they marry and attempt to make adjustments necessary for mutually satisfactory sexual relations.

Accurate information about the anatomy and physiology of the reproductive systems and a sincere desire to please one's partner in marriage do much to reduce difficulties in adjustment. The following discussion provides basic information for an understanding of the normal functioning of both male and female genital systems.

Male genitalia. The reproductive cell produced by the male is the spermatozoon, or *sperm.* The sperm cells are produced, a real example of mass production, in the paired sex glands, or testicles. The testicles are suspended in the scrotum, a saclike external structure behind the penis. These glands produce a sufficient number of spermatozoa to provide 200 million to 600 million or more of these cells for each normal ejaculation, or discharge.

The microscopic, tadpole-shaped sperm are formed within the minute, coiled tubes which make up the testicle. The newly formed cells are collected in the epididymis, where they are stored until discharged from the body.

Safeguarding the sperm. The spermatozoa are affected readily by adverse conditions. They lose their ability to fertilize an ovum, or egg, in a matter of hours (probably twenty-four to forty-eight hours at the most) even under favorable conditions.

The location of the testicles outside the body provides the lower temperature necessary for survival of the sperm. The male whose testicles fail to descend from the body cavity into the scrotum is sterile unless

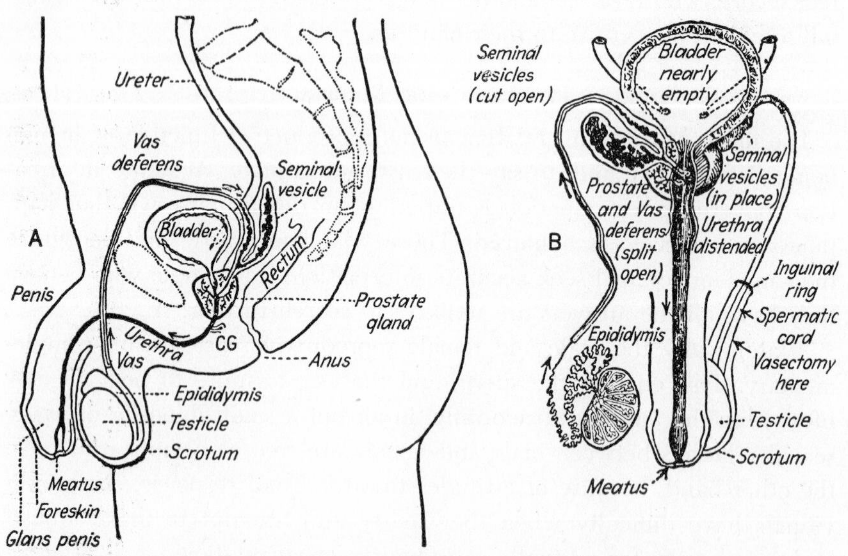

Fig. 7.3. The male reproductive system. (Henry A. Bowman, "Marriage for Moderns," 3d ed., p. 416. New York: McGraw-Hill Book Company, Inc., 1954.)

proper medical treatment is undertaken to cause the testicles to descend. Normally these glands pass down into the scrotum either before birth or soon after.

When discharged from the epididymis, the sperm are combined with the secretions from the seminal vesicles and the prostate gland to form the seminal fluid, or semen. In addition to providing an ideal environment, these fluids serve as a means of transportation for the sperm. The cells become activated when exposed to these secretions. The whiplike action of a sperm's tail helps to propel the cell when it is deposited on the surface of the vagina during intercourse.

Discharge of the sperm. The penis is composed of columns of erectile tissue which run lengthwise in the organ. In addition, the urethral canal extends the length of the penis, providing a passageway for the sperm and for the elimination of urine from the urinary bladder. During periods of sexual stimulation the penis becomes enlarged as a result of the increase of blood in the erectile tissue and thus becomes sufficiently rigid to enable it to enter the vagina during intercourse.

Continued stimulation during intercourse results in an orgasm. This is the climax of the stimulation and is accompanied by a series of contractions which force the seminal fluid out through the urethral canal. The discharge of semen from the penis is called an ejaculation.

The discharge may occur normally while the male is asleep. Orgasm which occurs in this manner is called a nocturnal emission, or "wet dream." This type of sexual outlet has been discussed in Chapter 5. It is important for the male approaching maturity to understand that this is a perfectly normal occurrence, along with growth of hair on the body, appearance of a beard, deepening of the voice, and broadening of the shoulders.

Self-stimuation, or masturbation, resulting in orgasm causes a discharge of semen just the same as during intercourse or wet dreams. The significance of masturbation also is discussed in Chapter 5. At this point it suffices to say that, although masturbation is not the ideal outlet for the sex drive, neither is it known to be physically harmful to the individual under most circumstances. However, guilt feelings associated with masturbation cause emotional difficulties for some individuals.

Circumcision. It is common practice at the present time to have the physician perform minor surgery to free the foreskin of the penis. If this is not done, the male may have difficulty due to irritation and infection around the head of the penis. Circumcision usually is performed within the first two weeks after the birth of the boy. The surgery is easier on the individual at this early age, but it may be performed at any age.

Female genitalia. The reproductive cell produced by the female is called the ovum, or egg. It is from this speck of protoplasm, barely visible to the human eye, that each human being grows and develops. Approximately 300 to 500 mature ova are produced by the average female during a lifetime. The maturation and release of one or more ova by the female sex glands or ovaries occur approximately every twenty-eight days. The almond-shaped ovaries, which are about 1 to 2 inches in length, are located within the abdominal cavity.

Only one ovum matures or ripens during each menstrual cycle under ordinary circumstances. This one ovum moves to the surface of the ovary and is enclosed in a saclike structure called a graafian follicle. The ovum is released when the follicle ruptures. In this way the egg is freed to start on its journey. The release of a mature ovum is called ovulation.

Mature ova are released regularly in most women for a period of approximately thirty years beginning with puberty and lasting until menopause.

The mature ovum, under normal circumstances, is drawn into the open end of the fallopian tube and gradually is moved down the tube toward the uterus, or womb. The uterus is a small, hollow, pear-shaped organ which has the ability, during pregnancy, to expand many times its normal

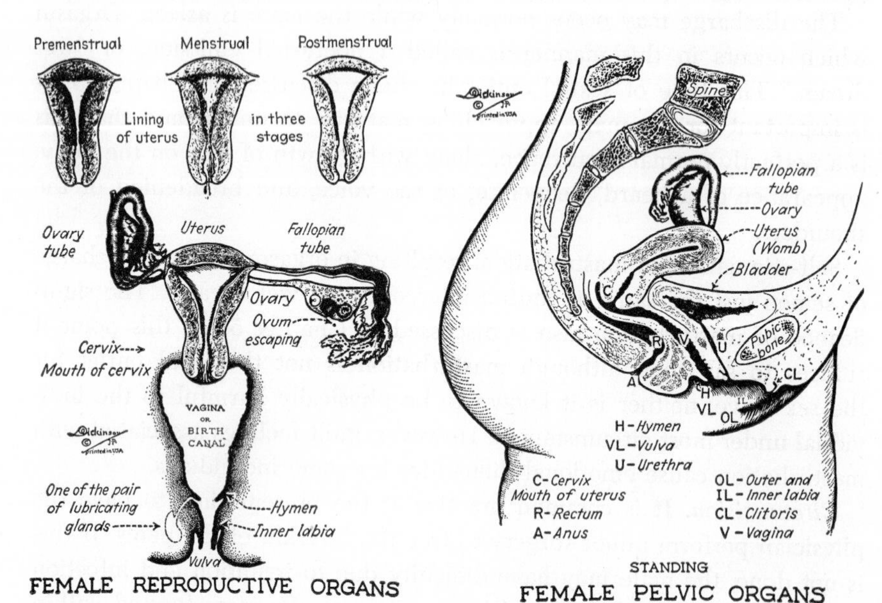

Fig. 7.4. The female reproductive organs. (*Copyright Robert Latou Dickinson, by permission from Educational Department, Tampax Incorporated.*)

size as the fetus grows and creates pressure from within. At the small end of the uterus, corresponding to the location of the stem of a pear, there is an opening of about the same diameter as the lead in an ordinary pencil. The small rounded end of the uterus, called the cervix, extends into the tubelike vagina, which in turn opens to the surface of the body. During intercourse the penis is inserted into the vagina, which stretches to allow its entrance. Semen is deposited at the mouth of the uterus. From this area the sperm make their way up through the uterus and into the fallopian tubes in search of an ovum to fertilize.

External genitalia. Observation of the diagram of the female genital system shows that, for the most part, the genital organs are located within the body. One of the structures located at or near the body surface is the hymen, or "maidenhead." This membrane, when present, stretches across the lower part of the vagina near the external opening. The extent of the membrane varies considerably with different women. It is negligible in many women and almost completely obstructs the opening in others. Because of its location and the nature of the membrane, the hymen is sometimes considered an indicator of virginity. It is important to understand, however, that the tissue can be broken down in other ways besides intercourse. Its presence or absence is not valid evidence as to whether or not the person has had intercourse at some previous time.

Intercourse may be difficult or impossible if the hymen obstructs the vaginal opening. For this reason, it is wise for the woman to have her physician examine this membrane during the premarital health examination. Correction under the physician's care is a simple matter if it is necessary. This correction prior to marriage aids the couple in making a satisfactory adjustment in their sexual relations during marriage.

The labia, or folds of skin, which extend over the vaginal opening also cover the clitoris and the urethral orifice, or opening, from the urinary bladder. The clitoris is the seat of much of the feeling or stimulation for the woman during sexual relations.

Menstrual cycle. Menstruation is one phase of the menstrual cycle. It is unfortunate that some women and men are unaware of the real significance of menstruation. The false ideas concerning this perfectly normal bodily process cause difficulty in adjustment for some individuals. The first and foremost idea to bear in mind is the fact that menstruation is not an illness. It is a normal function of the reproductive system and is one sign of increasing female maturity. Menstruation results when the egg produced by the ovary is not fertilized and the prepared uterine lining tissue is not needed.

Some days prior to ovulation the menstrual cycle is initiated by the production of a follicle-stimulating hormone by the anterior lobe of the pituitary gland. This hormone stimulates the maturation of an ovum. The ovum moves to the surface of the ovary and is enclosed in the graafian follicle. This follicle in turn secretes a hormone (estrogen) which causes changes in the lining of the uterus in preparation for the arrival of a fertilized egg. When ovulation occurs, the ovum leaves the follicle and the lining cells of this follicle change to form what is known as the corpus luteum. The corpus luteum functions as a source of still another hormone (progesterone). This hormone also stimulates the endometrium, or lining of the uterus, to further its preparations for receiving the fertilized egg.

The lining of the uterus, after a period of days, is in a full state of readiness for a fertilized egg. Theoretically if the implantation of a fertilized egg has not taken place within approximately fourteen days, the corpus luteum ceases to function. The lack of progesterone then leads to a disintegration of the endometrial tissue. The lining of the uterus gradually sloughs off, and some loss of blood occurs during the process. This passage of blood and lining cells of the uterus is called menstruation. The average duration of the menstrual flow is between three and six days for most women. Variations from this are perfectly normal for some individuals, however.

Following menstruation, the lining of the uterus returns to a quiescent or resting state until stimulation by endocrine secretions initiates the cycle once again. The average woman has a menstrual period approximately every twenty-eight days. Variation in length of time between menstrual periods is normal. For some women the time between periods is less than twenty-eight days, and for other women the time is longer.

Menarche. The first menses, for the average girl, occur between twelve and fourteen years of age; but menstruation may start as early as the ninth year or as late as the seventeenth or eighteenth year. Menstruation is only one of the indications of the onset of puberty. Enlargement of the pelvis, filling out of the breasts, and the appearance of pubic and axillary hair offer physical evidence that the girl is maturing.

The importance of properly preparing a girl for the first menses needs to be understood by all parents. The emotional effect of a first menstrual flow on an uninformed girl can be severe. The possibility of poor adjustment to the menstrual process is reduced by providing sound information for the girl prior to the onset of the menstrual periods.

Dysmenorrhea. Painful menstruation, or dysmenorrhea, is a problem to some women. Much can be done to alleviate this difficulty by developing proper attitudes concerning the normal function of menstruation and by seeking the assistance of a physician to correct remediable defects which exist.

Possible indications of a condition which needs correction are prolonged menstrual flow, irregularity in appearance of the menstrual period, and leukorrhea, or discharge. These symptoms are not always indicative of malfunction. However, it is advisable to seek the advice of one's physician when they occur. Infections or malignant growths sometimes are the cause of such symptoms, and early treatment is important to control these disorders.

Menopause. Whereas puberty refers to the beginning of the occurrence of the menstrual cycle, menopause refers to the period during which the decrease and cessation of menstruation occur. A gradual decrease in the function of the ovaries is the main characteristic of the menopause, or climacteric. Cessation of ovulation means the conclusion of the childbearing period for the woman. Menopause occurs in a majority of women sometime between the ages of forty-five and fifty-five years. Most women have no general disturbance in body function. However, emotional strain is a problem for some during this period of change. Poor attitudes regarding the change and an inadequate understanding of what is taking place are factors which contribute to the difficulties experienced by some women. Assistance by a gynecologist or by one's family physician can be helpful to a woman who experiences bodily disturbances due to endocrine imbalance.

In making and maintaining good adjustments in sexual relations it is important for the woman to understand that the end of the childbearing period does not mean the termination of normal sexual relations.

Unsatisfactory Marriages

Marriages are terminated in the divorce court because husband and wife fail to establish a mutually satisfactory relationship which they deem worth continuing. It is unfortunate that so many couples come to this conclusion. Just as unfortunate, or perhaps even more so in many instances, are the marriages in which individuals fail to attain a mutually desirable relationship and yet continue to remain together under extremely trying conditions over long periods of time.

It is unduly optimistic to expect every married couple to make all the adjustments discussed earlier in this chapter. It is too much to expect every marriage to be a completely happy and satisfying relationship for both partners. However, it is reasonable to expect all individuals who plan to marry to be prepared adequately for such an important undertaking. All couples are expected to make a wholehearted effort to accomplish the required adjustments.

Those who seek to escape from an unsatisfactory marriage through a divorce are not necessarily repudiating marriage. The fact that approximately one out of eight married women have been married previously is an indication that these women are not rejecting marriage because of one unsuccessful venture.

Marriage is not fulfilling its purposes if all possible resources are exhausted and the relationship continues to be unsatisfactory. To desert one's mate, to separate informally without dissolving a partnership which really is nonexistent, or to take a new mate without legally ending a former partnership is not a feasible solution if the sanctity of marriage is to be maintained. Divorce, as a commonly accepted means of terminating unsuccessful marriages, needs to be understood by members of society.

The following statement by Kingsley Davis[3] points out the necessity for understanding all aspects of divorce:

> Since divorce is an old institution and is embedded in the social structure in countless ways, there already exist agencies for handling its different aspects. First, divorce is a legal matter, with its elaborate legal machinery and a traditional legal philosophy for handling it. Second, it is a cultural and statistical fact, with certain hard realities. Third, it is an emotional and personal process, with psychologic and psychiatric ramifications. Finally, it is a moral fact, with official and unofficial attitudes toward it that are mutually opposed. All these aspects must be kept in mind if divorce is to be understood.

Divorce is not an easy way out. The individual who assumes that a divorce provides a simple solution to an unsatisfactory marriage can be badly mistaken. Many factors complicate the adjustments required by the termination of a marriage partnership. A few of these factors are considered in the following paragraphs.

Policies regarding divorce vary widely among the various religious groups. Some religious codes do not recognize divorce. For some individuals the church position in regard to divorce and remarriage proves to be an insurmountable obstacle.

Alimony payments can constitute a severe handicap to future adjustments by the man. Paying for a past mistake while attempting to make a new adjustment makes the latter extremely difficult.

The task of caring for children, unfortunate victims of an unsatisfactory marriage, presents one of the most difficult aspects of the adjustment following divorce. There is no single solution for the relationship between a divorced couple and their children. Each couple choosing divorce must come to some decision concerning their children. At best this is a difficult decision.

Finally, the individual has to make his personal adjustment to a society in which he has participated previously as a member of a marriage

[3] Kingsley Davis, "Divorce," in Morris Fishbein and Ernest Burgess (Eds.), *Successful Marriage*, p. 459. New York: Doubleday & Company, Inc., 1949.

partnership. Examination of our society shows that it is constructed primarily around the activities of married couples and their families. The adjustment to society without the benefit of the marriage partner is more difficult than many persons anticipate. This problem is a distinct handicap to those whose marriage partnership has been characterized by frequent associations with other married couples. The felt need for a partner to satisfy the demands of a "couple or family society" induces some to seek a new mate.

Help for those who need it. The trend toward establishing more qualified marriage counseling services offers hope in solving the problem of unsatisfactory marriages. These services provide help for many marriage partners who are having difficulties. Some couples are unable to work out all their own problems without the aid of trained personnel and need help in discovering the stumbling blocks and in planning the ways and means of surmounting the obstacles to successful marriage.

The need for qualified personnel to provide the required type of counseling service presents a problem. Many who offer such services are not qualified. Instead of providing assistance these counselors further complicate the difficulties confronting the marriage partners.

Following is a list of nationally known agencies furnishing information about persons or organizations qualified to provide marriage counseling services:

1. American Association of Marriage Counselors, 563 Park Ave., New York 21.
2. Family Welfare Association of America, 122 E. 22 St., New York 10.
3. National Association for Mental Health, 1790 Broadway, New York 19.
4. National Conference on Family Relations, 1126 E. 59 St., Chicago.
5. National Council on Family Relations, 1126 E. 59 St., Chicago.

Individuals are advised to be as careful in their selection of marriage counseling services as in the selection of health advisers.

Individuals Who Do Not Marry

The importance of planning for marriage has been stressed in the preceding pages. In addition, it is desirable to consider the importance of planning for life as an unmarried person. Some people do not marry and must therefore make adjustments as single individuals in an adult society which is organized basically around family groups. Some unmarried persons adjust in a completely satisfactory manner. Others are unable to accept their status as unmarried individuals and therefore fail to make desirable adjustments.

The factors which determine why the individual has not married are important in determining his ability to make the adjustment. The most frequently stated reasons for failure to marry are: (1) unhappy home experiences during childhood; (2) failure to achieve emotional independence; (3) inadequate development of love pattern—homosexuality; (4) unwillingness to accept obligations involved in marriage; (5) failure to meet members of the opposite sex; (6) failure to interest the opposite sex; (7) failure to take advantage of opportunities to marry; (8) careers and education delaying marriage too long; (9) physical or psychological defects [3, 9].

Those who desire marriage but fail to find a mate are most likely to have difficulty in making adjustments as unmarried adults. Persons who desire marriage should recognize some of the obstacles which confront them. It may be necessary to move to another geographical location in order to overcome the unequal distribution of the sexes. The occupation and also activities during leisure time determine the frequency with which eligible members of the opposite sex are encountered. Changing the occupation may be impractical, but planning for new leisure-time activities is advisable. A person who desires a mate should take advantage of every possible opportunity to meet eligible members of the opposite sex.

Those who do not marry have adjustments to make. There are no socially sanctioned sexual outlets for the unmarried in our culture. For this reason, satisfaction of the sex drive poses one of the major adjustment problems. The unmarried may achieve a normal satisfaction of their affectional needs through relationships with other members of their family group or with friends. They can direct their attention toward a successful career and achieve security in this manner. They can make a contribution to society by devoting a portion of their time to service clubs or charitable organizations.

Summary

Successful marriage is desired by most persons. Successful marriage is dependent upon the marriage partners making adjustments relating to mutual friends, in-law relationships, spending family income, social activities, religion, children, sex relations, and getting along with one another. Tact, intelligence, and a respect for the partner as an individual are basic to making successful adjustments in marriage.

Suggested Activities

1. Compare the regulations relating to premarital physical examinations in your state with regulations in the surrounding states. Compile a composite of the most important aspects from all these regulations. Suggest any additional regulations which you think might be valuable.

2. Compare the divorce regulations of the various states of the United States with regulations of a foreign country. Analyze the reasons for the differences which exist.

3. Compile a list of counseling services which are available to married couples in your school, in your local community, and in your home state. Analyze the qualifications of these agencies to offer such services.

4. Compile your own list of "musts" for your marriage from observations you have made of happily married couples and from your reading.

5. Summarize the advantages and disadvantages of being married in American society as it exists today.

6. List the groups of individuals who are prohibited from marrying in your state, and analyze the health reason or reasons for such restriction.

7. Make up regulations for marriage on the basis of current practices in your state and others, suggestions offered in material which you have read, and a consideration of the reasons for failure of marriages at the present time.

8. Visit a marriage counseling center or interview a marriage counselor in your community. Prepare a report summarizing the information received during the visit or interview.

9. Visit the local court which conducts divorce cases in your community. Report on the reasons given for divorce and whether or not marriage counseling services have been used by the couple.

10. Preview, show, and discuss audio-visual aids pertinent to family life such as the following: (1) *Marriage is a Partnership* (sound, 13 minutes), Coronet Films, 1951; (2) *Marriage Today* (sound, 22 minutes), McGraw-Hill Text-Film, 1950; (3) *Human Reproduction* (sound, 21 minutes), McGraw-Hill Text-Film; (4) *Who's Boss* (sound, 16 minutes), McGraw-Hill Text-Film, 1950.

Suggested Readings

1. Becker, Howard, and Reuben Hill, *Family, Marriage and Parenthood.* Boston: D. C. Heath and Company, 1948.

2. Bowman, Henry, *Marriage for Moderns,* 3d ed. New York: McGraw-Hill Book Company, Inc., 1954.

3. Duval, Evelyn Millis, and Reuben Hill, *When You Marry.* Boston: D. C. Heath and Company, 1953.

4. Fishbein, Morris, and Ernest Burgess (Eds.), *Successful Marriage.* New York: Doubleday & Company, Inc., 1949.

5. Foster, Robert G., *Marriage and Family Relationships*, rev. ed. New York: The Macmillan Company, 1950.

6. Kinsey, Alfred C., and others, *Sexual Behavior in the Human Female*. Philadelphia: W. B. Saunders Company, 1953.

7. Kinsey, Alfred C., W. B. Pomeroy, and Clyde Martin, *Sexual Behavior in the Human Male*. Philadelphia: W. B. Saunders Company, 1948.

8. Landis, Judson T., "Length of Time Required for Adjustment in Marriage," *American Sociological Review*, 2:668, December, 1946.

9. Landis, Judson T., and Mary G. Landis, *Building a Successful Marriage*, 2d ed. New York: Prentice-Hall, Inc., 1953.

10. Landis, Judson T., and Mary G. Landis, *Readings in Marriage and the Family*. New York: Prentice-Hall, Inc., 1952.

11. Landis, Paul H., *Your Marriage and Family Living*. New York: McGraw-Hill Book Company, Inc., 1946.

12. National Council on Family Relations, *Marriage and Family Living*. (Journal, published quarterly.)

13. Stone, Hannah M., and Abraham Stone, *A Marriage Manual*, rev. ed. New York: Simon and Schuster, Inc., 1952.

Popular Readings

14. Adams, Clifford R., and Vance O. Packard, *How to Pick a Mate*. New York: E. P. Dutton & Co., Inc., 1946.

15. Alsop, Gulielma Fell, and Mary F. McBride, *She's Off to Marriage*. New York: Vanguard Press, 1942.

16. Butterfield, Oliver M., *Sex Life in Marriage*. New York: Emerson Books, Inc., 1947.

17. Dublin, Louis I., *The Facts of Life from Birth to Death*. New York: The Macmillan Company, 1951.

18. Himes, Norman E., *Your Marriage. A Guide to Happiness*. New York: Farrar & Rinehart, Inc., 1940.

19. Popenoe, Paul, *Modern Marriage*. New York: The Macmillan Company, 1943.

20. Scheinfeld, Amram, *The New You and Heredity*. Philadelphia: J. B. Lippincott Company, 1951.

21. Scheinfeld, Amram, *Women and Men*. New York: Harcourt, Brace and Company, 1943.

8. Preparing for Responsibilities of Parenthood

There is nothing in the life of a man or a woman so important to them or to society as the achievement of healthy, happy parenthood. One may speak of wise parents, intelligent parents, or just plain parents; regardless of the name, mothers and fathers are the guardians of our way of life and architects of the future. This was true in the past, and it is true now. Present-day young men and women can and perhaps will do a superior job of being the parents of tomorrow. If traditions are to be maintained and our way of life preserved, they will have to do a superior job.

Most young people marry because they are in love. They wish to establish a happy home. They want children. They hope to rear their families so as to be a credit to themselves, to their community, and to the nation. These noble aspirations can be fulfilled. Understanding children and disciplining them wisely are important, but they are not innate characteristics of parenthood. Such achievements are the result of purposeful and diligent effort.

Facts about human conception, the hygiene of pregnancy, childbirth, the postnatal care of infants, and child behavior should be studied. Such studies need not stop with infancy and childhood. They should continue on through the physical, mental, social, and spiritual growth and development periods, including that interesting and often bewildering state called adolescence.

To stimulate an interest in and to satisfy the need for being an informed parent, professional groups have produced a wealth of pertinent materials. Many excellent books, pamphlets, motion pictures, and slides, as well as radio and television programs, are available to parents. Health agencies, state departments of education, colleges, and universities offer guidance in accepted methods of child rearing. There is a need for parent education, and, in a general sense, this need is being met.

An important fact about marriage and parenthood which sooner or later makes itself known is that, the more insight young men and women have into the status of marriage and parenthood, the happier and more secure their marriage can be made. When one purchases a new automobile, he discovers that the more he knows about its construction, operation, and maintenance the greater is his satisfaction in driving the car and the longer it is likely to give him good service. That is why a user's guide is provided with each new automobile: the manufacturer and the agent want to be sure they have a satisfied customer. Is there any doubt that understanding marriage and the subsequent shaping of the personality of a child are as complex, interesting, and important as understanding the structure, operation, and maintenance of an automobile? Can anyone logically question the importance of informing young people on successful methods of being a parent? American colleges and universities supply an answer in part. In most of the institutions of higher learning in this country there are qualified men and women teaching courses on marriage and parenthood. These courses seldom lack for students. They are popular because of the manner in which they are taught and because of a felt need on the part of young people for guidance in and preparation for marriage and parenthood.

It is not the purpose of this chapter to give a detailed discussion of all the factors which are important to harmonious marriage and good parenthood. From among many others the following questions stand out as being most important for the prospective parent to be prepared to answer: How is a baby conceived? What are the most significant aspects of the hygiene of pregnancy? How is a baby born? What care should be provided for infant and mother during the postnatal period? How should children be reared?

How a Baby Is Conceived

Human conception is one of nature's greatest achievements. The physical act which results in conception reaches a climax when the male deposits between 200 million and 600 million spermatozoa at the entrance of the uterus of the female. Under favorable conditions, these active, microscopic cells begin a "fishlike" movement which propels them through the cervix and the cavity of the uterus and into the fallopian tubes. The journey is likely to produce many casualties. Sperm that survive keep moving through the oviducts until they meet the ovum. At first the egg appears to resist their advance; however, after repeated attacks, a single sperm breaks through the weakened wall of the egg, and fertilization, or conception, takes place. At the moment the single sperm penetrates the egg, the remaining spermatozoa appear to be violently repulsed. They retire, making no further attempts to gain an entrance.

As soon as conception has been completed, cell division within the egg begins. After two to four days of continuous dividing, the new combination of cells, or zygote, has moved slowly along the oviduct to a specially prepared lining in the wall of the uterus. It is here the zygote comes to rest to be nourished and protected for approximately nine calendar months.

Hygiene of Pregnancy

Shortly after the zygote becomes implanted in the uterus, nature imparts this fact to the mother by a series of physical and emotional changes. Through the centuries, women have come to accept the following as signs of pregnancy [16]:

1. *Increase in nervous tension.* The mother is easily upset over minor disturbances. This is the earliest indication that she may be pregnant.
2. *Cessation of menstruation.* The failure of the menstrual period is accepted universally as an indication of pregnancy. (There are other causes of cessation, which include emotional disturbances, mental illness, exposure to cold, cysts in the ovary, and the like.)
3. *Morning sickness.* This symptom occurs about the fifth or sixth week after conception. It is common in more than half of all pregnancies.
4. *Changes in the breasts.* Usually by the fifth week the breasts begin to increase in size and firmness. They become tender to the touch and show dark about the nipples.
5. *Change in size of abdomen.* During the third or four month, the abdomen shows an increase in size.
6. *Sensation of movement.* About the fourth or fifth month, movement of the baby can be observed.
7. *Frequency of urination.* As the baby grows, pressure on the bladder increases, resulting in an increased desire to urinate.

It is obvious that the first three signs indicate a possible pregnancy and the other four more or less confirm it. However, to leave no doubt, the woman consults her physician. Aided by modern science, a physician can determine with reasonable accuracy whether or not the woman is pregnant. The tests most frequently used are the frog test, the Aschheim-Zondek test, and the Friedman test. In these tests the urine of the mother is injected into a frog, a mouse, or a rabbit. If there is a pregnancy, the injection causes changes to take place within the bodies of the animals. In late pregnancy, the baby's skeletal structure can be seen on an X-ray film, and the fetal heartbeat can be determined by the stethoscope. Once pregnancy has been confirmed, the mother should continue to be under the supervision of a physician.

Choice of a physician. The choice of a physician is important. He is the one who will guide the mother through the prenatal period. He will deliver the baby. He will probably give postnatal care to both mother and child, and he may be called upon to counsel the parents on rearing their progeny. It is not unusual for the family physician to render these services; however, should serious complications develop during pregnancy or at the time cf delivery, the added service of an obstetrician can prove of great importance.

It is possible that the family has no physician or is new in the community. If this is the case, the mother may find helpful counsel at the nearest approved hospital, local health center, or county medical society. For further information relative to choosing a physician, see Chapter 12.

Prenatal care of the mother. During the period of pregnancy, each member of the family assumes responsibilities a bit different from routine family life. The father experiences a stronger protective drive. He usually finds it brings greater happiness to himself and to his wife when he sublimates his sex urges, particularly during the latter part of the pregnancy. The wife, while she may dream about and plan for the baby, does not neglect her husband. She makes him feel that he, too, is important. As time passes, she finds her weight increasing, her breasts becoming larger and more sensitive, her walk or gait changing; and she may experience some degree of morning nausea.

After these early adjustments have been made, the mother-to-be generally enjoys a high degree of well-being. To ensure maximum health and happiness and to give the fetus its best chances to survive and grow, the prospective mother seeks and follows the advice of her physician in such matters as diet, exercise, travel, sexual intercourse, shoes, wearing apparel, smoking, drinking, the layette, and plans for the delivery. It is common practice for family physicians or obstetricians to provide their patients with a booklet of instructions covering these subjects. The teeth should be inspected frequently. Daily baths are encouraged. The wearing of high-heeled shoes may be dangerous; shoes having low, wide heels should be worn instead. Regular exercise such as light housework, walking, and swimming is encouraged. Automobile trips at high speed, over rough roads, or for long distances are discouraged. Sexual relations during the last two or three months of pregnancy usually are forbidden. Alcohol and smoking are usually looked on with disfavor, or their use is reduced or restricted. Apprehensive parents are told that it is impossible to "mark" the baby and that the sex of the child cannot be accurately determined before birth.

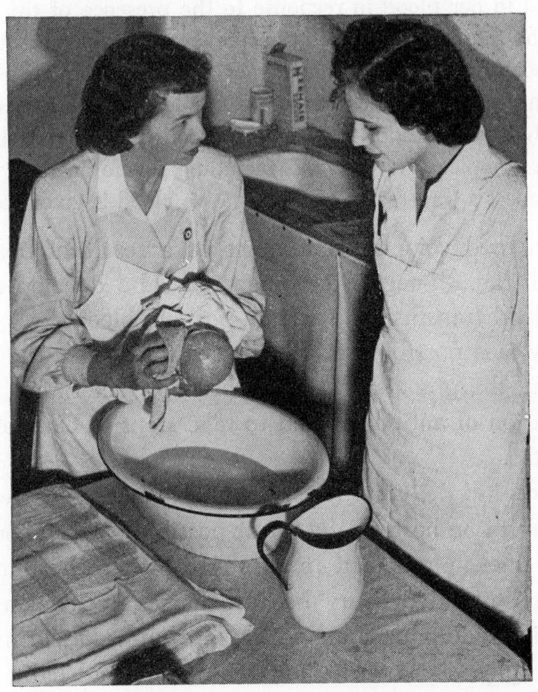

Fig. 8.1. A public health nurse demonstrates proper technique in bathing a baby as a part of prenatal care instruction. (*Los Angeles City Health Department.*)

Complications in pregnancy. Most women enjoy normal health during the period of pregnancy. Now and then, complications occur and should have immediate medical attention. A condition which often poses a problem for physician and patient alike is toxemia. This disease is characterized by nausea, vomiting, a rise in blood pressure, and albumin in the urine. Other danger signals are severe persistent or recurring headaches, blurring of vision, spots before the eyes, puffiness of face, hands, and feet, a marked reduction in the amount of urine passed, general depression, and excessive gain in weight. These symptoms are believed to result from the mother's failure to "throw off" the waste products of the fetus. If all pregnant women received adequate medical care, the mortality rate for this disease would cease to be serious.

The Rh factor. It was not until 1941 that Levine, Katzin, and Burnham discovered the cause of a circulatory disorder which proves fatal to some infants. Fishbein and Burgess[1] describe the general nature of the problem in the following statement:

> When an Rh-negative woman carries an Rh-positive fetus, an antibody is often produced in her blood in response to the presence of the Rh antigen in the blood of the fetus. This antibody accumulates slowly, but in certain cases, particularly second or third pregnancies of this type, enough of the antibody from the mother's blood passes over into the fetal blood to set up a violent reaction, involving destruction and agglutination of fetal red cells. The baby is born with a complex of symptoms, including severe anemia. The condition may be fatal unless a transfusion of Rh-negative blood is given soon after birth.

In addition to developing antibodies as a result of bearing an Rh-positive child, the Rh-negative woman may also develop antibodies as a result of blood transfusions with Rh-positive blood.

Fortunately it is possible for the obstetrician to test the blood of the woman during the prenatal period in order to determine the extent of the concentration of antibodies and to take steps to counteract the danger to the fetus.

Home or hospital delivery. If she had her choice, every woman would want her baby to be born in the safest possible place. There is no safer or more convenient place than an approved modern hospital. Most physicians prefer hospital delivery because nurses, technicians, specialists, modern medical equipment, and drugs are immediately available. Not only does the physician benefit, but the mother and baby have greater comfort and security because of these modern facilities. An approved hospital will always have on display a certificate of approval by the American Medical Association, the American College of Surgeons, or the American Hospital Association. Such a certificate is issued yearly.

Some women prefer to have their babies born at home. In England and Wales, 45 per cent of the babies are delivered in the home; in the United States, 13 per cent. There is much to be said in favor of having the baby born at home. Home deliveries can make the occasion a family affair. The baby is born into the family group and is accepted at once. The mother has her baby within arm's reach, and from the moment of

[1] Morris Fishbein and Ernest W. Burgess, *Successful Marriage,* p. 235. New York: Doubleday & Company, Inc., 1949.

birth she feels that he is really hers. The father is available to the mother and the family during the most crucial times. In choosing the place for birth of the child, these points cannot be treated lightly. However, births taking place in the home require special precautions for the protection of both mother and child [23]. Should complications arise, a home delivery can prove unsatisfactory, expensive, and even dangerous to both mother and child.

The Birth of the Baby

Birth is a natural process. To the baby, it happens but once; therefore, it must go well. To the mother, bearing her first child can be difficult, but, under wise and skillful handling, her preparation, labor, and delivery can be accomplished with a minimum of discomfort. To the father, his first child brings mixed emotions of pride and relief. To the physician, there is the great satisfaction of bringing into the world a new personality and at the same time providing a maximum of protection to both mother and child.

As the date of delivery grows near, the mother's discomfort may heighten. Visits to her physician increase in frequency. She is "tired of waiting" and looks forward to the birth of her baby. The first indication that the baby is ready to be born may be any one or all of the following: (1) abdominal pains appearing infrequently and at irregular intervals; (2) rupturing of the "water bag" which has surrounded the baby; (3) the "show," a discharge of thick mucus from the vagina. The appearance of any one of these signs is sufficient to warrant calling the physician. In the case of a woman having her first baby, sixteen to twenty hours may pass before the child is born. From the moment the fetus indicates a serious intent to leave the uterus until it is entirely free from its mother's body, the physician deals with three stages of action, or "labor."

The first stage is characterized by contractions in the abdomen. This is identified by weak and irregular pains which start in the lower back and move around to the lower part of the abdomen. These pains occur every fifteen to forty minutes. As this stage progresses, the contraction speeds up in frequency and intensity. The first stage of labor comes to an end when the cervix is sufficiently dilated to permit movement of the baby down the birth canal.

The second stage of labor consists in the actual passage of the baby from the body. As the cervix dilates, the baby's head moves into the pelvis. This places pressure on the lower bowel, and the desire to push and expel is given added impetus. For the first child, this second stage usually takes an hour and a half to two hours.

After the baby has been born, the umbilical cord is tied and severed. The physician clears the baby's throat, and, if it has not cried, he administers a gentle pat or pinch. As a precaution against possible disease such as gonorrhea, a weak solution of silver nitrate is placed in the child's eyes.

The final stage of labor for the mother consists in the expelling of the placenta and other membranes from the uterus and birth canal. Its duration is five to thirty minutes. This ends the birth process. The mother is very tired. The father is grateful and relieved. Everyone is happy.

Some fathers register temporary disappointment if the first child is a girl, although it is usually only a short time until they are completely captivated by the new daughter. There is a somewhat greater chance of having a boy than of having a girl: [2]

> Although according to the law of chance, there should be 100 boy babies born for every 100 girl babies, nature produces a slight excess of boys, and at birth there are actually about 105 boys for every 100 girls. The sperm cells containing Y chromosomes may be a little more active, or a little more successful in penetrating the wall of an ovum than are those with X chromosomes. No evidence, however, has ever been obtained which satisfactorily explains the preponderance of males over females at birth.

This brings up the question of sex determination. The method nature uses to determine the sex of the fetus has been a subject of speculation for centuries. Before modern science attacked the problem, all sorts of fantastic beliefs prevailed. For example, in France it was accepted that conception before midnight produced a boy and after midnight a girl. The Babylonian Talmud informed parents to be that the sex of the child depended upon the parent who could generate the greatest passion. There still persists, in the minds of many people, the idea that diet, the moon, acidity and alkalinity, and hot and cold weather influence the sex of the child.

It is believed by modern scientists that sex is established at the moment conception occurs and that it is the male reproductive cell that determines it. The genes in a special pair of chromosomes are responsible for the sex of the fetus. In the female the chromosomes are always xx; in the male they may be xx or xy. Some sperm cells contain x chro-

[2] Edith L. Potter, *Fundamentals of Human Reproduction,* p. 49. New York: McGraw-Hill Book Company, Inc., 1948.

mosomes. If the ovum carrying the x factor is fertilized by an x-bearing sperm, the child will always be a girl. If the sperm carries the y factor, it will be a boy. In other words, the y chromosome is the differential.

After the baby has been born, the mother is kept in the delivery room for fifteen or twenty minutes to be observed for unfavorable reactions. When her physician is satisfied that she is making a normal recovery, she is returned to her room for the well-earned rest and sleep. It is not uncommon for her to have mild discomfort for a few hours after delivery.

The length of time before the mother may leave her bed and walk varies with her condition. The day following a normal delivery patients are often permitted to sit up and later to walk about the room. Most obstetric patients return to their homes within four to five days after delivery.

Upon returning home, the mother is advised to keep up the "convalescent attitude" for two or possibly three weeks. This is a temporary health safeguard. Many women become depressed when they must resume household responsibilities immediately after returning home and at the same time assume the entire care of the new baby. For her future health, as well as her baby's, it is important that the mother resume home duties gradually and that she take regular periods of rest each day. The time which must elapse before she returns to social functions, automobile driving, and strenuous exercises varies with the individual. Special exercises are important to her recovery and will be ordered by her physician. Sexual relations usually are not resumed until after the physician declares her to be in a normal state of health.

To the mother who cannot breast-feed her baby, menstruation may return as early as six weeks after the birth. If, however, the child is breast-fed, the first menstruation usually begins three to four months after the birth.

Finally, it is important for the future well-being of both mother and child to establish the practice of having an annual health examination. Such a practice has strong backing from the family physician and the pediatrician. City and county health departments express their approval by providing for frequent child health conferences. All mothers in the community are encouraged to bring their babies for medical examinations and health supervision. Nutritional needs, health practices, mouth health, immunization against diphtheria, tetanus, and whooping cough, and vaccination for smallpox are among the major services given children up to five years of age. Many expectant mothers take advantage of the prenatal service offered by public health departments. These conferences are primarily for mothers unable to afford private medical care.

Multiple birth. Twins and triplets are of never-ending interest to most people. What are the chances of multiple birth? Potter[3] says:

> In one out of every eighty-five or ninety human pregnancies, more than one baby develops within the uterus. It has been calculated that twins occur about once in every eighty-eight pregnancies, triplets about once in 8,000 and quadruplets about once every 500,000. Prior to 1940, there were approximately forty-five seemingly authentic reports of quintuplet births, the Dionnes being the most famous. According to Professor Horatio Newman, who has spent many years studying multiple births, sextuplets have been recorded by reliable observers on only four occasions, and none of the children survived. No well-substantiated case of septuplets or pregnancy with a greater number of offspring has ever been reported.

Premature birth. Despite wishes, calendars, formulae, and science, no one can predict with accuracy the day a baby will be born. If the time of conception is unknown, physicians usually add seven days to the first day of the last normal menstruation and then subtract three months. This will not pin-point the date, but it will be very close. If the exact date of conception is known, by adding 266 days one can predict with reasonable accuracy the day labor will occur.

Regardless of predictions and precautions, babies are born prematurely. In this country there are about 150,000 such babies born each year. A baby whose birth weight is less than 5½ pounds or who is severely underdeveloped at birth is usually classified as premature [23].

Premature births have a number of causes. In many cases the cause can be controlled, while in others neither the physician nor the patient can prevent what happens. A woman who wishes to come to a normal term of delivery must exercise extreme care during the last three months of pregnancy. In spite of precautions and good care, premature births occur. Accidents and illnesses may precipitate them. Some of the typical causes of premature births are falls on stairways, on slippery floors, and in bathtubs. Conditions such as an Rh-negative mother and an Rh-positive father, pregnancy toxemia, high blood pressure, heart defects, and kidney diseases can also cause a premature birth.

A premature birth may take place anywhere. Outside of a hospital this can, and usually does, produce great excitement. Until a physician arrives, the most important things to remember are:

[3] *Ibid.*, p. 50.

First: Keep the baby warm. A constant room temperature of 80°F. is best. An incubator can be improvised from a bassinet or basket, or even a cardboard carton, lined with a large blanket and heated by hot-water bottles wrapped in towels. *Second:* Keep the air moist by evaporating water in the room. *Third:* Handle the baby as little as possible.

If it is decided to move him [the baby] to a hospital, do so in the improvised incubator in a heated car, or in a specially equipped ambulance if available. A baby weighing less than four pounds, or one who is "blue" and needs oxygen, will almost certainly be sent to a hospital by the physician in charge if at all possible.[4]

From the foregoing it is not difficult to understand why 87 per cent of the babies born in this country are delivered in hospitals.

Sterility

Because of inherited or acquired anomalies, it may be impossible for a man or a woman to produce a child. Most authorities agree that one out of nine marriages in this country is infertile. It is estimated that there are 2 million couples of child-producing age who are childless [10].

Some of the common causes of sterility in men and women are the following: (1) stricture or clogging of the fallopian tubes, which causes one-third of the cases of sterility among women; (2) stricture of the vas deferens (male); (3) postinfection state of the testicles or ovaries, which reduces or destroys their efficiency; (4) defective spermatozoa, the most common defect of the male; (5) lack of erection—rare; (6) failure of testes to descend, which is also rare; (7) emotional factors. Perhaps the best security against a childless marriage is a thorough premarital medical examination. Objective tests and counsel by the physician are available to determine presence or absence of fertility in the male and in the female.

Adoption of Children

Should a couple enter into a marriage and find themselves unable to produce children, there is always the possibility of adoption. The adoption of children is becoming increasingly popular. However, owing to the great interest in adoptions, at present there is but one child available for every ten couples who want to adopt a child. This shortage

[4] Lucile Nelson McMahon, "When a Baby's Premature," *Parents' Magazine*, 37:90–94, September, 1950.

has led to illegal adoption practices. To ensure adequate protection for foster parent and child, many states have enacted adoption legislation. These enactments cover such procedures as permitting children to be legally adopted through independent action, agency adoptions, adoption by stepparents, and adoption of an illegitimate child by the natural father.

Where can one find a child to adopt? The best plan is to go to a responsible licensed adoption or child-placing agency and place a request. State departments of public welfare and local councils of social agencies are prepared to give lists of licensed approved agencies. To avoid legal "headaches," it is best to choose an agency within one's own state.

The Growth and Development of Children

To the average parent, the new baby is a wonderful, bewildering speck of humanity—not well understood, often spoiled, but always loved. It is one thing to marry and produce a child and another to bring that child to his rightful potential. Educators, scientists, and physicians are well aware of this fact, but sometimes parents are not. As a result, there has been no field more carefully studied for the benefit of parents and children than that of the physical, social, mental, and emotional growth and development of boys and girls.

Research studies indicate that parents worry themselves needlessly because their child appears to be slow in growing. Children grow physically because of an innate urge to do so. Growth is continuous, orderly, and at an individualized rate. It is possible to change the rate and direction of growth, but it is not always wise to do so. When a child's environment fails to provide adequate nutrition, physical activity, sleep, motivation, affection, and discipline, his growth can be markedly changed. Heredity is also a factor in the rate of growth and development of children [1]. Studies by Gould [5] show clearly that there is a difference between fast- and slow-maturing families. Boas [6] made a study showing a similar family pattern in growth and height. Klein [7] has reported well-defined patterns in rate of tooth decay within families.

The three firsts. All parents show great interest in the "three firsts" of their babies—the first word, the first tooth, and the first step.

[5] H. N. Gould and M. R. Gould, "Age of First Menstruation in Mothers and Daughters," *Journal of the American Medical Association,* 98:1349–1352, April, 1932.

[6] F. Boas, "The Tempo of Growth of Fraternities," National Academy of Science, *Proceedings,* 21:413–418, July, 1935.

[7] H. Klein, "Experience in Parents and Offspring," *Journal of the American Dental Association,* 33:735–743, June, 1946.

The first clear verbalizing, such as "bye bye" and "ma ma," occurs by the fortieth week in most babies. At fifteen months, the vocabulary has increased to 5 or more words, including proper names. "Car car," "all gone," "bye bye," and other expressions are freely used by the year-and-a-half-old youngster. By the time the child is two, 3-word sentences are normally achieved. At five he has a vocabulary of about 2,000 words and

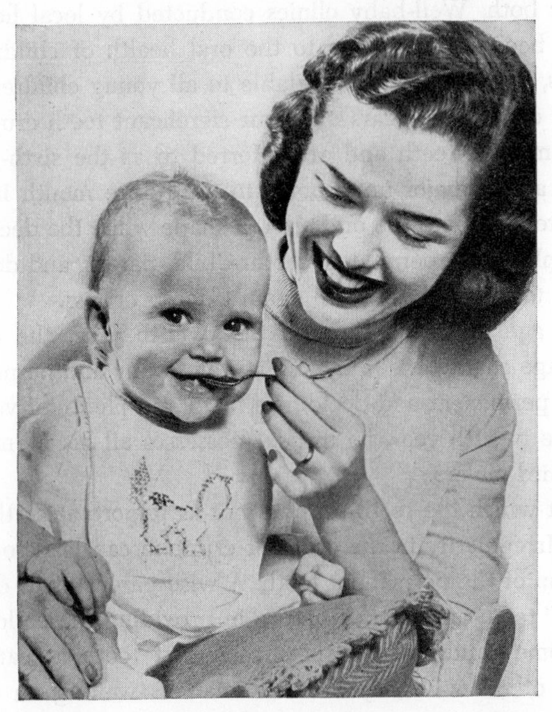

Fig. 8.2. It's that first tooth that causes so much pleasure and excitement. (*Kenyon and Eckhardt, Inc., New York.*)

uses them. The six-year-old youngster likes to use big words and enjoys speaking over the telephone. By the time the child reaches ten years, his language has become a tool and is used less to impress himself and others. Verbalization depends largely on temperament and example. The home environment and the speech of the parents tend to set the pattern. If a child is a late talker, he is only expressing his own rate of growth. At no time should he be hurried or placed in competition with other children. He should be given every chance to develop naturally [1, 4].

The appearance of baby's first tooth is cause for great excitement in the average family. It is a lone front tooth that is usually the center of the excitement. It usually erupts by the sixth month. During the following two or three years, all the "baby," or deciduous, teeth erupt. From then on until about the sixth year, there is little obvious dental activity. Wise parents make a practice of having routine examinations of their child's mouth beginning as early as two or three years of age. Such procedures serve to acquaint the child with the dentist and the dentist with the oral health of the child. It can be a happy and profitable experience for both. Well-baby clinics conducted by local health departments have been a great boon to the oral health of children. In most communities, such clinics are available to all young children.

When the child is six years old, four significant teeth erupt. They are the first permanent teeth and are referred to as the sixth-year molars. These teeth are of major importance to the future mouth health of the child. They tend to hold the oral arch in shape while the deciduous teeth are being replaced by permanent teeth. Child, parent, and dentist should form a team to guard these teeth against decay or loss.

From the age of six on through the twelfth year, the child passes through a stage characterized by a mixture of baby and permanent teeth. He has both permanent and deciduous teeth and plenty of vacant spaces [1]. After the twelfth year, he usually possesses all his permanent teeth except the third molars.

The age at which the teeth erupt is not as important as the sequence of eruption. Irregularity in the order of eruption can lead to irregularity in the position of the permanent teeth. A wise parent gives diligent care to the "baby" teeth and so aids nature in providing the child with good occlusion. Some children may show their first tooth as early as three months, and others will keep anxious relatives waiting an entire year. Tooth eruption is basically a matter of individual and family pattern and cannot be hurried [1].

As in the cases of delayed tooth eruption and delayed speech, there are children who are slow in beginning to walk. Locomotion should not be hurried, nor should the child be placed in competition. A baby will walk when he is ready to walk. By the end of the twelfth month, most children can walk if one hand is held. At fifteen months they are capable of taking a few steps alone. The average year-and-a-half-old child walks freely. By three years he walks erect and is sure of his movements. About the time he enters kindergarten, he walks with ease and has good control over his movements [1]. Spock [8] observes that:

[8] Benjamin Spock, *The Pocket Book of Baby and Child Care*, p. 147. New York: Pocket Books, Inc., 1950.

Lots of factors enter into the age when a baby walks alone: Ambition, heaviness, how well he can get places by creeping, illnesses, bad experiences. A baby just beginning to walk when an illness lays him up for two weeks may not try again for a month or more. Or one who is just learning and has a fall may refuse to let go with his hands again for many weeks.

Height and weight. Growth in height and weight are high on the priority of parental interests. Mothers and fathers write and speak with great pride about the birth length and weight of their babies. The "average" newborn baby measures about 21 inches and weighs about 7 pounds. Throughout the period of infancy his growth is very rapid. For example, during the first year the average male child grows nearly 10 inches in height and triples his birth weight. However, nature does not promote as rapid a growth as this for any length of time. After two years, the rate of growth slows down and levels off. From then on to the tenth or eleventh year, the child experiences a much slower growth. Starting at about ten years, the weight of the average girl increases in momentum until it reaches maximum acceleration at about the twelfth year. The average boy is slower and does not reach his greatest acceleration until he is fourteen. From this time on growth in weight slows and then tends to remain stable in the early twenties. Growth in height reaches its maximum acceleration at about twelve for the girl and at fourteen for the boy. As with weight, the growth in height finally stops between the sixteenth and twenty-third year [1, 4, 27].

It is a source of pleasure to most children to know that they are growing taller and heavier. It is their business to grow, and they should be able to measure their gains. Unfortunately, there are no 100 per cent accurate height-weight standards.

A few years ago an unusual system of assessing growth was advanced by Dr. N. C. Wetzel. He called this appraisal form the "Grid for Evaluating Physical Fitness." [9] By studying the charts of the Grid, it is noted that there are two sets of ruled lines. One set is for height and one for weight. By plotting one's height and weight, a physique channel is determined. The physique channels indicate body build and form the pattern by which one can chart the direction of the child's growth. A youngster who follows a given channel without deviation is following his own growth pattern. Should this growth pattern deviate from the channel, it is indicative of an important change and the child should be examined by his physician. This gives the Grid a predictive value. A condition can

[9] Norman C. Wetzel, *Grid for Evaluating Physical Fitness.* Cleveland, Ohio: N.E.A. Service, 1948.

be detected before it becomes a clinical case. The isodevelopmental lines help to chart the growth progress made by the child each year. They also show the speed of growth achieved. According to Wetzel, direction and speed of growth determine one's quality of growth.

Nutrition. A child may be a prize product of heredity, good breeding, culture, and material wealth, but unless he has good nutrition, these factors will profit him little. The nutritional problems of infants and young children are best met by the teamwork of parents, physicians, and nutritionists. Such a team can ensure wholesome physical growth to children by providing a balance of nutrients such as protein, carbohydrates, fats, minerals, vitamins, and water. The daily diet of the growing child should include meat, butter, milk, eggs, citrus fruits or tomatoes, whole-grain cereals, green or yellow vegetables, and raw leafy vegetables in proper proportion. Occasionally, a physician will advise the taking of food supplements to ensure an adequate vitamin supply. Now and then he will withhold certain foods during the transient period of allergies. At present information relative to allergies is undergoing a major change. Much new material is being incorporated into the diagnosis and treatment of children with allergies.

Another significant factor in sound nutrition is the emotional climate at the dining table: it can set the pattern for good or poor nutritional practices. Parents who provide wholesome foods, a happy social experience, and good fellowship, well mixed with a leisurely attitude while dining, are providing the child with the best possible opportunity for establishing wholesome eating practices. There are other factors which influence nutrition, such as adequate sleep and rest, wholesome physical activity, avoidance of overfatigue, and good elimination.

Posture. A happy, healthy, well-adjusted child has an enthusiasm for living and expresses this through a variety of body movements. When the control of his body is good, he grows in physical efficiency; when he is awkward or his muscles are weak, his physical efficiency is impaired. So-called "good" and "poor" postures have been fairly well established. For example, a good standing posture can be determined by using the plumb-line test. This test is conducted from a side view. The body is in good alignment if a straight line can be drawn from the ear through the shoulder, elbow, hip, and knee joints and to a point just in front of the ankle bone.

The posture of a baby is usually of little concern to the parent. However, babies do have bowed legs and knock knees. Fortunately, these conditions tend to correct themselves as the child begins to walk. By the time he is six years of age, his legs are usually straight. Sometimes parents become concerned because their child has a hollow back and a protruding abdomen. This condition is also transient. Because the pre-adolescent has a great desire for activity, he reduces this protruding abdomen in a natural way. By the age of ten, the average youngster carries his head, neck, and shoulders in good balance [4].

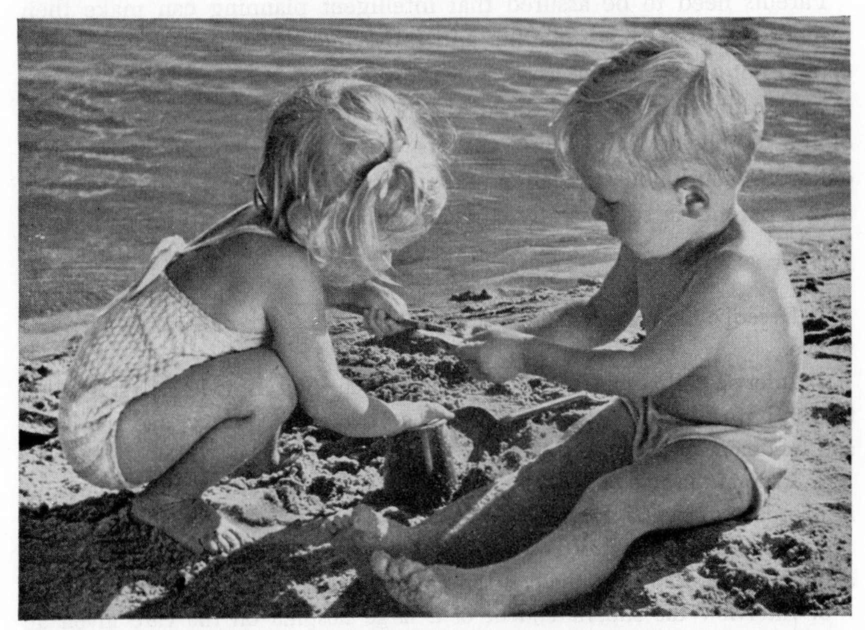

Fig. 8.3. Play is fun. Children become acquainted with their environment through perception. (*McGraw-Hill Text-Film Department, McGraw-Hill Book Company, Inc.*)

It is the posture of the adolescent that usually gives parents and teachers concern. Between the ages of twelve and seventeen, the boy and girl undergo a variety of changes. Their growth is rapid; their muscles range from weak to strong. They have feelings of security and insecurity, happiness and unhappiness. They make satisfactory and unsatisfactory social-emotional adjustments, and their personal regimen is good and again it is poor. These factors have much to do with posture.

Social-emotional adjustments. Of great significance to the immediate as well as the future happiness of both child and parent are the ways by which the emotional needs of children are met. Plant believes, as do other psychiatrists, that all children must have a feeling of belongingness or security; they must adjust to the world as it is; they must discover that they are like other people; they must have opportunities for creative expression and status within their own group [12]. How successfully parents meet these needs may make the difference between an efficient, well-adjusted personality and one who is unhappy and a source of trouble to himself and his fellows (see also the discussion of adjustment, Chapter 5).

Summary

Parents need to be assured that intelligent planning can make their responsibilities both stimulating and satisfying. Wise parenthood is concerned not only with the aspects of reproduction but also with the place in which the baby is to be born, the prenatal, natal, and postnatal care of the mother and child, and the growth and development patterns of children. Continuous guidance and supervision by the family physician assists parents in successfully carrying out the responsibilities of parenthood.

Suggested Activities

1. Describe the growth and development characteristics of children aged one to five.
2. Interview a prominent obstetrician on such subjects as home vs. hospital for the birth of a child, techniques for determining pregnancy, and the cause and treatment of pregnancy toxemia.
3. Explain the role of heredity in cases of incompatibility of blood types, as in reference to the Rh factor.
4. Study the problem of how to care for a woman giving birth to a child in an automobile. Report to the class on your findings.
5. Interview the superintendent of a large hospital on the care given an obstetrical patient from the time of arrival until she is ready to go home.
6. List the evidence for and against pregnant women smoking or drinking alcoholic beverages during the prenatal and lactation period.
7. Interview the city or county health officer on the well-baby services rendered by his health department.
8. Discuss natural childbirth.
9. Study the causes and treatment of sterility in both male and female. Report to the class on your findings.
10. Investigate the laws of your state pertaining to the adoption of children, and report on your findings.
11. Discuss services that can be rendered to underprivileged children by men and women who are unable to adopt children.
12. Visit a child care center in your community, and report on the methods being used to care for small children.
13. Start a Wetzel Grid Chart on a brother or sister or on a child of your acquaintance, and keep a record noting his growth at regular intervals.

14. Work out a sociodrama answering this question of a five-year-old boy: "Where do babies come from?"

15. Organize a panel discussion on an "ideal" family life.

16. Survey the facilities in your community available for maternal and child welfare.

17. Work out what you consider an ideal plan for counseling college students on preparation for parenthood.

18. View and discuss the following films: (*a*) *Heredity and Prenatal Development* (sound, 21 minutes), McGraw-Hill Text-Film, 1951; (*b*) *Human Reproduction* (sound, 21 minutes), McGraw-Hill Text-Film, 1947; (*c*) *Children's Emotions* (sound, 22 minutes), McGraw-Hill Text-Film; (*d*) *That Mothers Might Live* (sound, 10 minutes), M.G.M.

Suggested Readings

1. Breckenridge, Marian E. and E. Lee Vincent, *Child Development.* Philadelphia: W. B. Saunders Company, 1949.

2. Boas, F., "The Tempo of Growth of Fraternities," National Academy of Science, *Proceedings,* 21:413–418, July, 1935.

3. Fishbein, Morris, and Ernest W. Burgess, *Successful Marriage.* New York: Doubleday & Company, Inc., 1949.

4. Gesell, Arnold, and Frances L. Ilg, *The Child from Five to Ten.* New York: Harper & Brothers, 1946.

5. Gould, H. N., and M. R. Gould, "Age of First Menstruation in Mothers and Daughters," *Journal of the American Medical Association,* 98:1349–1352, Apr. 16, 1932.

6. Klein, H. "Experience in Parents and Offspring," *Journal of the American Dental Association,* 33:735–743, June, 1946.

7. Kris, Mariana, *When Children Ask about Sex.* New York: The Child Study Association of America, 1953.

8. Landis, Paul H., *Your Marriage and Family Living.* New York: McGraw-Hill Book Company, Inc., 1946.

9. Lockridge, Frances, *Adopting a Child.* New York: Greenberg: Publisher, Inc., 1947.

10. Meaker, S. R., *Human Sterility.* Baltimore: The Williams & Wilkins Company, 1934.

11. Newman, H. H., *Multiple Human Births.* New York: Doubleday & Company, Inc., 1940.

12. Plant, James S., *Personality and the Cultural Pattern,* New York: Commonwealth Fund, Division of Publication, 1937.

13. Potter, Edith L. *Fundamentals of Human Reproduction.* New York: McGraw-Hill Book Company, Inc., 1948.

14. Strain, Frances B., *Sex Guidance in Family Life Education.* New York: The Macmillan Company, 1950.

15. Wedberg, Alma, *Help Them to Speak.* Los Angeles: Los Angeles County Board of Education, 1951.

16. Williams, Jennie, *Family Health.* Philadelphia: J. B. Lippincott Company, 1945.

Popular Readings

17. deSchweinitz, Karl, *Growing Up.* New York: The Macmillan Company, 1945.

18. Dublin, Louis I., *The Facts of Life from Birth to Death.* New York: The Macmillan Company, 1952.

19. Foster, Robert G., *Marriage and Family Relationships,* rev. ed. New York: The Macmillan Company, 1950.

20. Gruenberg, Sidonie, *The Wonderful Story of How You Were Born.* New York: Doubleday & Company, Inc., 1952.

21. Hohman, L. B., *As the Twig Is Bent.* New York: The Macmillan Company, 1940.

22. Jenkins, Gladys G., Helen Schacter, and W. W. Bauer, *These Are Your Children.* Chicago: Scott, Foresman & Company, 1953.

23. McMahon, Lucile Nelson, "When a Baby's Premature," *Parents' Magazine,* 25:90–91, September, 1950.

24. Prentice, Carol S., *An Adopted Child Looks at Adoptions.* New York: Appleton-Century-Crofts, Inc., 1940.

25. Pulford, G. S., "The Rh Factor," *Today's Health,* 29:27–28, November, 1951.

26. Redl, Fritz, "The Technique of Sex Information," *Child Study,* January, 1939.

27. Spock, Benjamin, *The Pocket Book of Baby and Child Care.* New York: Pocket Books, Inc., 1950.

PART FOUR

Developing and Maintaining Health

9. Maintaining a Healthy and Attractive Body

The concept of wholeness is reaffirmed when the healthy, attractive body is considered. One's facial expression, for example, shows the interrelationship of personality traits and physical make-up. One's physical appearance has a definite effect upon others. Size and strength often are reasons for a man's social acceptance, while women think of good looks as a key to social success. The fat man is classed frequently as the jolly, good-natured type of individual and the square-jawed man as one of firm will. One's own body is a factor in the judgments and the attitudes of others.

The physically fit, well-developed human body is nature's supreme creation. The body begins when two microscopic cells unite. It grows, develops, and finally becomes a compact, coordinated organism composed of trillions of cells. It is capable of reproducing itself; of giving protection to its vital organs; of repairing much of its injured tissue; of maintaining a constant temperature; of skillfully neutralizing disease germs and their by-products; of converting food into energy and tissue—in short, of an amazing number of psychic and biological phenomena, some known, but many yet to be discovered.

Being physically fit is a relative term. Physical fitness is a condition, a state of readiness, of preparation to do a job. It is a desirable state in which the body is prepared to meet effectively the requirements of the environment in which it is placed.

A discussion of the following questions is presented to help the student gain an appreciation of his body: (1) What are the predominant body types? (2) How should one care for the body? (3) How can one use the body wisely? (4) What are the characteristics of a physically fit individual? (5) How does one develop and maintain physical fitness?

Body Types

Almost everyone would like to have an attractive figure. For women, this means being truly feminine; for men, masculine and athletic. Contrary to common belief, participation in vigorous games and sports by women does not result in a "masculine build" [13].

Many studies of body builds have been made, and some have resulted in rigid typing. For example, some authorities have classified all people into one of the following types: (1) the linear type, with slender body; (2) the lateral type, with a broad body build; (3) an average build somewhere between the first two.

Constitutional factors. Sheldon made a contribution with his study of constitutional factors and somatotypes.[1] In his study he photographed the posture of 4,000 college students. He made a classification of body types and studied personality traits characteristic of these types. He bases his classification on the three layers of the human embryo: (1) the endoderm, an inner layer of cells from which develop the organs of digestion; (2) the mesoderm, a middle layer which produces the skeletal, muscular, and circulatory systems; (3) the ectoderm, the outermost layer, predominating in the production of the skin, hair, nails, and nervous system. According to Sheldon's system, individuals are classified as *endomorphs, mesomorphs,* and *ectomorphs.* This is not a rigid classification, since allowance is made for each individual with his unique body build. Each component of the embryonic layers is found in everyone, but in varying proportions, which may be denoted numerically. Thus, for the somatotype classed as 7-3-1, the figure 7 indicates a predominance of endomorph, the 3 indicates some degree of mesomorph, and the 1 shows a very small proportion of ectomorph.

The *endomorph* is a viscerotonic person who is generally relaxed and loves comfort and sociability. He is fond of food and needs companionship. This type of individual has large digestive organs and weak, undeveloped muscular tissue. He is generally fat.

The *mesomorph,* the somatotonic individual, is the athletic type with hard, firm muscle. He is energetic and muscularly active, with vigor and push. His corresponding personality traits are adventurous, competitive, and aggressive. The mesomorph has a direct manner; also, he shows a

[1] W. H. Sheldon, "Constitutional Factors in Personality," in J. McV. Hunt (Ed.), *Personality and the Behavior Disorders,* Vol. 1, pp. 526–545. New York: The Ronald Press Company, 1944.

need for and an enjoyment of exercise. He is oriented toward his goals and needs action when troubled.

The *ectomorph,* or cerebrotonic person, is characterized by restraint and tightness in posture and movement. He is quick to react, mentally overintense, and self-conscious, loves privacy, fears people, and seeks solitude when troubled. In build he is tall and slender, with fragile bones and stooped, hesitant posture, rather restrained in movement.

Sheldon's study obviously is not the complete answer, but it does point the way for an understanding of body-type–personality relationships. His studies are continuing at the Constitutional Laboratory at Columbia University and in other institutions financed by foundational grants.

Studies indicate that constitutional factors influence adjustment to life situations, primarily in relation to stress, though many mental mechanisms, such as compensation and substitution, also play an important part. The constitutional factors seem to be closely related to the personality traits of courage and morale and to the motivational forces such as the will to live. Sheldon believes that, with further standardization of constitutional types, his methods promise to be useful in isolating and controlling the constitutional diseases such as cancer, ulcer, epilepsy, tuberculosis, and hereditary mental afflictions. At present his findings are in the experimental stage. However, the constitutional factors present another example of the unifying relationship of mental and physical functions.

Body structure and performance. Variation in body structure usually means varying abilities in performance. For example: "When the anatomical structure is particularly advantageous for strength, it is disadvantageous for speed. Large joints are strong, but they also may limit motion. Long distance runners are observed to have the flattest longitudinal arches and sprinters have smaller feet and higher arches." [2]

The Body as a Medium for Self-expression

The versatility of the human body has no counterpart in the animal world. Within a remarkably short interval of time, as well as space, one can run or walk, skip or gallop, jump or leap, glide or slide, crawl or roll, push or pull, dive or swim. One can perform most of these activities forward or backward, fast or slow, for long or short periods and, at the same time, smile or frown, cry or laugh, shout or be just plain sober. A variety of professions are based on this versatility. The entire field of

[2] Laurence E. Morehouse and Augustus T. Miller, Jr., *Physiology of Exercise,* p. 313. St. Louis: The C. V. Mosby Company, Medical Publishers, 1952.

athletic performance is an example of it. Portraying character through posture forms, which is fundamental to the ballet, modern dancing, and the drama, is another illustration. In short, the body is truly a medium of expressing the self, the total personality.

The Need for Physical Activity

If one looks in the right places and at the right time, he can find people of his own age engaged in a variety of athletic sports and games. He also finds spectators. If it were possible to obtain a composite picture of the physical fitness of those who engage in regular physical activity and a picture of those who are satisfied always to sit in the bleachers and watch, the contrast would be revealing. The physically fit men and women have a "lower oxygen consumption, slower pulse rate during work, large stroke volume of the heart, lower blood lactate during work and faster return of blood pressure and heart rate to normal after work." [3] This means that the physically fit person is able to perform work for longer periods of time with less exhaustion. To the college man and woman, beset by long hours of both mental and physical work, it means greater opportunity for success.

In primitive times, as well as in the days of the early settlers of this country, there were few, if any, spectators. It was a time of action for all. In those days, physical weakness invited disaster. It was only the vigorous and the alert who survived to reproduce and to pass on our present-day inheritance. It appears that the strength of that inheritance is fast diminishing. If this nation is to remain physically strong, and at this period in mid-century anything else is unthinkable, the desire for soft living and soft thinking must be replaced by more of the spirit and action of vigorous men and women of earlier days. Physical fitness can be a reality for all. It results from a combination of native equipment, opportunity, and discipline.

Characteristics of a physically fit person. The following characteristics of a physically fit person may serve as a helpful guide. The physically fit person:

1. Possesses sufficient muscular strength to maintain good posture and to meet emergencies and other physical demands on the body.
2. Functions as a total person with efficiency and without discomfort.
3. Meets the requirements of the environment through efficient functioning of his sense organs.

[3] *Ibid.*, p. 5.

4. Possesses the resilience to recover rapidly from fatigue and tension without the aid of stimulants.
5. Sleeps well at night and is fit and alert for the job ahead.

How to Care for the Body

The human body is a precision instrument, capable of great achievements. It is delicately adjusted and easily put out of order, yet is exceedingly tough and resilient. For example, the eyes, capable of a great number of accurate adjustments each minute for near or far seeing, are also liable to a variety of disorders of the muscles, iris, lens, retina, cornea, and humors. The ears, capable of transmitting 12,000 to 41,000 vibrations per second, often fail in their function because of preventable pathology or because of excessive wax in the outer ear. The skin and hair, important for their effect on the personality and also effective agents of protection, are affected by such undesirable conditions as boils, carbuncles, hives, eczema, and acne. The heart, a tough muscular organ with great capacity for work, is subject to a variety of organic and functional disorders, diseases, mechanical derangements, blockage of its own blood supply, and toxins. The kidneys, composed of millions of cells which filter all the blood of the body every few minutes, are subject to conditions such as nephritis, abscesses, tumors, tuberculosis, and kidney stones. The digestive system is essential to health; yet dyspepsia, gallstones, constipation, diarrhea, and various infections may be developed. The reproductive organs, both male and female, vital as they are to procreation, are sometimes rendered ineffective by cancer, venereal disease, tumors, and functional disorders. This brief positive-negative résumé of the body emphasizes the fact that the student has a wonderfully made instrument at his command. If given the right care, it is capable of high achievement; if allowed to become ill or to degenerate, it can be the source of inefficiency and unhappiness.

Few people have a perfect body. Almost everyone has one or more physical imperfections. The important point is to recognize these imperfections, to make the most of what one has, and to continue to strive for high achievement.

Developing and maintaining a healthy body. Physical fitness and personal attractiveness are assets to the student. They can be realized in varying degree by nearly everyone. To the individual who wants to improve his well-being and to gain the satisfactions which accompany physical fitness, the following suggestions may be helpful:

Begin by recognizing, in a functional way, one's physical capacities. It may be necessary to accept the fact that there are limitations. If this is the case, then plan to compensate for these shortcomings by engaging in the activities best suited for one's own capacities. The following example emphasizes the importance of constructive adjustments to a physical handicap: At the conclusion of his entrance medical examination, a college student with severe postpolio scars amazed the chief examiner when he scorned the suggestion that he register in a restricted form of physical activity, saying: "I am capable of playing handball, and that is where I want to be." And that is where he was assigned.

The modern physical education department provides activities for all students. Whether one is normal or handicapped, permission to register in a physical activity class is based on the findings of thorough medical examination.

Whether one is engaged in a physical program or not, it is a good practice to have a complete medical and dental examination at least once a year. Because hearing and vision are so essential to learning, special attention should be given to these sense organs.

Though participation in physical activity is only a part of fitness, it is difficult to imagine being physically fit and not following a program of physical exercise. Deep within the nervous system there is a fundamental urge for movement. This is seen in the newborn baby as he twists and wriggles; in the supercharged action of the athlete; in the middle-aged person trying to stave off the paunch of his prototype; and in the elderly person exercising for the sake of circulation. What is common to each is that some form of physical exercise seems necessary to every age, and the college student is no exception. As a result of a balanced program of physical exercise engaged in regularly, several days each week, he can expect to make important gains as follows: The student can gain:

1. In muscular strength. This, however, is dependent upon the vigor, frequency, and tempo of the exercise [12]. Games, sports and other activities which can favorably influence muscular strength are swimming, water polo, wrestling, basketball, soccer, speedball, gymnastics, weight lifting, rowing, tumbling, football, volleyball, and tennis.

2. In strength and efficiency of the heart, arteries, and veins. This is dependent upon the manner in which he exercises, the condition of the heart and blood vessels, the tonus of the skeletal muscles surrounding the veins, and the strength of the muscles of the abdomen as they influence the return of blood to the heart [13]. Activities which favorably influence the circulatory system are similar to those influencing gains in muscular strength. Some examples in-

clude baseball, dancing, gymnastic games, golf, "lifesaving," softball, aquatics, and track and field events.

3. In respiratory efficiency. This favorably influences the oxygen–carbon dioxide exchange in the blood. Physical exercise tends to increase the ability to expand the chest muscles, making respiration easier and more effective. Activities which aid this increase are the same as those which promote muscular growth and circulatory efficiency. Artificial deep-breathing exercises have no significant value for the normal person over the natural deep breathing induced by games and sports [12, 13].

4. By improving his metabolic activity. Through the stimulation of vigorous games and sports all body processes are integrated. The result of such activity is the sensation of feeling "good all over," as though the body were in tune [12, 13].

Developing a balanced program. The physically fit person balances his program of work with rest, sleep, and recreation. Purposeful and enjoyable work contributes much to total well-being. Rest and sleep provide opportunities to recover from fatigue and tension. Recreation is the "spice" that adds flavor and richness to living (see Chapter 10 for further discussion of sleep, rest, and recreation).

In discussing sleep, Jacobson describes two types, light, or restless, sleep and relaxed sleep. The restless sleeper shifts his position frequently, breathes irregularly, and fails to relax completely. The relaxed sleeper lies quietly, shifts his position but slightly, and is completely relaxed. For the student who finds it difficult to relax, Jacobson suggests six exercises:

1. Lie on the back, arms at sides, legs straight; rest for a few minutes. Stretch both arms upward (vertically), hands closed tightly—hold for a minute. Let arms fall limply to the sides; repeat exercise; concentrate on relaxing the arms.

2. The next night, lie quiet, eyes closed, legs straight; extend the feet and toes, and hold this position. Relax. Point the toes and hold, relax, rest. Repeat the exercise; then relax the arms and legs.

3. Take the same position on the third night. Breathe deeply, and expel the air. Relax the chest as completely as possible. Breathe normally. Relax arms and legs.

4. On the fourth night assume the resting position, close the eyes, tense the forehead, hold it for a few minutes, relax, and then repeat. Relax arms, legs, chest, and forehead.

5. On the fifth night, begin by closing the eyes and relaxing the body for several minutes. Open the eyes, and look to the right. Close eyes, and relax

them. Allow the lids to droop—close the eyes. Relax the forehead, the eyes, arms, legs, and chest.

6. The sixth night lie quietly. Begin counting audibly without using the lips; relax the lips, the tongue, and throat. Now relax all parts of the body. Lie in the most comfortable position, and *sleep well* [10].

Relaxation and attractiveness seem to go together. For a graphic example of this, stand before a mirror, tense the facial muscles, clench the teeth, cause the eyes to squint and contract the neck and throat areas. The image reflected is not a pleasant one. It shows facial tension at its maximum. Now relax each group of muscles, and keep the lips lightly touching. This image is more pleasant and takes far less energy to produce.

Campus life includes both times of happiness and times of stress. Times of stress produce or increase tensions. Knowing the causes of tension, being able to recognize them, and then "consciously changing the mental and physical pattern reaction, so as to redirect the body into purposeful activity," [4] is perhaps the secret of efficient and relaxed living.

Personal appearance. An attractive, healthy body plays a major part in good personal appearance. Among the constitutional factors related to personal appearance are nutritional status, weight, skin, hair, teeth, vision, grooming, build, posture, and height. A few of these are selected for brief discussion. Others may be studied by referring to the Suggested Readings.

Nutritional status. The basic functions of nutrition in effective living are developed in Chapter 11. However, a brief account of nutrition in relation to physique is presented here.

The endomorph likes comfort and is fond of food. His digestive organs are large and weak, and his muscles are soft and flabby. This type needs a diet with more bulk and one low in caloric value to keep from adding more weight. The program of exercise and diet should be directed by a physician.

The mesomorph, the athletic type, is characterized by energy and muscular activity, with vigor and push. He has good circulation and digestion. He can eat almost any food. He usually is a hurried eater. He needs a well-balanced diet for energy, growth and repair of tissues, and regulation of body processes.

The ectomorph, the slender person with the long, narrow chest, has

[4] Eleanor Metheny, *Body Dynamics*, p. 75. New York: McGraw-Hill Book Company, Inc., 1952.

poor circulation. Often he is poorly nourished because of lack of proper assimilation. As a result he has decreased vitality and a tendency to chronic fatigue and nervous indigestion. It is difficult for this type to put on weight regardless of how much he eats. However, he needs a nutritious, concentrated, well-prepared diet. The ectomorph may fare better by eating four or five small meals rather than three larger ones each day [2].

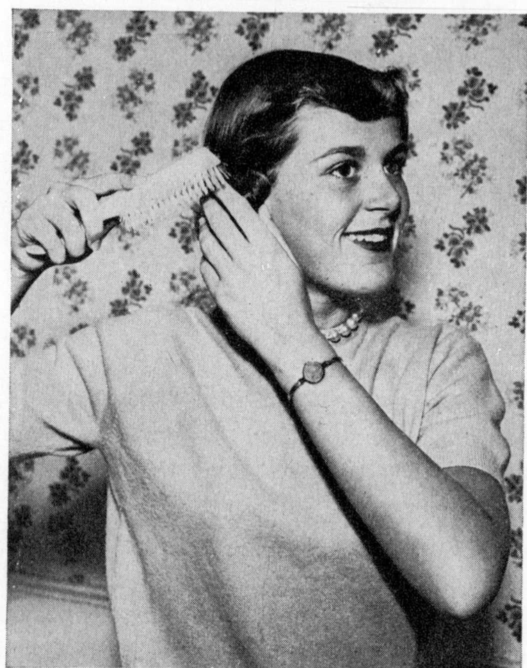

Fig. 9.1. Good grooming is basic to an attractive, healthy body. (*Photo by Lee Hansen.*)

Weight. When a man or a woman is physically fit and within the normal weight range for his height, age, body type, and race, he looks better, feels better, and reflects this attitude in his behavior. Excess weight produces a feeling of ineptness and unhappiness, which may lead to eating between meals and more weight. Thus the problem is often a psychosomatic one. The reduction of excess weight is both a psychological and a physiological undertaking [2, 29].

Skin. Someone has remarked that women would rather be beautiful than healthy. He might have added that they can be both. A healthy, attractive skin is desirable for men as well as for women.

In infancy, one of the first responsibilities of the mother is to ensure for her baby a soft, fresh, delicate skin. Proper external care by means of baths and cleansing creams and oils and proper internal care by means of good nutrition help to retain this fresh look even into adulthood.

About the time a young person enters adolescence, he may have trouble with a common skin disorder called acne, which is an inflammation of the ducts of the skin glands. Self-diagnosis and -treatment of acne are a waste of time and may be dangerous. When acne begins to show, it is wise to consult a skin specialist. He may regulate the diet, use antibiotics or ultraviolet light, or in severe cases use X-ray and hormone therapy. The important point is that he can be of great assistance.

Hair. Goodman writes that man has been interested in his hair from the earliest times. Here are a few of the strange customs and beliefs listed by him [6]:

1. It was believed that, if a magpie built her nest with recently discarded hair, the owner of the hair would die.
2. In Sumatra, only women with long hair were permitted to sow rice—this would ensure abundant crops with long stalks.
3. The early Greeks washed gray hair with the eggs of ravens, to restore the dark color.
4. Haircutting in some of the ancient tribes of Fiji was a sacred ceremony. The chief of the tribe always ate human flesh during the cutting of his hair.
5. In old Dutch courts of law, confessions were obtained by threatening to cut the hair of the prisoners.

Realistically, hair on the head has one primary function, and that is protection. Remove the hair, and the head becomes vulnerable to sun, wind, rain, cold, and insects. Retain it, and one has not only protection but an important factor in a good appearance. A question frequently asked by men is, How can I keep from becoming bald? If it gives any comfort, this question has intrigued mankind since the earliest times. One of the first prescriptions known to medicine was used by the ancient Egyptians in an effort to grow new hair. It was based on the fats of snakes, geese, lions, the hippopotamus, and the crocodile [6]. Up to the present time, hundreds of remedies as useless as this one have been tried, none of which have proved effective.

A complete medical examination by the family or college physician is the first step to take when one discovers he is losing his hair. Developing cases of baldness have been stopped by prompt treatment of infections and glandular disorders. Superfluous hair is thought to be inherited. The secretions of the endocrine glands, particularly the thyroid and pituitary glands, may have something to do with both the amount and the quality of hair [6].

The problems of milady's hair are too complicated for this short discussion. Books like *Your Hair* [5] give constructive answers to questions about dandruff, shampooing, superfluous hair, hair dyes, waving, permanents, and nutrition of the hair.

Teeth. Teeth have three primary functions, (1) masticating food, (2) assisting good speech, and (3) contributing to the personal appearance. To make sure that these can be fulfilled, teeth should always be kept clean and in good repair. The following suggestions for maintaining sound oral health may seem simple, but they are nevertheless highly effective:

1. Have a complete dental examination at least once a year.
2. Have all repair work promptly done by a competent dentist.
3. Faithfully practice a daily regimen which includes:
   a. A balanced diet with emphasis on calcium, phosphorus, vitamins A, D, and C, hard breads, and raw, crisp fresh vegetables.
   b. A diet that minimizes refined starches and sugars in the form of white flour, soft drinks, and candy.
   c. Brushing the teeth and gums *after each meal* when possible.
   d. Rinsing the mouth with water after eating (that is, if brushing is impossible).
   e. Avoiding the crushing of hard substances with the teeth.

Dental caries is probably the most common of all human ailments. It is caused by acid resulting from bacteria acting on fermentable carbohydrates. The greatest damage to the teeth appears to occur a few minutes after eating. Therefore, brushing of the teeth soon after food is eaten is a very important preventive measure. Another preventive agent is sodium fluoride. It is used in two ways: (1) by fluoridation—the addition of fluoride in community water supplies; (2) by topical application—direct to the teeth by a dentist. The caries-prevention effect of adequate fluoride intake is conferred principally upon children up to twelve years of age. This increased resistance to caries is carried over into later life to an appreciable degree. Both methods have been tested by the dental profession and found effective as preventive agents [3].

Vision. It is fun to see and to see well. It always is interesting to greet a friend and watch how the eyes reflect his emotions. In fact, when two people are talking face to face, they are actually talking eye to eye. What better reason is there for taking proper care of the eyes?

Of course, the eyes are significant socially, but they are also important to the student's scholastic achievement. The functions of the eyes are

[5] Herman Goodman, *Your Hair.* New York: Emerson Books, Inc., 1950.

(1) to see accurately, (2) to record depth, and (3) to fuse two images into one image in the brain. Both binocular vision and depth perception appear to be mastered early in childhood. After this, change in vision depends a great deal on age and how well the eyes are cared for. Binocular vision, or the fusing of two images into one in the brain, can be made easier by good illumination. "It takes but a fraction of a second to fuse the images of both eyes when the illumination is favorable, but it takes several seconds with poor illumination." [6] As was indicated in Chapter 3, Exploring the College Health Program, 30 foot-candles is recommended for ordinary visual tasks.

To ensure good service from normal eyes or those with good correction, the student will find the following helpful:

1. Practice the principles of good nutrition, since an adequate, balanced diet is important to good sight.
2. Determine the best light for a given type of work, and meet the requirement.
3. Avoid using the eyes for difficult work when fatigued.
4. Avoid lengthy reading periods when lying down.
5. Have the eyes examined by an eye specialist at regular intervals. Wear glasses if prescribed, and keep them clean.
6. While studying, occasionally rest the eyes by looking at distant objects.

Grooming. A well-groomed person is usually a happy person. He is self-confident, he has poise, he is pleasing to others. Grooming involves such matters as physical fitness, care of the skin, hands, and hair, maintaining a good posture, and proper selection of clothes.

Summary

To develop and maintain a physically fit body, one should:

1. Have a thorough medical and dental examination annually.
2. Employ good practices in nutrition.
3. Engage in appropriate physical exercise regularly.
4. Establish a balanced program of work, rest, sleep, and recreation.
5. Establish a daily regime of sound hygienic care of the body.

Suggested Activities

1. Make a study of members of athletic teams. Choose one sport, and classify each member of the team as to his body build.

[6] Gerhard A. Brecher, "How We Learn to See," *Today's Health*, January, 1952, p. 58.

2. Plan a physical exercise program for a postpolio patient, a postsurgery patient, one who is overweight, and an underdeveloped person.

3. Discuss the role of the medical and dental examination in the physical fitness program.

4. What is meant by physical fitness, and how does one know when he is physically fit?

5. List and describe a number of functional tests by which physical fitness is determined.

6. Describe the effects of training on the body.

7. Experiment with one or two restless sleepers to determine the effectiveness of Jacobson's six suggestions for reducing tension [8].

8. The solution of the excess-weight problem is often more psychological than physiological. Discuss and illustrate.

9. Discuss the philosophy used by Dr. Goodman in meeting the problem of baldness [6].

10. Set up an ideal study room, from the point of view of furniture, light, ventilation, and noise.

11. Pick out several well-groomed acquaintances, and describe their technique.

12. List the arguments in favor of placing fluorides in drinking water.

13. View and discuss the following films: (*a*) *Body Care and Grooming* (sound, 17 minutes), McGraw-Hill Text-Film; (*b*) *The Nose, Throat, and Ears* (sound, 11 minutes), McGraw-Hill Text-Film; (*c*) *Sport Stamina* (sound, 9 minutes), Teaching Film Custodians, New York; (*d*) *Circulation* (sound, 16 minutes), Encyclopaedia Britannica.

SUGGESTED READINGS

1. Brecher, G. A., "How We Learn to See," *Today's Health,* 30:58, January, 1952.

2. Bogert, L. J., *Nutrition and Physical Fitness,* 5th ed. Philadelphia: W. B. Saunders Company, 1950.

3. Cady, F. C., "Fluorides and Teeth," *Today's Health,* 30:50, February, 1952.

4. Derrick, Vail, *The Truth about Your Eyes.* New York: Farrar, Straus & Young, 1950.

5. Dimmick, F. L., "The Dependence of Auditory Experience upon Wave Amplitude," *American Journal of Psychology,* 12:463–470, 1933.

6. Goodman, Herman, *Your Hair.* New York: Emerson Books, Inc., 1950.

7. *Handbook of Human Engineering Data for Design Engineers.* Medford, Mass.: Tufts College Institute for Applied Experimental Psychology, 1949.

8. Jacobson, Edmund, *You Can Sleep Well.* New York: McGraw-Hill Book Company, Inc., 1938.

9. Laird, Donald, *Increasing Personal Efficiency.* New York: Harper & Brothers, 1952.

10. Marsh, Hattie M., *Building Your Personality.* New York: Prentice-Hall, Inc., 1949.

11. "The Measure of the Effects of Noise on Working Efficiency," *Journal of Industrial Hygiene,* 9:431–434, 1927.

12. Metheny, Eleanor, *Body Dynamics.* New York: McGraw-Hill Book Company, Inc., 1952.

13. Morehouse, Laurence E., and Augustus T. Miller, Jr., *Physiology of Exercise.* St. Louis: The C. V. Mosby Company, Medical Publishers, 1948.

14. Rathbone, Josephine, *Relaxation.* New York: Teachers College, Columbia University, 1943.

15. Sonders, V. L. "The Physiological Basis of Visual Acuity," *Psychological Bulletin,* pp. 465–490, 1948.

16. Tebbel, John, *Your Body.* New York: Harper & Brothers, 1951.

Popular Readings

17. Bond, Estelle, "Dictionary of Dentists," *Today's Health.* 29:21–22, June, 1951.

18. Brooks, Esther E., *You and Your Personality.* New York: Harper & Brothers, 1949.

19. Clendenning, Logan, *The Human Body.* New York: Alfred A. Knopf, Inc., 1948.

20. Conley, Veronica L., "Lipstick for That Touch of Color," *Today's Health,* 30:51–52, February, 1952.

21. Carson, Byrta, *How You Look and Dress.* New York: McGraw-Hill Book Company, Inc., 1949.

22. Dublin, Louis I., *The Facts of Life from Birth to Death.* New York: The Macmillan Company, 1952.

23. King, Eleanore, *Your Face Value.* Los Angeles: National Press Service, 1942.

24. Kisker, George W., "Learn to Relax," *Today's Health,* 29:22–23, November, 1931.

25. Lane, Janet, *Your Carriage, Madam!* New York: John Wiley & Sons, Inc., 1947.

26. Spencer, S. M., "This Screaming World," *The Saturday Evening Post,* Aug. 15, 1953.

27. Stafford, George T., *Exercise during Convalescence.* New York: A. S. Barnes and Company, 1947.

28. Stratton, Dorothy C., and Helen B. Schleman, *Your Best Foot Forward.* New York: McGraw-Hill Book Company, Inc., 1940.

10. Utilizing Opportunities for Rest and Recreation

How many students have stopped long enough in their drive for achievement to sit down and attempt to "let down" and have found to their surprise that this is more difficult than they thought? What they discover is that, in meeting the demands of the college program and possibly in spending some hours earning a few dollars, they have developed tensions which do not subside automatically. Is this condition undesirable? To the normally active student, with reasonably good resilience, a temporary state of tension probably does him little harm and often helps accomplish considerable work. However, excess tension accompanied by fatigue which persists day after day is not desirable and can lead to serious conditions.

Throughout life the individual moves in a pattern which is fundamentally rhythmic. He experiences the flow of seasons, day and night, hunger and food, fatigue and recovery, cardiac and respiratory regularity, and muscle-nerve coordination, all of which give balance, understanding, and beauty to his utilitarian, cultural, and creative efforts.

Such a rhythmic pattern exists for all the dynamics of life. Whether one is a day laborer or a student in an institution of higher learning, the sooner he makes a conscious effort to integrate a pattern of balance into his daily living, the more tranquil, harmonious, and constructive will be his periods of work, exercise, rest, sleep, and recreation.

The principle of balance between work, rest, and recreation is not new; it has been employed in all successful business and industrial institutions for many years.

Laban's concept of this principle implies the economy of human effort. One aspect of his theory includes placing the best-trained individual where his talents count most. Then he is instructed in the values of a rhythmized program. Such a combination offers the satisfying experience of perfect performance, with the capacity for further achievement fully sustained [8].

This principle of balance or rhythm in the daily program has great significance for the college student. It is important for him in this time of preparation to put into practice a schedule or plan which assures him a smooth transition into the business world. Such a plan starts with the daily program of activities, which provides time for work, relaxation, recreation, rest, and sleep.

The discussion that follows is organized to help the student arrive at answers to such questions as: (1) What are the characteristics of a relaxed person? (2) How should one plan his daily program so as to make the most effective use of his time? (3) How significant is it to avoid overfatigue and how does one guard against it? (4) Is sleep an acquired practice or a physiological necessity? (5) Where are the opportunities in the daily program for rest, relaxation, and recreation?

Characteristics of a Relaxed Person

Skill in relaxing mind and body helps sustain efficiency. A person who is relaxed:

1. Moves with ease and with freedom of all parts of the body.
2. Shows no extra motility—that is, has no nervous mannerisms.
3. Maintains body postures that permit him to function effectively.
4. Has good mobility in the joints, especially in the spine.
5. Has no difficulties with the respiratory system (asthma, irregular breathing, etc.).
6. Has normal blood circulation (extremities not cold, no excessive sweating, cramps, or flushing of skin).
7. Has no discomfort from the visceral organs (no constipation, diarrhea, or indigestion).
8. Has no exceptional or unusual urinary action.
9. Has a normal menstrual period (women).
10. Has skeletal muscles which function easily without discomfort.
11. Makes wholesome adjustments to irritating factors in his environment (people, noise, criticism).
12. Enjoys periods of rest, and finds it easy to reduce his tensions.
13. Has no difficulty in going to sleep, and sleeps well.
14. Has a feeling of security.
15. Adjusts quickly to the demands of his job.
16. Avoids the stamp of perfectionism and is satisfied with reasonable accomplishments.
17. Creates time for recreation and hobbies.

18. Finds happiness in things of beauty.
19. Finds satisfaction in spiritual things [12].

The well-adjusted student should approximate these characteristics. If, however, "the score is low," it may be time to readjust one's goals as well as one's daily program. Perhaps it will be necessary to increase the opportunities for rest, relaxation, and recreation. Once these periods are firmly established and a rhythmized program is functioning, excessive tension and fatigue are less likely to occur.

The Daily Program

There is one thing a student can be sure of during his college life, and that is a daily program of activities. Experience has shown that a schedule can become a ruthless, tireless taskmaster, a producer of fatigue, discouragement, illness, and inefficiency; or it can be an orderly disciplinarian, holding a balance between work, relaxation, recreation, rest, and sleep. At best it is demanding and fatiguing; however, schedules are a combination of faculty and student planning and can be constructed in keeping with student needs and interests. Table 1 illustrates a sample daily program of a freshman majoring in business administration. It is not a perfect schedule, but it is functional and illustrates a broad pattern of work, then rest; work, then recreation; work, then rest and sleep. Each twenty-four hours provides four hours for class work, seven hours for rest, recreation, and meals, five hours for study, and eight hours for sleep. To the healthy student this twenty-four-hour schedule, consistently employed, provides a means of achieving scholastic excellence, with no neglect of his social and physical activities and with a minimal drain on his energies.

It would be naïve to believe that such a schedule is inviolate. Unforeseen happenings and just plain desire to change the pace are to be expected. In fact, once in a while it is good to break with routine. Such a break can be stimulating, and it does not defeat the rhythm principle. Some people are temperamentally unsuited to a regular routine and find it difficult to follow it. However, dangerous wear and tear occur when there is little opportunity for repair of body tissues and when the pace or rhythm of daily living is irregular, with constant fluctuation. For example, in the case of a given student the suggested schedule may be followed on Monday, but on Tuesday classes are missed, lunch taken on the run, rest and recreation disregarded, dinner gulped, all for the sake of concentrated study. On Wednesday a tired student sleeps in

Table 1. Sample Daily Program

Major—Business Administration Freshman or 13th Year

	Time	*Monday*	*Tuesday*	*Wednesday*	*Thursday*	*Friday*
Classwork	8	Business math		Business math		Business math
	9	English	Physical education	English	Physical education	English
	10	Economics	American political institutions	Economics	American political institutions	Economics
Free time	11					
Lunch	12	Lunch	Lunch	Lunch	Lunch	Lunch
Classwork	1	Psychology	Orientation	Psychology		Psychology
	2		Health education		Health education	
Free time	3					
	4					
	5					
Dinner	6					
	7					
Study	8					
	9					
	10					
Sleep	11 P.M. to 7 A.M.	Retiring at 11 and arising at 7 provides 8 hours of sleep				

classes, cuts out recreation, and in the evening turns completely to social activities. Thursday, a desperate effort is made to return to the schedule, with some success. Friday, the desire to get away from it all results in cutting classes and much play, followed by a great desire to sleep. It is this kind of irregularity repeated often which produces physical and emotional disharmonies, tension, chronic fatigue, irritability, lack of interest in schoolwork, and, eventually, scholastic failure.

Prevention of Overfatigue

Activity, then recuperation, are part of the rhythmic cycle of daily living. The threat to attaining one's academic goals is too much fatigue. When one arises tired after eight to ten hours of sleep morning after morning, he is in all probability in a state of overfatigue or chronic fatigue. In the athletic world this is called staleness. The symptoms are easily observed; some of the most typical are (1) lack of interest in almost everything, even food; (2) loss of weight; (3) a feeling of exhaustion at the end of the day; (4) constipation; (5) an increased feeling of irritability; (6) lowered resistance to infection; (7) a desire to be alone; (8) restlessness; (9) paleness; (10) loss of interest in studies and social events; (11) shortness of breath on exertion; (12) sleep disturbed by dreams, a tendency to awaken early in the morning; (13) an increasing desire to adjust through excessive use of coffee, tobacco, or beverage alcohol.

The causes of such a condition are constant irregularity in living, fear, worry, tension, and a failure to make satisfying adjustments. Prevention lies in developing a balanced program of activities. The correction of the already existing situation involves breaking the irregular rhythm which produced the difficulty and rebuilding the daily program to include a balanced routine. Such constructive effort requires intelligent recognition of the job to be done and organizing and budgeting adequate time for work, recreation, rest, and sleep.

Sleep

During the summer months, in the temperate zone, there occurs a cycle of about fifteen hours of daylight and nine hours of darkness. In the winter, the ratio is reversed, with fifteen hours of darkness and nine hours of daylight. This natural arrangement of light and dark has been functioning since the creation of time and for a purpose. Early man established his living schedule by it. The behavior pattern of people up to modern times was influenced by it. However, today, by the flip of a switch or the pressure of a finger, there is no darkness. Modern man has broken the cycle. He turns night into day. He changes the work and play patterns of his fellow man. He is in full control of what was once nature's business. However, man still needs, at regular intervals, opportunities to withdraw from activity and seek the quiet seclusion of darkness, to rest and sleep.

Scientists agree that natural sleep is the most satisfying form of recuperation from fatigue. During sleep and rest, all vital functions of the body are reduced. Body cells which have been used during activity are repaired. The metabolic rate is lowered, and energy is restored.

"How are you?" and "How did you sleep last night?" are probably the two most popular questions in the English language. Questions such as these are asked because of interest in and real concern for the well-being of friends and relatives. In health education classes, students often ask questions about sleep such as: What is the purpose of sleep? How much sleep should I get? Would it hurt me to study all night? Will my efficiency be impaired if I go without much sleep? Is it normal to twist and turn during sleep?

Present-day research can give partial answers to these queries. Sleep has been established as a normal state which "periodically interrupts waking activities" [5]. During this interval the body rests, and the conscious mind becomes unconscious. Students have been known to do quite well on 6 hours of sleep nightly. However, Barry's studies indicate that students who sleep 8 hours "feel better" than those who sleep 6. Those who sleep 9 do not feel so good as those who sleep 8 hours [2].

Research by Tyler indicates that after 200 hours of induced insomnia there was no significant physiological change [15]. Many people can testify that during World War II men went 48 to 72 hours without sleep and made normal recoveries after 10 to 12 hours of rest and sleep.

Edwards studied the effects of loss of sleep on visual acuity and found that, after 100 hours of remaining awake, students showed no significant change in the visual-sense function [4]. Tyler found no significant change in the auditory acuity of his subjects after they had gone 200 hours without sleep [15]. Kleitman, experimenting with students who had gone 60 hours without sleep, observed that the only significant sensory reaction was a progressively lowered threshold for pain reception. Visual and auditory acuity remained unchanged [7].

Kleitman also found a decreasing ability at mental arithmetic and at naming opposites, but no change in ability to name colors [7].

As to the effect of the amount of sleep on how one feels, Edwards observed that, after 100 hours of wakefulness, his subjects were irritable and restless and suffered from headaches. It took 7 days of normal living and sleeping for them to return to the pretest status [4]. Kleitman found that in his subjects, the feeling of drowsiness came in waves, the most difficult periods occurring at 3 A.M. and 6 A.M. [7].

Kleitman reports that normal people move many times during the course of a night's sleep. He observed, however, that not over 30 seconds per hour is consumed in these movements [7].

Some studies have been made as to the influence of the seasons of the year on sleep. Laird reports that one is apt to sleep less well in spring than in autumn. He believes that this is due to calcium metabolism, which appears to be at its lowest during the spring months [9]. Kleitman believes that in the spring of the year one falls asleep with greater ease and has less motility (movement) [7].

From these findings it is noted that normal sleep provides a great margin of safety, not only for these experiments but for emergency situations as well. After as much as 200 hours without sleep the danger areas have not been reached. However, it must be remembered that the total "cost to the body" does not show up in these short performance tests that follow sleeplessness.

In view of this research, the physically well student can take comfort in the fact that occasional loss of sleep is not necessarily harmful to his health or to his efficiency. It is the continuous loss which produces chronic fatigue and can be harmful to health.

There are times, however, when it is difficult to reduce body tension enough so that one can go to sleep. Such a state is not uncommon and, as previously stated, is no cause for alarm. A restful night's sleep can be induced (1) by the use of drugs or (2) by following a planned routine for relaxing the body in a natural manner. At this point it is well to give one word of caution regarding sleep induced by drugs. The practice of using sleeping pills (barbituric acid) can be harmful to effective living. Health authorities condemn the unrestricted use of all forms of barbituric acid derivatives (see Chapter 15, Understanding Depressants and Stimulants). Toxic effects of a serious nature can follow the undisciplined use of these drugs. Sleeping pills should be used only in an emergency and then only upon the advice of a reputable physician.

Perhaps the most frequent reason for failure to go to sleep within a reasonable time is fatigue and tension. As stated, drugs can be employed to stupefy the conscious areas of the brain. However, they are crutches and as such should never be used except in an emergency. Sleep or unconsciousness is as natural a state as is consciousness. If given a chance, the body responds to the need for sleep in a natural and satisfying way. The individual who is not suffering pain may find the following suggestions beneficial in achieving a restful night's sleep:

1. Establish a regular hour for going to bed.
2. Avoid all forms of stimulation before retiring.
3. Prepare in a leisurely manner for retiring.
4. Take a warm, not hot, tub bath or shower; it can be helpful.
5. Make sure that irritations are reduced to a minimum (noise, lights, insects, extremes of temperature).
6. Take a few long, slow, deep inhalations and exhalations while in bed; this helps to reduce tensions.
7. Read for a brief period some interesting literature.
8. Do not recapitulate past activities or rehearse coming events.
9. Lie quiet, with covering adjusted and lights out, and begin to relax the entire body: let the head fall from the shoulders (figuratively); relax the scalp, the forehead, the eyes and eyelids, the jaw, the tongue, the right arm, hand, fingers; relax the left arm, hand, fingers; relax the right leg, foot, toes—the left leg, foot, toes.
10. Finally, create a feeling of great space, drift into it, and sleep.

Jacobson lists ways by which one can reduce tensions and induce sleep. He works on the principle of first contracting muscle groups so that one becomes aware of tension, then relaxing. He places great emphasis on learning how to relax the arms, the legs, the breathing apparatus, the forehead and brow, the eyes, and then the speech muscles [5].

Rest, Relaxation, and Recreation

The daily program previously discussed suggests not only time for work and sleep but a total of seven hours out of each twenty-four for periods of rest, relaxation, and recreation. Authorities believe such a schedule is beneficial [6]. In present-day society, the pace at which people live is rapid and sustained. Competition is part of every waking hour. And when a job depends equally upon personality and skill, extreme pressure can be inflicted and severe tension develop. Without some planned form of release, rest, relaxation, and recreation, ill health and inefficiency may result.

The modern college campus, wonderful as it is, is an environment in which tensions are produced. Unless the student is on guard, he can find much to harass him and build up fatigue. Long and late hours of study, problems about finances and grades, lack of sleep, illness, conflicts, and dates are tension-producing factors. However, it must be pointed out that tensions are not all bad. In fact, to reach top performance in almost any physical or mental pursuit, it is necessary to develop a certain amount of neuromuscular tension. But such tensions cannot be maintained indefinitely; there must be a letdown, a release, or ultimately there results a slow but profound accumulation of fatigue, irritability, loss of efficiency, and illness. The letdown, or period of rest, is a specific antidote to excessive tension and chronic fatigue.

Rest. If tensions are the by-products of curricular pursuits, and they probably are, rest is both a healer and a deterrent and can help to balance a strenuous schedule.

In rest there is a diminishing or cutting down of sensory and motor stimulation. There is no activity. The purpose of rest is to reduce tension —to recover from fatigue. The length of the rest period should be in proportion to the length and type of exertion. A tennis, handball, or basketball player, who is participating for fun, finds it necessary to take periods of rest. As the game progresses, he takes more time-out periods. He finishes the game tired, but never exhausted. A student studying uninterruptedly for two to three hours builds up a substantial amount of fatigue. It is better to employ rest periods at thirty-minute intervals.

A busy day on the campus does not afford many opportunities for rest. However, there are times when rest can be taken, and with profit. The time between classes offers a few minutes' letdown. Some colleges provide rooms where students can pause for quiet and meditation. Musical or motion-picture presentations offer periods for rest during the noon hour. The time prior to and immediately after lunch or dinner may be used for rest and quiet.

Rest is necessary to all forms of animal life. Even plants and trees have periods in which they are dormant. It is a wise student who understands and recognizes his need for rest and who consciously employs techniques to enjoy it each day.

Relaxation. Relaxation differs from rest. In rest, there is no obvious activity, while in relaxation the individual reduces action without abolishing the tension necessary for a good performance [8].

Relaxation is derived from a variety of activities; it is not always the same for all people or for all occasions. Newspapermen covering the White House report that President Eisenhower finds relaxation through painting, cooking, playing golf, or simply changing his attitude toward his work. A well-known surgeon found it important to leave his office at lunch time to seek the seclusion of a darkened motion-picture theater. A business executive found that driving slowly along a highway adjacent to the ocean relaxed and refreshed him. Rathbone believes that simply changing the pace is not enough. Along with the change of pace, she believes that rhythmic exercise, constructed specifically for tension reduction, should be employed. In her book *Relaxation,* she suggests techniques for accomplishing this. She describes a series of rhythmic exercises which permit the arms and the legs to swing freely; the spine to "sway," to twist, and to move backward and forward; the tissues of the joints to be fully stretched; and restrictions to normal breathing to be released. These exercises are worth the attention of the student [12].

Jacobson believes that by lying quiet and comfortable, then tensing muscle groups, tension can be reduced—for example, tensing muscles in the hand, then relaxing them. This is then repeated for muscles of the neck and of the abdomen. He also illustrates methods of relaxing while active. In fact, he states that one can relax most of the muscles of the body while reading or writing. Relaxation is a matter of training [6].

Relaxing the skeletal muscles at will is difficult at first. It requires many hours of work under the direction of well-qualified personnel. Most college physical education departments provide the student body with this kind of instruction. Students lie on mats or firm cots in a comfortable position. The room is quiet. Instructions are given slowly, rhythmically, in a low, pleasant voice, often accompanied with soft music.

The lying-on-the-back position can be very comfortable and should encourage total relaxation. A small support to the neck and one to the lower back can add to one's comfort. The knees should be raised slightly, supported by rolls if necessary. The thighs should be permitted to rotate outward. The arms lie parallel to the body. Instruction in relaxing isolated muscles may then follow.

Recreation. Whereas rest precludes activity and relaxation involves action on a sliding scale, recreation is activity. It is activity motivated by freedom and joy and expressed through mind and body with revitalizing effects.

Recreation is many things to many people. It varies with needs and interests. That which brings joy and satisfaction to one may be hard work and a backache to another. Gardening can be fun or just plain drudgery. Fishing is often acclaimed as the king of recreational sports, but those who think of a stream, lake, or ocean as something to swim in, ride on, or photograph are left cold by thoughts of a fishing trip. An art gallery

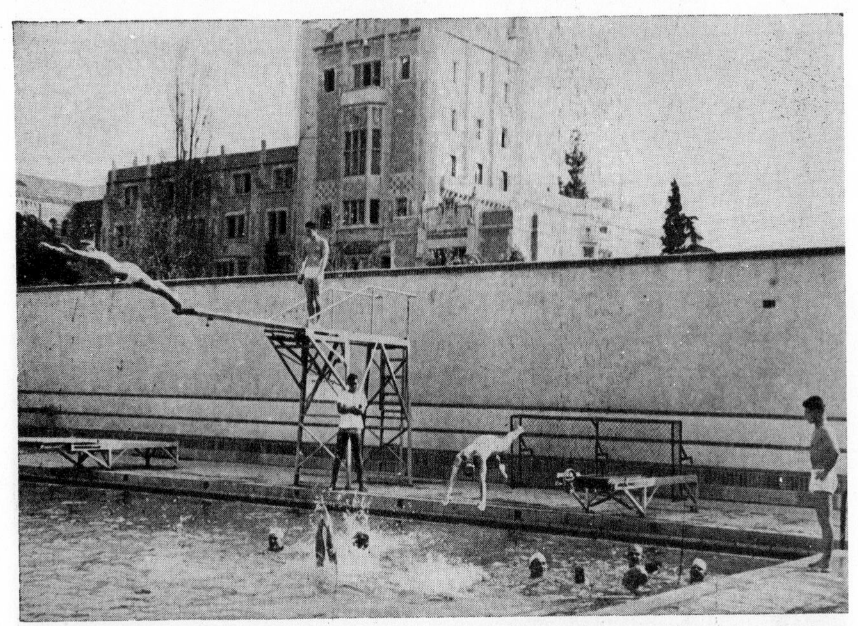

Fig. 10.1. Swimming is a popular recreational activity among college students. (*Photo by Lee Hansen.*)

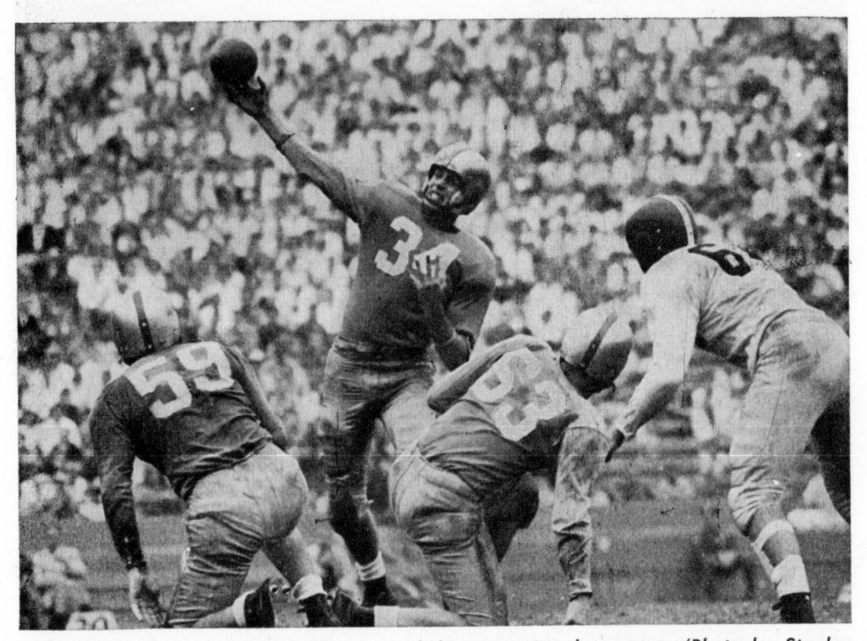

Fig. 10-2. Spectator sports may be part of the recreational program. (*Photo by Stanley Troutman.*)

or a modern dance concert can bring release, happiness, and spiritual uplift, or it can bore, fatigue, and induce a spirit of derision. Evenings of social, square, and folk dancing, satisfying and popular as they are to some, are times of torture and embarrassment for others. Carpentry and home hobbies of the craft type give hours of satisfaction and pleasure to the skilled or to those with an aptitude for them and produce feelings

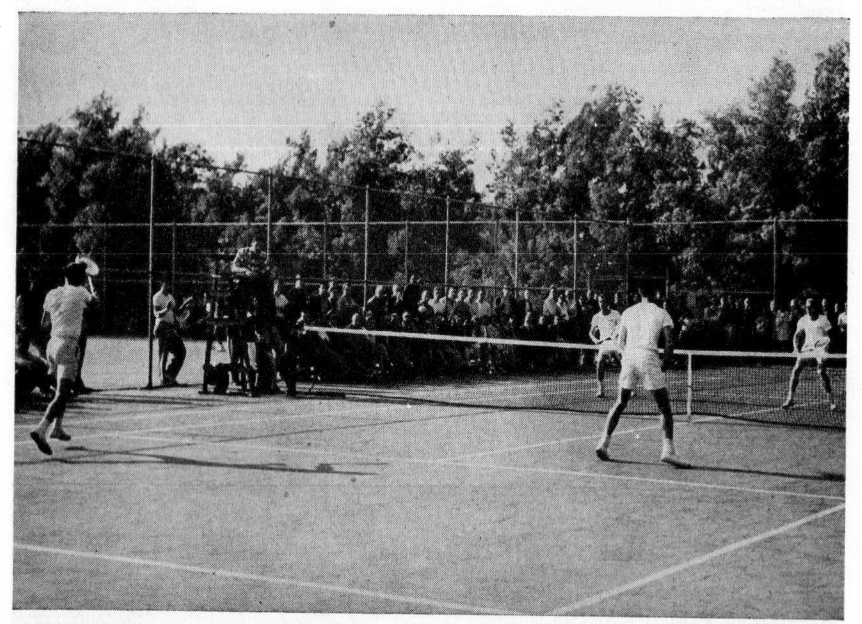

Fig. 10.3. Tennis is fun for both players and spectators. (*Photo by Stanley Troutman.*)

of guilt and frustration in the unskilled. Watching games and sports either at the scene or on television passes many interesting hours and provides conversational topics at business or social gatherings to most men. To some women they offer little that is revitalizing.

Reading, running the scale from comic books to classics, holds priority over most indoor pastimes. Singing, playing a musical instrument, or listening to music can afford experiences of great spiritual depth.

In short, any force that helps to expand, to enrich human personality by developing potentialities and giving them quality and direction is a major factor in the ultimate success and happiness of the individual [14]. This is recreation. The college student is in a strategic place to take full advantage of such forces. Recreational skills learned during student days not only give satisfaction then but tend to ensure the future for effective living.

One of the great tragedies of life occurs when an individual reaches the age of sixty-five, is retired, and finds himself with leisure time but with no skills or interests beyond the scope of his former job. William P. Shepard, of the Metropolitan Life Insurance Co., addressing the 1953 National Industrial Health Conference, said: "A fellow who never has

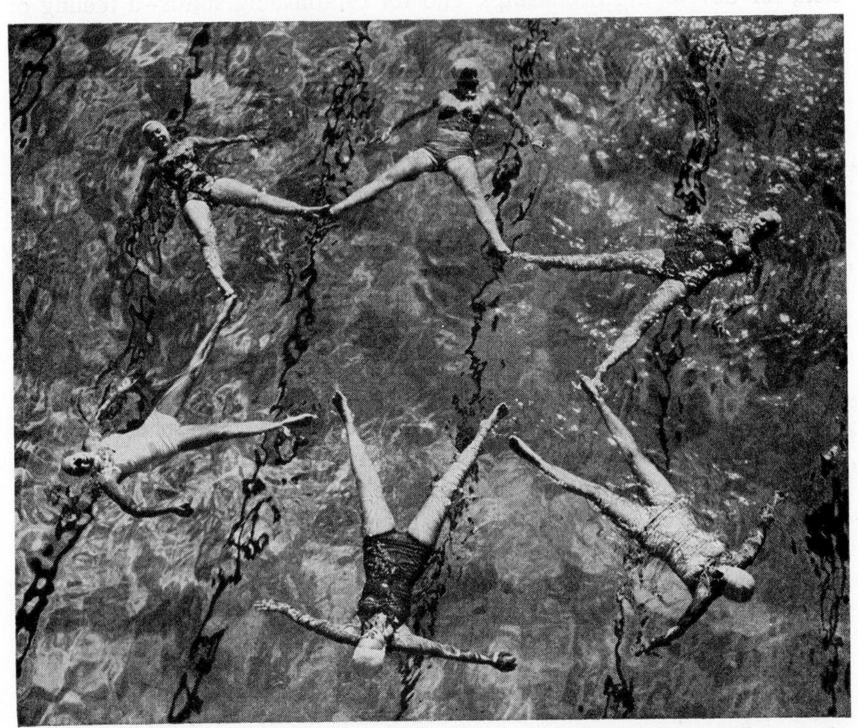

Fig. 10.4. A college or university recreation association swimming club can entertain the public as well as provide wholesome activity for its members. (*Photo by Stanley Troutman.*)

had any other interests but his job suddenly dries up and blows away when he is retired. But people who have a number of outside interests live to a ripe old age."

During the past few years, colleges and universities in this country have made available time, space, equipment, and recreational leadership so that their students can develop these "outside interests." Campus recreation associations are now integral parts of the college program. Students are encouraged by faculty and fellow students to become participating members of recreation clubs devoted to such interests as badminton, boxing, bridge, bowling, ceramics and other crafts, cycling, dancing, fencing, fiction, flying, fishing, golf, gardening, hiking, polo, painting and allied art work, photography, rod and gun, riding, skating, singing, swimming, sailing, tennis, and wrestling. Experience has shown that, where these clubs are cooperatively controlled, students find unexcelled opportunities for improving their recreation skills under expert instruction, for developing friendships, and for establishing status—a feeling of belonging.

The scope of activities is so impressive and broad that a choice may constitute a problem in making a selection of recreational activities for the first time. The following points should be given consideration by the student: (1) What is the initial cost of the equipment? (2) Is the activity primarily group or individual? (3) Is the program made up of active or passive activity or both? (4) Is it convenient to my program?

A brief consideration of each of these four points may be helpful in making wise selections.

1. *The initial cost of the equipment.* Most equipment for recreation of the active type is expensive. However, it is not necessary to purchase the most expensive or the newest equipment, and it is possible that the school may furnish part of it. Good equipment is essential to efficient performance. If an activity is worth participating in, it is wise to purchase the best equipment within one's means.

2. *Individual or group activity.* The choice between joining a club which emphasizes group or individual activity is made on the basis of interest, friendships, and the desire to acquire a new skill. During the four or five years in college it is a good practice to have experiences in both group and individual activity.

3. *Active or passive activity.* There are times in life when participation in vigorous recreational games and sports is impossible. It is then that skills in the less active or passive form pay dividends. Before graduation the student should have participated in both types of activity.

4. *Application to one's program.* Earlier in the chapter, emphasis was placed on the importance of balance so that the student's daily program conforms to some type of broad, harmonious rhythmic pattern. The advantages of such a pattern, including time for work, recreation, rest, and sleep, previously have been emphasized. In constructing the first program of the year, it will pay to make adequate place for the three R's—rest, relaxation, and recreation.

Summary

Rest, relaxation, and recreation are the important revitalizing elements in the routine daily program. Each must be given consideration. Together with adequate sleep, they form the main line of defense in maintaining total fitness. Also, separately and collectively, they are vital factors in developing and maintaining effective living.

Suggested Activities

1. Refer to your record of activities prepared in appraising your health needs as suggested in Chapter 2. Prepare a balanced daily program for yourself. Explain how it meets the needs for rest, relaxation, and recreation.
2. Reconstruct the daily programs of two or three friends on the basis of balance in work, rest, relaxation, and recreation. Compare them with yours.
3. How can overfatigue be prevented? Explain.
4. Discuss sleep from a physiological basis. Explain your favorite method of going to sleep. Prepare a sociodrama on recommended methods of going to sleep.
5. Review and report on Jacobson's book *You Must Relax.*
6. Observe a class in relaxation in the physical education department. Describe the procedures used. Interview the instructor on how one can employ techniques for relaxing both in class and at home.
7. List the recreational opportunities provided by the recreational association on your campus. Discuss them from the point of view of organization, leadership, equipment, and program.
8. Investigate the recreational programs provided for the employees of large industrial or business concerns within your city or state.
9. List both on- and off-campus recreational opportunities for students. Costs and equipment should be covered.
10. Explain the steps one has to take in joining a campus recreational club.
11. Make a brief survey of the local community recreation department. Report findings to the class. What activities are available for college students?
12. View and discuss the following films: (*a*) *Nine Bad Shots of Golf* (sound, 10 minutes), McGraw-Hill Text-Film; (*b*) *Follow the Arrow* (sound, 10 minutes), M.G.M.; *Tennis Tactics* (sound, 11 minutes), M.G.M.; (*d*) *Good Badminton* (sound, 10 minutes), Warner; (*e*) *Ski Flight* (sound, 10 minutes), Warner.

Suggested Readings

1. Ainsworth, Dorothy, *Individual Sports for Women.* Philadelphia: W. P. Saunders Company, 1946.
2. Barry, H., Jr. and W. A. Bousfield, "A Quantitative Determination of Euphoria and Its Relation to Sleep," *Journal of Abnormal and Social Psychology,* 29:385–389, 1933.
3. Benedict, Agnes E., and Adele Franklin, *The Happy Home: A Guide to Living.* New York: Appleton-Century-Crofts, Inc., 1949.

4. Edwards, A. S., "Effects of the Loss of One Hundred Hours of Sleep," *American Journal of Psychology,* 54:80–91, 1941.

5. Jacobson, Edmund, *You Can Sleep Well.* New York: McGraw-Hill Book Company, Inc., 1938.

6. Jacobson, Edmund, *You Must Relax,* 3d ed. New York: McGraw-Hill Book Company, Inc., 1948.

7. Kleitman, N., *Sleep and Wakefulness.* Chicago: University of Chicago Press, 1939.

8. Laban, R., and F. C. Lawrence, *Effort.* London: MacDonald and Evans, 1947.

9. Laird, D. A., and W. Wheeler, "What It Costs to Lose Sleep," *Industrial Psychology,* 1:694–696, 1941.

10. Metheny, Eleanor, *Body Dynamics.* New York: McGraw-Hill Book Company, Inc., 1952.

11. Neumeyer, M. H., and E. S. Neumeyer, *Leisure and Recreation.* New York: A. S. Barnes and Company, 1949.

12. Rathbone, Josephine L., *Relaxation.* New York: Teachers College, Columbia University, 1943.

13. *Recreation,* current issues. National Recreation Association.

14. Slavson, S. R., *Recreation and the Total Personality.* New York: Association Press, 1946.

15. Tyler, D. B., J. Goodman, and T. Rothman, "The Effect of Experimental Insomnia on the Rate of Potential Changes in the Brain," *American Journal of Psychology,* 149:185–193, 1947.

Popular Readings

16. Fink, D. H., *Release from Nervous Tensions.* New York: Simon and Schuster, Inc., 1943.

17. Greenbie, M. B., *The Art of Leisure.* New York: McGraw-Hill Book Company, Inc., 1935.

18. Hausman, Leon A., *Bird Hiking.* New Brunswick, N.J.: Rutgers University Press, 1949.

19. Loveless, James C., and Esther G. Post, "The College Outing Club," *Recreation,* March, 1951.

20. Menninger, William C., *Enjoying Leisure Time.* Chicago: Science Research Associates, Inc., 1950.

21. Micolean, Tyler, *Power Skiing Illustrated.* New York: A. S. Barnes and Company, 1949.

22. Pitkin, Walter, *Take It Easy.* New York: Simon and Schuster, Inc., 1935.

23. Roland, Geist, "How to Start a Bicycle Club in Schools and Colleges," *Recreation,* October, 1949.

24. Nichols, W. S., "Fly-tying for Recreation," *Recreation,* April, 1947.

25. Richardson, F. H., "Retirement: Tonic or Slow Poison?" *Today's Health*, 31:18, May, 1953.

26. Shaughnessey, Dick, *Skeet and Trapshooting*. New York: A. S. Barnes and Company, 1950.

27. Springman, O. I., *Photography Afield*. Harrisburg, Pa.: Stackpole Sons, 1953.

11. Selecting and Eating Wholesome Foods

During the course of a lifetime many hours are devoted to the eating of a variety of foods. Efficiency and pleasure during the remaining hours are influenced to a great extent by the food consumed. Many persons have what may be termed a passable state of health; they have no pronounced disease symptoms. Too few, however, have the sparkling, buoyant state of health or quality of life which is so desirable for effective living. For many, a diet inadequate in quality, more frequently than in quantity, is the basic reason for their failure to live effectively.

When an individual eats something which upsets his digestive system, he is likely to become suddenly and unpleasantly aware of the fact. Unfortunately, he is much less likely to be aware of the effects of *something he didn't eat.* Deficiency diseases are observed frequently in countries where the population is large and the food supply is limited in both quality and quantity. In the United States the deficiency diseases in their advanced stages seldom are observed. More frequently, Americans suffer from an insufficiency which decreases effectiveness physically, mentally, emotionally, and socially but does not result in acute deficiency symptoms.

The selecting of an adequate diet and the establishing of good eating habits help the individual live most effectively and happily. What are the most common weaknesses in the diet of the American people? What are the body needs which must be satisfied through the food one eats? What is a scientific, practical basis for selecting foods to meet one's needs? What effect does improper preparation have on the nutrient value of foods? To what extent does overweight or underweight influence one's health? What are some of the common food fads and fallacies which should be recognized in order that they may be avoided? Answers to such questions provide the basis for selecting and eating wholesome foods.

Nutritional Status of the American People

Studies carried on to determine the eating habits of American people indicate that many individuals do a poor job of selecting and eating wholesome foods. Low income is one cause of poor nutrition, but adequate purchasing power does not guarantee a good diet. American people on the average are well-fed, but there are many families and individuals for whom this is not true.

One of the most comprehensive studies of the eating habits of a selected group of families and the effect of diet on their general health was conducted at Pennsylvania State College [11]. The families included in the study were selected with certain limitations: each family agreed to cooperate, each family member was in apparent good health, each family had sufficient means to purchase food recommended by the consultants, each had sufficient educational background to understand the basic principles of nutrition which were presented to them, and all were urban families. On the basis of these criteria, the families selected were considered as being above average for American families, and yet the following information was discovered during the thorough health examinations which were undergone at the beginning of the study: [1]

> Several individuals in the group were found . . . by gastrointestinal x-rays . . . to have unsuspected digestive disorders of nutritional origin of major or near-major proportions.
>
> One person was found to have long standing nutritional deficiencies, accentuated by diabetes mellitus and nervous tension . . . *entirely unsuspected.*
>
> Most individuals exhibited at least minor nutritional deficiencies which neither they nor their families had ever suspected. Though these deficiencies were not serious at the time of the investigation they gave definite evidence of under-par condition which might have been avoided by consistent proper eating . . . or might easily become serious by consistent improper eating.
>
> Fatigue and nervous habits were common. . . . Although not serious in themselves these symptoms are danger signals of more serious conditions which might follow. Nor do they further family harmony . . . or enjoyment of life.

After one year of proper nutrition under the guidance of consultants, these individuals showed great improvement in their over-all health. Improvement in the condition of skin, gums, and tongue and in the reflexes, absence of fatigue and of nervous habits, fewer colds, better child

[1] Ellen H. Richards Institute, Pennsylvania State College, *They Never Suspected! Factual Report on a Family Nutrition Study,* p. 14. Mansfield, Ohio: Westinghouse Electric Corporation, Home Economics Institute, 1948.

growth, and improved weight status were some specific favorable changes noted in their medical ratings.

Findings of a one-day study of the food intake of over 8,000 men and women show a marked inadequacy in milk and in fruits and vegetables containing ascorbic acid or vitamin C and significant shortages in the fruits and vegetables containing carotene or vitamin A [12]. The summary of findings is shown in Table 2.

Table 2. Summary of New York State Nutrition Survey *

	1,567 *pregnant women,* %	5,368 *homemakers,* %	1,189 *industrial workers,* %
Protein intake satisfactory	20	40	47 (women) 85 (men)
Milk intake satisfactory	20	33	50
Fruits and vegetables high in ascorbic acid	25	50	40
Fruits and vegetables high in carotene	70	70	50

Percentages listed for each group are those whose intake was equivalent to the recommendations suggested by the National Research Council.

* Prepared from information reported by Martha Trulson and others, "New York State Nutrition Survey," *Journal of the American Dietetic Association*, 25:669–676, August, 1949.

The summary report of a study based on food consumption surveys under the auspices of the Bureau of Human Nutrition and Home Economics of the United States Department of Agriculture suggests the following characteristics of diets of city dwellers [20].

1. More families are short in calcium than in any of the other nutrients. Only about six out of ten city families include sufficient calcium to meet recommended allowances.
2. Although more high- than low-income families have good diets, even high-income families do have diets low in some essentials.
3. Higher nutrition levels are recorded for 1948 than for 1942.
4. Bread and flour enrichment are responsible for the greatest improvement between 1942 and 1948 in iron and the three B vitamins.
5. Greater improvement in diets is noted for the low-income families than for the high-income families.
6. Vitamin A more frequently is found to have a seasonal variability in diets than is any other of the nutrients included in the study.
7. The homemaker who has some college education is more likely to provide

a nutritionally satisfactory diet than one who has only elementary or high school education.

8. For the same income levels the quality of diet is higher for the higher educational group.

A study of food habits of a group of college students provides some interesting and challenging information. Approximately 80 per cent of the group of 595 students had their meals at boardinghouses, while 18 per cent ate in private homes. Of the total group only 76 per cent ate breakfast daily. The average intake of sweets was equivalent to 2 candy bars weekly, but the range was from none up to 28 per week. Carbonated beverages were used at an average rate of 3 glasses per week, the extremes ranging from none up to 21 glasses in a week. The over-all analysis of the group showed that 19 per cent had good diets, 64 per cent had fair diets, and 17 per cent had poor diets. The diets of the men, on the average, were rated superior to those of the women [13].

One characteristically bad habit of many Americans indicated in this study of college students is the failure to provide an adequate breakfast with which to start the day [13]. Additional confirmation is found in the Pennsylvania State study, which shows that 9 per cent of the persons omitted breakfast most of the time, 23 per cent either omitted breakfast occasionally or ate a sketchy breakfast which made little contribution to their daily needs, and only 14 per cent regularly took time to eat a good breakfast which supplied approximately one-third of their dietary needs per day [11]. On the basis of current findings which stress the need for protein foods at breakfast time to assist in maintaining a satisfactory blood-sugar level, inadequate breakfasts are one of the outstanding weaknesses in the eating habits of Americans.

Basis for Planning One's Diet

Many individuals realize that their diet is not adequate, but they are unable to establish a plan for selecting a well-balanced diet. During World War II, when the American people were being prepared for any eventuality, considerable emphasis was placed on the problem of conserving food and, at the same time, being certain that the diet was adequate. As a result of the research carried on, the Basic Seven food groups were widely publicized as a sound basis for meal planning. This guide is helpful to the homemaker who prepares meals for her family and to the individual who selects his own diet at public eating places.

The Basic Seven food groups. The Basic Seven food groups are illustrated in Figure 11.1. Despite the fact that recent scientific studies demonstrate the importance of specific substances not known at the time the Basic Seven was evolved, these food groups still provide a sound basis for planning for the daily dietary needs [7, 24].

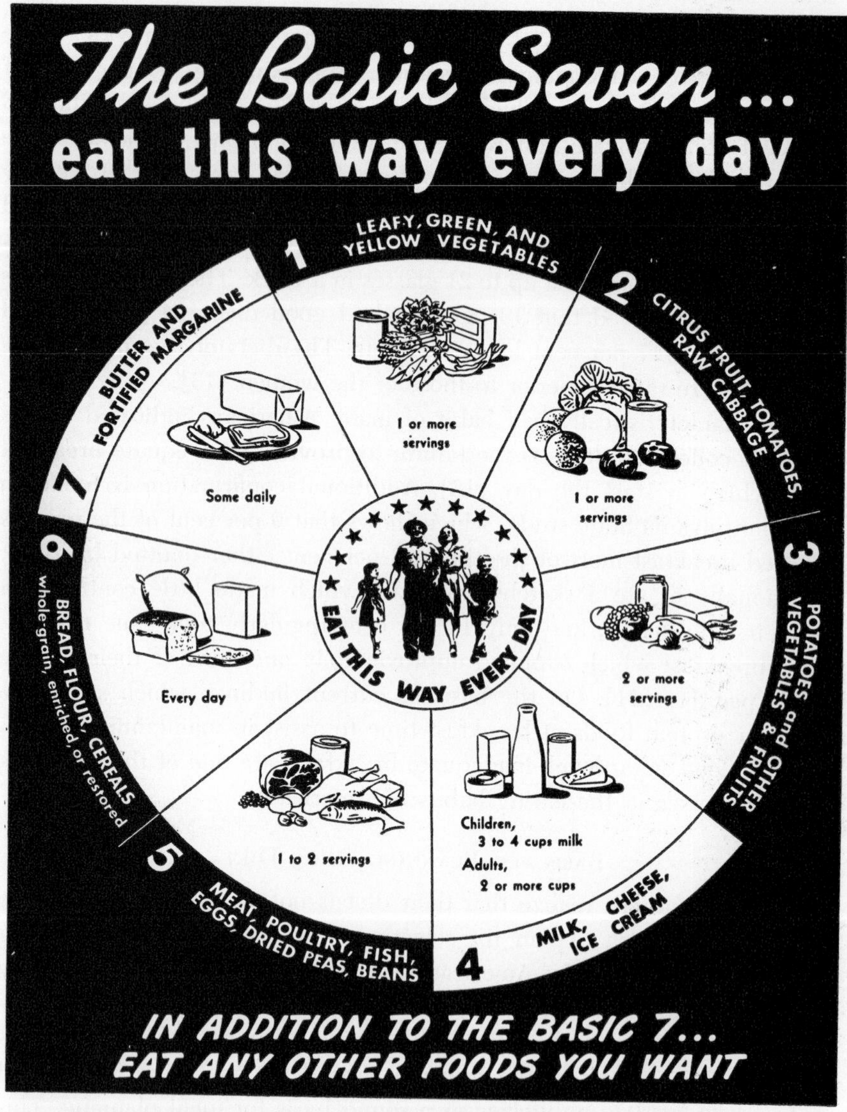

Fig. 11.1. The Basic Seven food groups. (*U.S. Department of Agriculture.*)

Many who speak glibly about vitamins and minerals actually understand little about these nutrients or about the best food sources for obtaining them. Fortunately, it is not essential to know one vitamin from

Table 3. A Food Plan for Good Nutrition *

(Quantities for 1 week)

Kinds of foods	For children 1–6 *years*	For children 7–12 *years*	*For girls* 13–20 *years*	*For boys* 13–20 *years*	*For women*		*For men, all activities*	*Total suggested for your family*
					All activities	*Pregnant and nursing*		
Leafy, green, and yellow vegetables	2–2½ lb.	2½–3 lb.	3½ lb.	3½–4 lb.	3½–4 lb.	4 lb.	3½–4 lb.	
Citrus fruits, tomatoes	2–2½ lb.	2½–3 lb.	3 lb.	3–3½ lb.	2½–3 lb.	3½–4½ lb.	2½–3½ lb.	
Potatoes, sweet potatoes Other vegetables and fruits	½–1 lb. 2 lb.	1½–2 lb. 2½ lb.	2½ lb. 3½ lb.	3½–4½ lb. 3½ lb.	2–3 lb. 3–4 lb.	2–3 lb. 3–3½ lb.	3–5 lb. 3–4 lb.	
Milk, cheese, ice cream (milk equivalent)	6 qt.	7 qt.	6–7 qt.†	7 qt.	5 qt.	7½–10½ qt.	5 qt.	
Meat, poultry, fish ‡ Eggs Dry beans and peas, nuts	1–1¼ lb. 6–7 eggs 1 oz.	2 lb. 7 eggs 2 oz.	2½–3 lb. 7 eggs 2 oz.	3 lb. 7 eggs 4–6 oz.	2½–3 lb. 6–7 eggs 2–4 oz.	3 lb. 7 eggs 2 oz.	3–3½ lb. 6–7 eggs 4 oz.	
Baked goods, flour, cereals (flour equivalent), whole-grain, enriched, or restored	1–1½ lb.	2–3 lb.	2½–3 lb.†	4–5 lb.	2–4 lb.	2–2½ lb.	3–7 lb.	
Fats, oils	½ lb.	½–1 lb.	¾ lb.	1–1½ lb.	¾–1 lb.	¾ lb.	1–2 lb.	
Sugar, sirups, preserves	¼–½ lb.	¾ lb.	1 lb.	1–1½ lb.	¾–1 lb.	¾ lb.	1–1½ lb.	

* U.S. Department of Agriculture, "Family Fare," *Home and Garden Bulletin* 1, pp. 14–15. Washington: Government Printing Office, 1950.

† Larger quantities are for younger girls.

‡ To meet the iron allowance needed by children 1 to 6 years, girls 13 to 20, and pregnant and nursing women, include 1 large or 2 small servings of liver or other organ meats.

another. The Basic Seven food groups are planned to include all the essential nutrients which the body requires.

Unlike the rigid diet prescribed by a physician for a patient with some specific ailment, the Basic Seven provides a wide range of choices within the various groups. It is difficult to conceive of an individual who cannot find foods to fit his taste as well as his needs.

One of the best statements relative to the value of the Basic Seven comes from Hawley and Carden [2] as they point out a common fallacy in evaluating the daily intake of food in respect to calories only: "Counting calories is not enough. Certain basic food elements must be included regularly in the diet. The 'basic seven' has become a popular, valuable, and practical working outline."

Functions of Food in the Body

The food one eats fulfills certain essential functions within the human body. The Basic Seven provides for foods which serve each of the functions essential to optimum efficiency of the body. The three general purposes for which foods must be provided in adequate amounts are:

1. Fuel to provide energy and warmth.
2. Materials for the building of new tissues and the repair of old tissues.
3. Regulating substances to control the complex functioning of the body.

Wisely selected foods provide the raw materials which can be converted by the body into substances which satisfy these requirements.

Fuel. For an individual to move, he must have fuel which can be oxidized by the body tissues to produce energy, which in turn results in motion. Motion is not limited, however, to external movements such as walking, writing, or talking. Activity goes on continuously within the body as long as a spark of life remains.

Internal activities which require energy include the beating of the heart, the communication functions of the nervous system, the contraction and relaxation of the breathing muscles, the peristaltic movements of the digestive tract, the filtering activities of the kidneys, and the hormone-producing activities of the endocrine glands. There is a constant demand for energy to maintain "muscle tone" in the skeletal muscles of the body. The energy demands of activities which go on continuously, whether the individual is awake or asleep, are referred to as one's basal metabolism.

[2] Estelle E. Hawley and Grace Carden, *The Art and Science of Nutrition,* p. 22. St. Louis: The C. V. Mosby Company, Medical Publishers, 1949.

Basal metabolism. The basal metabolic rate, or the basal rate of energy expenditure, can be computed. This may provide evidence of malfunction of the human organism to the physician who is qualified to interpret the information recorded. For example, an excessively high basal metabolic rate is associated with an overproduction of thyroxin, a hormone secreted by the thyroid gland, and a subsequent speeding up of the chemical processes of the body. Overproduction of thyroxin is called hyperthyroidism. The reverse of this condition, hypothyroidism, in which there is an underactivity of the thyroid gland, produces a lowered metabolic rate.

Basal metabolic rate is influenced by several factors. It is slightly higher for males than for females, and it shows a gradual decrease with age. It is influenced by the current rate of growth. The effect of endocrine secretions has been suggested earlier. As a point of interest, the influence of mental activity on metabolic rate has been measured and an amusing interpretation of the results made. The scholar who devotes an hour to intense mental effort may be surprised to discover that his energy expenditure for this is satisfied by eating half a salted peanut [2].

In addition to the aforementioned general variable factors, an individual's basal metabolic rate is modified by physical activity, the ingestion of food, and exposure to cold. A fifteen- to eighteen-hour period of no food intake and a period of complete rest under normal temperature conditions prior to and during the measurement of the metabolic rate reduce the influence of these factors. Measurement of the amount of oxygen used by the individual provides the basis for determining his BMR (basal metabolic rate). Oxygen consumption indicates the number of calories of heat produced, and the BMR is expressed in terms of calories per square meter of the body surface per hour.

Calories. Heat produced by oxidation of food is measured in calories. A calorie (large calorie) is the amount of heat (energy) required to raise the temperature of one kilogram of water one degree centigrade.

The number of calories required by an individual is computed by measuring his basal metabolism and by estimating the amount of activity in which he engages to determine the additional calories required. Table 4 shows the energy requirement in calories per pound per hour which are required for various types of activity.

Excess supplies of fuel. If an individual takes in fuel foods in excess of his body demands for energy and warmth, the additional amounts may be converted into body fats and stored for future use. This is of great importance to those who have difficulty in maintaining their body weight

Table 4. Requirement for Different Degrees of Activity per Unit of Body Weight *

Activity	*Calories per Pound per Hour*
Sleeping	0.43
Awake, lying still (with food)	0.50
Sitting at rest	0.65
Standing relaxed	0.69
Light exercise	1.10
Moderate exercise	1.56
Active exercise	1.88
Severe exercise	3.70

* L. Jean Bogert, *Nutrition and Physical Fitness*, p. 142. Philadelphia: W. B. Saunders Company, 1950.

within a normal range. In a discussion of weight control later in the chapter, the significance of this point is considered in greater detail.

Building and repair of tissues. The human organism is composed of cells of different sizes, shapes, and functions. Cells are the building blocks of the body, and to be strong they must be provided with proper amounts of protein, minerals, water, fat, carbohydrate, and other constituents of which they are composed.

It is obvious that the greatest need for building new cells occurs during the periods of most rapid growth, which for the woman includes the period of pregnancy. It must not be assumed, however, that with the cessation of growth and the attainment of maturity the need for building materials comes to an end. Cells continue to wear out as long as life continues. Replacement of worn-out cells is a requirement for maintaining life. For this reason, an older person must avoid reducing his intake of building substances, such as protein, below the level of his bodily needs.

Regulating body activities. Control of the complex activities of the human body requires an extremely fine balance of the regulating substances. Minute amounts of a substance can upset the balance and result in either minor or extreme divergences in the normal growth or activity pattern of the organism.

Hypothyroidism, underactivity of the thyroid gland, illustrates an inadequacy of one of these regulating substances. An insufficient supply of thyroxin causes a decreased rate of basal metabolism, which in turn results in other disturbances in body function. Hormones such as thyroxin exert their influence on various body activities. Excessive production of a growth hormone by the pituitary gland prior to the period of puberty results in gigantism. An insufficient production of insulin by the islands of Langerhans in the pancreas makes it impossible for the body to oxidize sugar properly, and diabetes mellitus results. The menstrual cycle in the female is largely controlled by hormones secreted by the pituitary gland and the ovaries.

It is amazing indeed that such infinitesimal amounts of these regulating substances are able to exert such a profound influence upon the body activities. It is even more amazing that the body remains in a normal state of balance to the extent that it does. It is essential that ingested foods contain the raw materials from which the body tissues can secure the components to make up the various regulating substances which can be manufactured by the tissues. Other substances, such as certain amino acids, must be obtained from food sources because the body is unable to manufacture them.

Essential Body Nutrients

The food groupings of the Basic Seven are organized according to primary contributions which foods make to the body for use as fuel, in building and repair, or for regulating functions. The specific nutrients included in foods are over forty in number, but they are classified conveniently as carbohydrates, fats, proteins, minerals, vitamins, and water. Although it has no nutrient value as such, roughage sometimes is added as a separate heading because of its regulating effect in the elimination of waste from the alimentary canal. The following discussion considers the nutrients in relation to functions which they serve in the body and foods from which they are derived.

Carbohydrates. Carbohydrates are composed of carbon, hydrogen, and oxygen. The combination of these three elements to form either sugars or starches provides a primary source of fuel for the body. Carbohydrates are chiefly of plant origin. Milk sugar, or lactose, is an exception, being an animal product.

The Basic Seven food groups which supply carbohydrates include the vegetable and fruit groups and the cereal and bread group. In addition, the average person obtains more carbohydrates from sirups, preserves, and brown or white sugar, which constitute regular "extras" in the typical American diet. These extras are not essential in the diet, but they do add to the enjoyment of meals. Because of the danger of increased tooth decay, moderate use of the extras is advisable.

The carbohydrates, along with fats, supply most of the calories which the body needs. Approximately two-thirds of the calories should be sup-

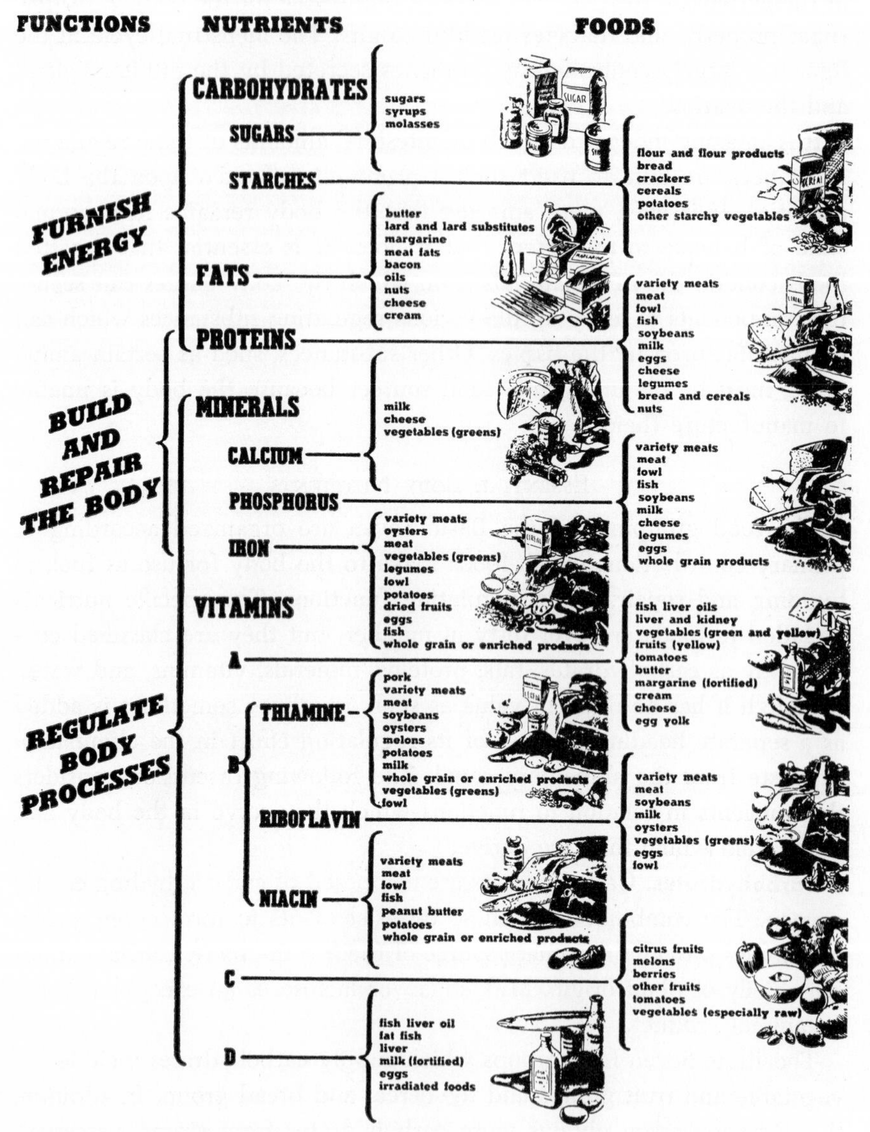

Fig. 11.2. Functions of food in nutrition. (*National Livestock and Meat Board.*)

plied by carbohydrates. In addition, the carbohydrates frequently supply calories which the body does not need. A wise practice relative to the choice of carbohydrate foods is to select calories on the basis of the company they keep [22]. Carbohydrate foods, such as whole-grain cereals, potatoes, starchy vegetables, and ripe fruits, supply calories and at the same time provide minerals and vitamins.

Fats. Although fats are composed of the same elements as carbohydrates, the carbon, hydrogen, and oxygen composition of fats is more complex. Whereas the carbohydrates are almost exclusively of plant origin, fats are the primary storage material of animals and therefore are obtained to a large extent from animal products. Certain essential fatty acids are synthesized slowly or not at all in the animal body, and it is recommended that individuals obtain some of their fats from plant products which contain these essential substances [7]. Whole wheat, soybeans, peanut oil, and olive oil are among the good plant sources of fats.

Bogert suggests three uses of fat in the diet: (1) as a highly concentrated form of fuel; (2) for flavoring and a lasting feeling of satisfaction; (3) as a bearer of vitamin A [3].

The fuel value of fats is approximately 9 calories per gram as compared with 4 calories per gram for carbohydrates. For an individual who wishes to put on weight, the energy value of the diet may easily be increased by addition of larger helpings of fatty foods, such as butter or margarine, richer milk, and mayonnaise. The danger of adding weight through eating excess amounts of fatty foods should be recognized by an overweight individual.

Inclusion of fats with other foods slows down the rate at which the food leaves the stomach. This tends to delay the gnawing pangs of hunger, which come on so quickly following some meals. During World War II it was found in many countries that the limited supply of fats which was allowed on wartime rations was one of the most distressing limitations.

Approximately one-fourth of the calories needed by the body should be provided by fats [9]. It is recommended, however, that excessive quantities of fat-rich foods at a single meal be avoided because of the added difficulty of digestion which results.

Proteins. In addition to the carbon, hydrogen, and oxygen found in fats and carbohydrates, the proteins also provide our only source of nitrogen and small amounts of sulfur. Some of the proteins also contain phosphorus and iron. The proteins are found in adequate amounts in both the animal and plant kingdoms.

Proteins are essential constituents of the cells of all living tissues. The word "protein" is derived from a Greek word meaning "primary," which suggests its importance to life. Proteins are necessary for the body to

Table 5. Recommended Daily Dietary Allowances *†

	Age, years	Weight, kg. (lb.)	Height, cm. (in.)	Calories	Protein, g.	Calcium, g.	Iron, mg.	Vitamin A, I.U.	Thiamine, mg.	Riboflavin, mg.	Niacin, mg.	Ascorbic acid, mg.	Vitamin D, I.U.
Men.....	25	65 (143)	170 (67)	3,200 ‡	65	0.8	12	5,000	1.6	1.6	16	75	
	45	65 (143)	170 (67)	2,900	65	0.8	12	5,000	1.4	1.6	14	75	
	65	65 (143)	170 (67)	2,600	65	0.8	12	5,000	1.2	1.6	12	75	
Women...	25	55 (121)	157 (62)	2,300 ‡	55	0.8	12	5,000	1.2	1.4	12	70	
	45	55 (121)	157 (62)	2,100	55	0.8	12	5,000	1.0	1.4	10	70	
	65	55 (121)	157 (62)	1,800	55	0.8	12	5,000	1.0	1.4	10	70	
	Pregnant (3d trimester)	...	...	Add 400	80	1.5	15	6,000	1.5	2.0	15	100	400
	Lactating (850) ml. daily	...	...	Add 1,000	100	2.0	15	8,000	1.5	2.5	15	150	400
Infants §..	1/12–3/12	6 (13)	60 (24)	kg. × 120	kg. × 3.5	0.6	6	1,500	0.4	0.5	4	30	400
	4/12–9/12	9 (20)	70 (28)	kg. × 110	kg. × 3.5	0.8	6	1,500	0.5	0.8	5	30	400
	10/12–1	10 (22)	75 (30)	kg. × 100	kg. × 3.5	1.0	6	1,500	0.5	0.9	5	30	400
Children..	1–3	12 (27)	87 (34)	1,200	40	1.0	7	2,000	0.6	1.0	6	35	400
	4–6	18 (40)	109 (43)	1,600	50	1.0	8	2,500	0.8	1.2	8	50	400
	7–9	27 (59)	129 (51)	2,000	60	1.0	10	3,500	1.0	1.5	10	60	400
Boys.....	10–12	35 (78)	144 (57)	2,500	70	1.2	12	4,500	1.3	1.8	13	75	400
	13–15	49 (108)	163 (64)	3.200	85	1.4	15	5,000	1.6	2.1	16	90	400
	16–20	63 (139)	175 (69)	3,800	100	1.4	15	5,000	1.9	2.5	19	100	400
Girls.....	10–12	36 (79)	144 (57)	2,300	70	1.2	12	4,500	1.2	1.8	12	75	400
	13–15	49 (108)	160 (63)	2,500	80	1.3	15	5,000	1.3	2.0	13	80	400
	16–20	54 (120)	162 (64)	2,400	75	1.3	15	5,000	1.2	1.9	12	80	400

* Courtesy of Food and Nutrition Board, National Research Council, Washington, D.C. Revised 1953.

† In planning practical dietaries, the recommended allowances can be attained with a variety of common foods which will also provide other nutrient requirements less well known; the allowance levels are considered to cover individual variations among normal persons as they live in the United States subjected to ordinary environmental stresses common thereto.

‡ These calorie recommendations apply to the degree of activity for the reference man and woman described. For the urban "white-collar" worker they are probably excessive. In any case, the calorie allowance must be adjusted to the actual needs of the individual as required to achieve and maintain his desirable weight.

§ The recommendations for infants pertain to nutrients derived primarily from cow's milk or commercial milk preparations. There should be no question that human milk is a desirable source of nutrients for infants, although it may not provide the recommended levels of certain nutrients, *e.g.*, protein, calcium, thiamine, and riboflavin.

build new tissues and repair those tissues which wear out. They are not stored in the human body as are carbohydrates and fats but must be supplied regularly by eating animal or plant foods which contain them. In addition to their function in building and repairing tissues, proteins are needed in manufacturing regulating substances which control the complex functioning of the body. Excess amounts of protein serve in an additional capacity. They are converted and utilized as a source of energy. Approximately 10 to 15 per cent of the daily calorie requirement should be provided by protein foods.

Amino acids. Proteins are made up of substances called amino acids. More than twenty of these amino acids have been identified. Proteins are of different quality according to the combination of amino acids from which they are made. At least eight of the amino acids cannot be synthesized within the body but must be supplied directly from an external source. Proteins containing all these essential amino acids are referred to as complete proteins. Complete proteins provide all the amino acids needed by the body to manufacture the proteins required for growth and repair. Incomplete proteins must be supplemented by complete proteins to provide all the amino acids needed by the individual.

Animal and plant sources. Gelatin is the only animal protein which is incomplete. Because many of the plant proteins are incomplete, it is generally recognized that animal sources of protein are most satisfactory. It should be noted, however, that with careful selection an individual is able to obtain all the protein requirements without making use of animal sources.

In the Basic Seven the meat, fish, poultry, and egg group, which is the primary source of proteins, also includes some plant sources. Soybeans, dried beans, peas, and nuts or peanut butter are considered to be the best plant sources of proteins.

Protein requirements of the body. The greatest demand for protein comes during the periods of most rapid growth. During the first year of life, the protein requirement per kilogram of body weight is greater than at any other time. One must not forget, however, the maintenance requirement for protein which persists throughout life. Table 5 lists the recommended protein intake for individuals. When one ceases to grow, there is still a need for protein to repair or replace tissues. Chaney and Alborn indicate that there is no adequate proof that a high-protein diet is harmful to a healthy human being [5]. Excess amounts may, however, be harmful in some cases of kidney malfunction.

Minerals. The minerals required by the body are used for building and repair of body tissues and for regulating body activities. Some of the regulating functions are to (1) influence the contractility of muscles; (2) determine the irritability of nerves; (3) control the movement of fluids in the body; (4) aid in coagulation or clotting of the blood; (5) assist in the formation and functioning of digestive juices and hormones; (6) maintain the acid-alkaline balance in the body; (7) transport oxygen and carbon dioxide; and (8) assist in all normal cell functions of oxidation, secretion, development, and reproduction [3, 6].

Calcium, phosphorus, iron, and iodine are the minerals most likely to be inadequately supplied in one's diet. Relatively small amounts of sodium, potassium, magnesium, manganese, sulfur, chlorine, fluorine, and copper are required, but even in small amounts they serve important functions. Only traces of cobalt, silicon, nickel, aluminum, and zinc are found in the body tissues, and it is questionable that all of them are essential in the diet.

Calcium and phosphorus. Both calcium and phosphorus are required for proper bone and tooth development as they are the chief mineral constituents of these tissues. Calcium in the blood is essential for clotting, normal function of the nerves, and good muscle tone. Phosphorus is an essential constituent of muscles and nerves as well as blood.

Increased amounts of both minerals are required for the skeletal structure, particularly during periods of rapid growth. Likewise, the woman who is pregnant or who is producing milk to nurse an infant is in need of additional supplies of calcium and phosphorus. Marked effects of deficiencies are most likely to be noted during such times (see Table 5 for recommended daily allowances of calcium).

Calcium is unevenly furnished in foods, and calcium absorption from the digestive tract is poor compared with absorption of other nutrients. The best single source of calcium comes from the Basic Seven food group of milk and milk products. The second best source is green, leafy vegetables, but depending upon this source alone is not advisable because of the relatively small amounts of calcium as compared with the large amounts available in milk.

Calcium utilization by the body is dependent primarily upon the presence of phosphorus and of vitamin D. Vitamins A and C and perhaps other vitamins also promote more favorable utilization of calcium. Phosphorus is amply provided in protein-rich foods and in cereal products. A diet which includes these substances affords adequate amounts of phosphorus to meet one's needs.

The inclusion of recommended amounts of milk and milk products in the daily diet is advisable if one wishes to be assured of an adequate supply of calcium. Milk also supplies appreciable quantities of many of the other nutrients and is considered to be the most nearly perfect single food.

Iron and copper. The body is dependent upon iron and copper for the oxygen-transporting function of the blood. Hemoglobin in the red cells serves as the vehicle for carrying oxygen. Iron is a basic constituent of hemoglobin. Hemoglobin combines with oxygen in the lungs and transports it to the cells, where it is needed for the oxidation of fuel provided by the carbohydrates, fats, and proteins. It also carries carbon dioxide back to the lungs for elimination. Although copper is not a part of the chemical make-up of hemoglobin, it is essential for its formation.

Iron may be stored by the body. Most of the iron not in the hemoglobin is found in the liver, spleen, or bone marrow, where it is available for use when needed. Additional amounts of iron are found as a part of all cells of the body.

The standard allowance for iron as recommended in Table 5 provides a liberal supply. The best sources of iron are organ meats (liver and heart), egg yolk, whole grains, and dried fruits. Other foods, such as green, leafy vegetables, contain relatively high amounts of iron, but it is questionable that this iron is as readily available for use by the body.

Anemia is a condition in which the blood is unable to carry sufficient amounts of oxygen. An inadequate supply of iron in the diet can result in anemia due to the lack of hemoglobin. Specific disease conditions likewise cause anemia. The best insurance against nutritional anemia is to eat adequate amounts of foods which supply bodily needs for iron. The treatment of anemia is a medical problem because of the many possible causes other than insufficient iron intake in the diet.

Iodine. The fact that iodine constitutes only about 3 parts per million of the body weight does not minimize its importance. The striking effects of iodine inadequacy on the function of the thyroid gland provide sufficient evidence of the essential nature of this substance. Insufficient amounts of iodine cause a decreased production of thyroxin by the thyroid gland. The decrease in thyroxin results in a reduced metabolic rate. Enlargement of the thyroid gland to compensate for the reduced production of thyroxin is called simple goiter. Iodine in the diet will prevent such a condition from occurring. Other types of goiter or evidence of thyroid malfunction are not traced primarily to dietary inadequacy.

In some parts of the country the amounts of iodine in the drinking water or in the soil are insufficient to supply human needs. In such an area the regular diet may have to be supplemented. The use of iodized salt is generally accepted as being an economical and efficient way of providing for adequate amounts of iodine in the diet. Such use is especially important during the period of adolescence and during pregnancy.

Other minerals. Because of the limited knowledge about the function of many of the other minerals and because of their availability in a typical diet, little need be said about these substances. The importance of fluorine in preventing dental caries in children is recognized, and fluoridation of drinking water is practiced in an increasing number of communities. Sodium, potassium, magnesium, iron, and calcium as basic or alkaline elements and phosphorus, sulfur, and chlorine as acidic elements are important in maintaining a normal acid-alkaline balance. The body must maintain such a balance in order to live. Despite the misleading claims made for many products, the chemical balance of the body in terms of acid and base does not require the intake of particular neutralizing substances. The use of such substances is best left to the judgment of one's physician.

Vitamins. Discovery of the existence of body-regulating substances, now called vitamins, marks an important milestone in the understanding of nutrition. The barrage of advertising claims designed to establish the virtues of a particular vitamin preparation tends to distort their true value. The average person is often on the horns of a dilemma as he attempts to determine how to satisfy his own need for vitamins. Many questions relating to individual requirements for vitamins are as yet unanswered, but essential facts are known which are helpful to a person as he plans his diet.

The vitamins are required in extremely small amounts. They are essential for normal growth and for regulation of body activities. Animals, including human beings, are not capable of synthesizing some of the vitamins within their bodies and must depend upon foods to furnish them. The chemical make-up and the physiological effect vary with different vitamins. It is difficult to generalize about vitamins except to indicate that they exert a regulating effect similar to that of the hormones produced by the endocrine glands and by minerals such as copper and iodine.

Vitamins are available in varying amounts in most plants which are used as sources of food. Foods derived from animals also provide good sources of some of the vitamins. In addition, vitamin preparations provide an excellent source for supplementing the diet. In general, however, it is recommended that vitamin preparations be used only on the advice of a physician. Most individuals who select and eat a balanced diet have no need for supplementary vitamins. There is no scientifically established evidence that additional doses of vitamins increase general health or build up resistance to disease.

Vitamins are identified both by an alphabetical designation and by their chemical names. The alphabetical designations do not indicate the order in which these substances have been discovered. The terms "vitamin C" and "ascorbic acid" are used interchangeably, as are "vitamin B_1" and "thiamine" and "vitamin B_2" and "riboflavin."

Isolation of vitamins as pure substances makes it possible for research workers to measure the amount of a vitamin required to obtain a given nutritional response. Two units of measurement commonly used to designate the daily allowance of vitamins (see Table 5) are the actual weight in milligrams or the number of international units (I.U.). For most vitamins the amounts are stated in weight units such as milligrams. The recommended allowances in Table 5 are well above the minimum amounts required by the body, as these are standards designed to improve the quality of the diet of American people.

The Basic Seven provides an excellent guide for the selection of foods providing adequate amounts of the various vitamins. It is worth noting that some foods which in their natural state may be good sources of minerals and vitamins are deprived of some of their food value during the process of preparation for consumption. To compensate for the loss of nutrients during preparation the enrichment and fortification of foods are being practiced. Examples of fortification of foods recognized as desirable by the Council on Foods and Nutrition of the American Medical Association are not more than 400 units of vitamin D to a quart of milk, vitamin A to margarine not to exceed the amount in butter, iodine to table salt not in excess of 1 part of sodium or potassium iodide to 5,000 parts of salt, and the enrichment of white bread, flour, and cereal according to a prescribed formula [23].

Vitamin insufficiencies rather than extreme deficiencies are typical of the American population. Scurvy from vitamin C deficiency and beriberi resulting from thiamine or vitamin B_1 deficiency rarely occur in the United States at present. The symptoms of an insufficient supply are observed more frequently.

Fat-soluble vitamins. The fat-soluble vitamins are A, D, K, and E. The vitamins in this group are not all single substances. The identifying letter refers to a group of substances with a similar vitamin function. The fat-soluble vitamins are characterized by the presence of precursors, sometimes called provitamins. These substances are not active vitamins but are converted to vitamins in the body. Vitamin A, for example, has four precursors of which beta-carotene is superior. The vitamin D precursor found in the skin in converted to vitamin D by the action of sunlight on the skin. An additional characteristic of the fat-soluble vitamins is the fact that they are stored by the body to a greater extent than are water-soluble vitamins.

Water-soluble vitamins. Vitamin C and the B-complex vitamins are included among the water-soluble vitamins. Thiamine (B_1), riboflavin (B_2), and niacin, or nicotinic acid, are vitamins in this group best known to lay persons. Thiamine is one of the nutrients least likely to be provided in adequate amounts in diets of Americans [20].

Water. Water is the most important component of the human body if actual weight is the basis for evaluation. It comprises approximately two-thirds of body weight.

Some of the main functions of water in the body include being a solvent for innumerable substances, serving as a vehicle for transporting nutrients and waste materials, aiding in the regulation of body temperature, acting as a cushion to protect organs from external shocks, serving as a lubricant to facilitate movement of the joints, and being a fundamental substance in building and repairing tissues.

The body uses water for its normal processes and excretes water as urine from the kidneys, with the fecal discharge from the intestinal tract, as perspiration from the skin, and in the air discharged from the lungs. The water needed by the body to replace that which is used up or excreted is secured through the fluids which are drunk, the water contained in solid foods which are eaten, and water formed in the body tissues as a result of the combustion of foods.

The amount of water lost through excretion is regulated, to a degree, by the availability of water in the body. A scarcity of urine may be noted when fluid intake is cut down.

It is generally accepted that thirst is a satisfactory guide to adequate fluid intake for the normal adult person. It is, on the other hand, recommended that one drink five or six glasses of water per day to ensure sufficient amounts for normal functioning of the body [3]. Excess amounts of water are unlikely as the water not needed is excreted by the body.

Roughage. Roughage or vegetable fiber is not an essential nutrient in the same sense as carbohydrates, fats, proteins, vitamins, minerals, and water. It does, however, have a regulatory function in elimination of solid waste material from the alimentary canal.

Because of the rather complete digestion and absorption of most of the nutrient substances, there is little residue left in the alimentary tract except for the presence of vegetable fiber, or cellulose. In the absence of this bulk, the amount of residue in the canal or tract is so small that the stimulus to peristaltic action by muscles in the tract is inhibited and normal excretion is less likely.

Fiber is provided in a diet which contains recommended amounts of fruits, vegetables, and whole grains. The use of bran or other such substance is best left to the judgment of a physician as harm can result from the excessive use of these substances.

Preparation of Foods to Conserve Nutrient Value

Man's taste in foods does not always agree with an evaluation of food on the basis of contribution to the needs of the body. Unfortunately, many Americans have learned to prefer the taste of white bread to that of whole-grain bread. In the preparation of white flour, milling processes eliminate portions of the grain containing minerals and vitamins. Grain products which are thus refined provide little more than calories. Although through enrichment or fortification some of the lost nutrients are being replaced after the milling process, because the replacement of nutrients is only partial it is recommended that whole-grain products be included in the daily diet. Labels on packaged grain products provide information as a guide to selection.

The loss of some nutrient content is preventable by the manner in which food is handled and prepared for home consumption. Keeping vegetables too long before serving, storing fruits and vegetables improperly, throwing away the greens and skins of vegetables, using large amounts of cooking water, and overcooking of vegetables are some of the wasteful practices in the preparation of foods.

Overweight and Underweight

Underweight persons are malnourished. On the other hand, it is a fallacy to assume that all malnourished persons are underweight. It is possible to be overweight and, at the same time, inadequately supplied with minerals, vitamins, or even proteins. The individual who permits himself to become either excessively overweight or exceedingly underweight is placing a burden upon his body functions.

Overweight. The determination of normal weight for individuals is difficult because of variations in body build. For practical purposes, however, it is possible to determine whether or not an individual is obese. Metropolitan Life Insurance Co. statisticians define an overweight person as one with a deviation of 10 per cent or more above his ideal weight. On the basis of a 10 per cent deviation above ideal weight, it is estimated that at least one-fifth of the population over the age of thirty is overweight. On the basis of 20 per cent or more above ideal weight being considered obese, there are an estimated 5 million obese adults in the United States [1].

A comprehensive study on the influence of overweight on health clearly indicates that mortality rates for overweight persons exceed those for standard-weight persons [8]. The implications of overweight in the occurrence of degenerative disorders are considered in Chapter 14.

Causes of overweight. Most cases of overweight are due to one factor, overeating. One authority suggests that at least 95 per cent of overweight cases are due to this factor [1]. Inactivity and abnormal functioning of the endocrine glands are factors in some cases.

The reasons for overeating are varied. Some of the more common reasons are as follows: Good food and plenty of it are a tradition in some families. Some individuals eat to excess to be sociable. Rich foods are considered a symbol of success or social standing. Overeating is started during pregnancy or during convalescence following an illness. Some individuals eat because they are bored and eating is pleasant; others feel lonely or unloved or discontented about money, job, family relationships, or social standing [17]. Whatever the reason, the immediate concern is with the fact that overeating results in overweight.

Reducing safely. Obesity is a major health problem. It is advisable for the obese individual to consult his physician and to follow his suggestions for protecting his health while weight is being reduced. He should beware of the glittering promises made in advertising simple, safe methods of losing weight without changing eating habits. Drugs used in reducing compounds can injure the health. The best way to lose weight is to take in less calories than the body requires. Body fat is then used to supply the extra calories, and weight is decreased. However, a safe diet does not omit all carbohydrates or all fats or all of anything. The individual should be certain that all the nutrients are supplied in required amounts. As suggested earlier, he should choose his calories by the company they keep. Calorie sources should also provide minerals and vitamins.

Frequently, exercise is suggested as a good way to lose weight. However, additional exercise usually results in increased hunger, and this in turn leads to more food being eaten. In the final analysis, exercise is a poor way of eliminating the pounds of fat which one has stored [15, 18]. Note, however, that Chapter 9 considers other values of exercise in effective living.

It is easier to keep the pounds off than it is to take the pounds off. Perhaps the one exercise which an overweight individual should put into practice immediately is to push away from the table when the second helping of calorie-rich foods is passed his way.

Underweight. The individual more than 10 per cent under his ideal weight is likely to be functioning at a level somewhat below his optimum. The reduced vitality and stamina consequent to such a condition may be dangerous to his health.

Bogert suggests that some disadvantages of being slightly underweight include a scrawny appearance and a tendency to chill easily as a result of inadequate subcutaneous fat, irritability, lack of ambition, inability to concentrate, a tendency to tire easily, a tendency to digestive disorders and constipation, and general susceptibility to respiratory-tract infections [3]. The underweight individual needs the advice of his physician in order to determine whether or not the condition is due to an organic cause. If the condition is simply a matter of an insufficient supply of nutrients to meet the needs of the body, he can add more of these nutrients to the daily intake of food. High calorie content is a primary objective of a diet to increase the weight, but added amounts of protein, minerals, and vitamins are equally important.

One of the basic objectives of meal planning is to provide a diet which enables ideal weight to be maintained and at the same time adequate amounts of all necessary nutrients to be included.

Converting Food for Body Functions

The digestive system converts raw materials into substances which the body can absorb and use. A general understanding of the processes of digestion and elimination provides a sound basis for developing practices which promote proper functioning of the alimentary canal.

Digestion of foods. Digestion of food is both mechanical and chemical in nature. The mechanical portion of digestion begins in the mouth with the action of the teeth and the tongue serving to break the food into smaller physical components. Progressive constriction of muscles in the wall of the alimentary canal produces a series of wavelike contractions called peristalsis. The peristaltic action of these muscles serves to mix the contents thoroughly and to move them along.

The chemical phase of the digestive process is somewhat more complex in nature. Numerous chemical substances are involved, and each has a specific effect on the food. Chemical action is initiated in the mouth as salivary secretions mix with the food during mastication and begin the breakdown of carbohydrates.

The food passes down the esophagus into the stomach, where digestive juices are added and the mixture is reduced to a semifluid consistency by muscle action of the stomach. The digestion of proteins and milk is initiated in the stomach, and carbohydrate digestion is continued.

The length of time required for foods to pass through the stomach into the small intestine is influenced by the nature of the food itself, as well as by emotional factors and physical activity. In general, the stomach requires three to five hours to empty itself following a meal. Fluids pass through the stomach in a matter of minutes. Carbohydrates tend to be emptied from the stomach more quickly than proteins, which in turn pass through more rapidly than do fats. Combinations of fats and proteins leave the stomach more slowly than does either of these nutrients alone. Persistent feelings of hunger, which cause some to overeat, can be relieved partially by eating foods which do not leave the stomach too quickly. Carbohydrates contain a rich supply of calories and by themselves do not satisfy one's hunger for a great length of time. Herein lies one of the reasons for those added pounds.

Bands of muscles, called sphincters, form valves at the upper and lower end of the stomach. The valve at the upper end normally prevents the acid contents of the stomach from moving back into the esophagus. The pyloric sphincter at the lower end of the stomach controls the flow of material from the stomach into the duodenum, the first section of the small intestine.

In the small intestine, food is acted upon by additional digestive juices. Some of these substances are produced by glands in the intestinal wall, and others are produced by special glands apart from the alimentary tract, the pancreas and the liver being two examples.

Digestion in the large intestine is produced by action of the digestive juices brought from the small intestine. There are no secretions of digestive enzymes into the large intestine.

Products of digestion. As a result of the digestive process, foods are converted into substances which the body is able to absorb. Carbohydrates are broken down into simple sugars. Fats are converted to fatty acids and glycerin. Proteins are reduced to their component amino acids. The vitamins and minerals are freed so that they can be absorbed.

Absorption. The passage of food substances through the epithelial cells of alimentary canal into the blood or the lymph is called absorption. Food is transported by these fluids to the various tissues where it is to serve its function as a source of fuel, for building and repair, or in the regulation of body activities.

The primary place for absorption is within the small intestine, little absorption taking place in the stomach. An exception to this is the absorption of alcohol, which explains the immediate effects of alcohol, particularly when one has not eaten for several hours.

Because of the length of the small intestine, the numerous folds, and the small, fingerlike villi which project from the lining of the intestinal wall, the surface available for absorption is extensive. Differences in the rate and degree of absorption due to variations in body build may be a factor in determining the ability to maintain normal weight. The movement of food as a result of peristaltic action brings it into contact with the lining of the intestine and facilitates the process of absorption.

The simple sugars and the amino acids are absorbed directly into the blood. The fatty acids and glycerin must be re-formed into tiny fat globules, which in turn are taken into the lymphatic system. The lymph fluid eventually empties into the blood stream, and the fat products are distributed to the tissues, where they are utilized.

Absorption in the large intestine is confined to removing the excess amounts of water. The residue is left as a semisolid waste.

Elimination of waste. The fiber, or roughage, part of the ingested food remains as a major portion of the residue after digestion and absorption are completed. This residue passes through the large intestine and is eliminated as solid waste material called feces, or fecal matter.

Disorders of the Digestive System

It is a rare individual who does not at some time suffer from a disturbance in the function of the digestive system. The pain or discomfort may be short-lived, or it may be a persistent or chronic ailment. The discomfort may be only mildly irritating, or it may be extremely painful. The degree of pain or discomfort does not necessarily indicate the seriousness of the disorder. Any abdominal pain which persists for a period of time should be brought to the attention of a physician, who is best qualified to determine the cause and to recommend the treatment. Effective treatment for one disorder can be dangerous if used for another ailment.

Indigestion, or dyspepsia. Indigestion, or dyspepsia, is a symptom of a disorder in the digestive tract. Simple indigestion is the result of a functional rather than an organic condition. Functional nervous indigestion is a distressing condition which frequently is caused by faulty eating habits. For some the symptoms are brought on by overeating. Irritating substances, such as alcohol, may produce the symptoms in others. Emotional states, such as fear, anger, or worry, commonly are associated with disturbances in function of the alimentary tract with the resulting discomfort of indigestion.

Advertisers are doing an effective job of convincing the consumer that he is suffering from "acid stomach." This should not be too difficult, because the contents of the stomach are normally acid in nature. An unfortunate aspect of such advertising is the claim that a certain preparation is needed in order to relieve the condition. The correction of persistent indigestion should not be attempted by the use of preparations selected from the well-stocked shelf of the corner drugstore. The assistance of a physician is needed to determine and treat the cause and not just the symptoms. Ulcers, gallbladder disorders, cancer, and appendicitis are common disorders of the digestive tract which produce symptoms often associated with simple indigestion.

Ulcers. Peptic ulcers affect as many as 5 per cent of the population [21]. They are associated with pepsin, a substance found in the stomach digestive juices, and are found in the stomach and also in the duodenum, or first part of the small intestine. Nine out of ten are found in the duodenal area, perhaps because the tissue lining this area is less resistant to the action of the digestive juices [14].

The exact cause of an ulcer is not known. Alvarez suggests that heredity plays an important part in determining whether or not an individual develops an ulcer [14]. Most persons who have duodenal ulcers tend to have a higher gastric acidity than normal, but many who have extremely high concentrations of gastric acidity do not have such ulcers. Nervous conditions frequently are associated with ulcers, but many nervous persons do not develop them. It is interesting to note that more men than women suffer from ulcers.

Despite the fact that the specific cause of ulcers is not understood completely, it is known that strong emotional tensions and high gastric acidity are associated with them. The gastric secretions literally eat the wall of the stomach or the duodenum, and unless treatment is undertaken, a hemorrhage or a perforation of the wall occurs.

Persistent indigestion or pain which tends to occur as the stomach becomes empty may indicate the presence of an ulcer. Treatment of ulcers is a medical problem. The advice of a physician regarding diet or other treatment should be followed carefully. Fortunately, most ulcers can be kept under control by medication and diet.

Gallbladder disorders. Disorders of the gallbladder can produce symptoms such as heartburn, bloating after meals, nausea and vomiting, and, in some cases, pain in the upper right quadrant of the abdominal area. Because of the function of bile in the digestion of fats, the intake of foods rich in fats tends to aggravate the symptoms.

Disorders of the gallbladder require the care of a physician. In some cases the disorders respond to diet and medication, and in some instances surgery is necessary to correct the difficulty. In any case, early treatment of the condition is more likely to produce favorable results. Self-treatment of symptoms with liver pills or other such remedies seldom gets at the cause of the symptoms. It is much better to have a physician determine the cause and prescribe treatment before the disorder becomes severe.

Cancer. Cancer of the digestive tract accounts for more cancer deaths than does a malignant condition in any other organ or system of the body, for it is frequently undiscovered until it is too late to treat it effectively. Persistent indigestion or change in normal bowel habits may be the only early sign of cancer of the digestive tract. The importance of having a physician determine whether or not persistent indigestion is an early indication of cancer cannot be overstressed. A more detailed discussion of cancer is found in Chapter 14.

Appendicitis. Acute appendicitis—inflammation of the vermiform appendix on the colon near the juncture of the small and large intestine—produces symptoms similar to some other digestive disturbances. Severe abdominal pain may be felt in other areas of the abdominal cavity, but eventually the pain usually localizes in the lower right quadrant. Nausea and vomiting may occur as the condition becomes worse. Rupture of the appendix can cause peritonitis, which reduces the chance for recovery. Self-treatment for abdominal pain resulting from appendicitis, particularly if it involves the use of laxatives, can cause the appendix to rupture.

Constipation. Constipation is a condition in which excretion of fecal matter from the large intestine is delayed. Interference with the normal elimination of waste material results in considerable discomfort. In extreme cases of constipation, there is extensive irritation of the large intestine.

The sales of laxatives, a 100 million dollar a year business in the United States, would seem to indicate that constipation is the most common of physical disorders [4]. Laxatives produce their results in different ways. Some are drugs which stimulate peristaltic action of the muscles of the intestinal tract, some increase the bulk content by use of substances which swell up when combined with fluids, some contain salts to increase the fluid content, and others lubricate the lining of the tract by use of such substances as mineral oil.

In most cases, laxatives do not get at the cause of constipation. They are used to treat symptoms, and their excessive use adds to one's difficulties rather than eliminating them. The use of mineral oil interferes with absorption of fat-soluble vitamins in the intestinal tract. Drugs which stimulate peristaltic action can become habit-forming. Continued self-treatment with laxatives can result in a delay in the diagnosis of a serious disorder of the digestive tract.

Proper elimination is promoted by a well-balanced diet, such as that suggested in the Basic Seven, sufficient intake of fluids, physical activity, good posture, and a regular time for daily bowel movement. In general, laxatives should be used only when recommended by a physician.

Food Fads and Fallacies

Extravagant claims for any single food should arouse suspicions regarding the value of the food or the purpose of the person making the claim. With the exception of the very early period of life, when milk serves as the only source of nourishment, there is no single food which has super qualities of the kind that faddists claim for their favorite products. Milk is considered to be the most nearly perfect food, but milk alone provides an inadequate diet for anyone but a very young infant. The Basic Seven is suggested as a guide for selecting a well-balanced diet because of the need for a variety of foods to ensure that all the nutrients needed for body functions are obtained.

Why food faddists? Food faddists make their claims for a variety of reasons. Some are firmly convinced that they have an idea which is of benefit to mankind; unfortunately, though they have little scientific evidence to support their claims, they do have sufficient persuasive power to convince many of the gullible to take their advice. Others undertake the promotion of a particular product from the motive of personal gain.

The persuasive power of this group is no less effective than that of the righteous crusaders.

Bogert suggests three groupings of individuals according to their reaction to propaganda or advice regarding foods: (1) those who disregard all advice and eat whatever they wish; (2) those who attempt to follow anyone who offers such advice, with the result that they constantly switch allegiance; (3) those who become convinced of the value of a particular fad and become its wholehearted supporters [3]. As long as the latter two groups exist, food faddists have a fertile field for their endeavors. However, through a sound educational program the number of persons subscribing to such beliefs is decreasing.

At best, it is unfortunate for a healthy person to fall under the influence of the food faddist. For one who has undetected ulcers, cancer, diabetes, or heart condition the advice of the faddist can delay diagnosis until it is too late for the physician to effect a cure. A more detailed discussion of quacks and nostrums is found in Chapter 12.

Common food fads. Food fads change with the times. A consideration of some of the fads which have been prevalent in the past or which exist at the present time is helpful in illustrating the nature of the claims made by faddists.

Claims for specific foods. Various claims have been made for specific foods at different times. The stress on fish as a brain food, celery as a nerve tonic, and onions to cure a cold are examples of exaggerated claims made for specific foods. The more recent claims for yoghurt as a super food provide an excellent illustration. Yoghurt is made from milk and has whatever nutrient value can be derived from milk itself. Because it consists of milk alone, it provides only those substances found in milk. But the price of yoghurt makes it a rather expensive source of nutrients which are available in milk or other milk products [25].

Considerable caution should be exercised in accepting sweeping claims about specific food products. Sound, scientific information should be available relative to such products before one decides to use them to the exclusion of other foods.

Claims regarding combinations of foods. Certain foods when combined in the stomach are claimed to have reactions detrimental to health. Milk with cherries, fruits with vegetables, and two starches at the same time have been condemned because of their supposed detrimental effect when ingested together. Perhaps the reason for such claims is the fact that a given food may be difficult to digest and when two such foods are taken at the same time the results can be very annoying. There is no basis for the belief that foods will react with such other and "explode." A balance in the foods selected and eaten is essential to health. It is better to be less concerned with the combination at any given time and more concerned with securing a well-balanced and varied diet such as that provided for in the Basic Seven.

Raw foods as opposed to cooked foods. Fortunately, the answer to the problem of raw foods as opposed to cooked foods is, not one or the other, but a combination. Some foods are more readily digested when cooked properly. Some foods tend to lose part of their nutrient value when cooked. The general opinion of authorities is that the diet can profitably include some cooked and some raw fruits and vegetables.

Vitamin preparations. If the opinion of those who have vitamin preparations to sell be accepted, it can be assumed that it is impossible to obtain an adequate supply of vitamins through the daily food intake. The virtues of such products are extolled in a most convincing manner. The shelf space devoted to vitamin preparations in the neighborhood drugstore is evidence of a modern, convincing sales campaign. In the opinion of authorities, however, it is possible to obtain an ample supply of all nutrients from the diet without supplementing that diet with vitamin or mineral preparations.

Summary

Early in life, the individual depends upon other persons for the selection of foods to provide for energy, growth and repair, and regulation of body activities. In general, he eats whatever his mother, the dormitory cook, or some other person prepares for him. Many college students, however, are or soon will be completely responsible for selecting all the foods which they eat. This chapter gives the information necessary to select an adequate diet.

Some of the steps which the college student or any other person can take to develop the state of health or quality of life necessary for effective living include (1) checking the daily diet for a period of time by using the Basic Seven food groups as a guide; (2) taking advantage of "snack periods" to supplement the diet with fruit, milk, or other foods supplying nutrients lacking in the diet; (3) maintaining the weight at or near normal for age, sex, and body build; (4) practicing eating habits conducive to good digestion and waste elimination; (5) seeking the advice of a physician regarding persistent symptoms of body malfunction; and (6) assisting others to understand the basic concepts relative to proper nutrition.

Suggested Activities

1. Refer to the diet record compiled during the study of needs suggested in Chapter 2. Use this record of food intake to assess the adequacy of that daily diet. Base your evaluation on the suggestions included in the Basic Seven food groups. Repeat the evaluation of your daily diet after the study of nutrition is completed, and compare your findings. Indicate changes to be made in order to provide essential nutrients.

2. Survey the eating habits of your classmates or of some other student group. List the weaknesses and strengths of the eating habits of the group. Suggest changes which should be made.

3. Prepare a bulletin-board display to stimulate student interest concerning the selection of proper foods, the desirability of good eating habits, and the need for evaluating claims made for special foods.

4. Obtain information from campus sources and near-campus sources to show the consumption of candy and cola drinks by the college students. Prepare posters to inform students about the extent of the use of such substances, and include information showing the food values contained and the dangers of excessive usage.

5. Prepare illustrated information for use in campus eating places to stimulate student interest in selecting well-balanced meals.

6. Obtain advertisements, labels, or folders containing information about foods recommended as having special values as a source of nutrients. Evaluate the claims made, and determine the benefits to be derived from, as well as the dangers which may be associated with, the use of the substances. Consider the comparable cost of the substance with other food sources of equivalent nutritional value.

7. Accumulate information on dieting as suggested in the daily newspaper, magazines, and advertising circulars and by means of radio and television. Evaluate the information on the basis of findings included in this chapter and in other recommended sources. What are some of the prevalent, misleading claims in reference to dieting? What are some of the dangers of indiscriminate use of products advertised to assist in control of weight?

8. Observe and record some of the common practices in food preparation which tend to reduce the nutrient value of foods. Recommend procedures which are helpful in maintaining the nutrient value of foods.

9. Collect advertisements concerning various laxative products. What are some of the misleading claims included in such advertisements? In what way do the various preparations function to stimulate the elimination of waste from the digestive tract? What are dangers associated with the indiscriminate use of laxative substances?

10. List some of the common food fads or fallacies you have observed as

influencing your family or your friends. Explain the basis for the claims made. Explain the fallacy of the claims.

11. Preview, show, and discuss audio-visual aids which are pertinent to nutrition, such as the following: (1) *Losing to Win* (sound, 11 minutes), Metropolitan Life Insurance Co.; (2) *Foods and Nutrition* (sound, 11 minutes), Encyclopaedia Britannica Films; and (3) *Something You Didn't Eat* (sound, 9 minutes), United States Department of Agriculture.

Suggested Readings

1. Armstrong, Donald B., and others, "Obesity and Its Relation to Health and Disease," *Journal of the American Medical Association*, 147:1007–1014, Nov. 10, 1951.

2. Benedict, F. G., and C. G. Benedict, "The Energy Requirement of Intense Mental Effort," *Science*, 71:567, May 30, 1930.

3. Bogert, L. Jean, *Nutrition and Physical Fitness*. Philadelphia: W. B. Saunders Company, 1950.

4. Byrd, Oliver E., *Health Instruction Yearbook*. Stanford, Calif.: Stanford University Press, 1951. (Published annually.)

5. Chaney, Margaret S., and Margaret Ahlborn, *Nutrition*. Boston: Houghton Mifflin Company, 1949.

6. Cooper, Lenna F., and others, *Nutrition in Health and Disease*. Philadelphia: J. B. Lippincott Company, 1947.

7. Hawley, Estelle E., and Grace Carden, *The Art and Science of Nutrition*, 3d ed. St. Louis: The C. V. Mosby Company, Medical Publishers, 1949.

8. *Influence of Overweight on Health and Disease*. New York: Metropolitan Life Insurance Co., 1951. (Reprinted from *Postgraduate Medicine*, Vol. 10, November, 1951.)

9. National Research Council, Food and Nutrition Board, "*Recommended Daily Dietary Allowance, Revised, 1953*." Washington, 1953.

10. Sherman, Henry C., and Caroline Sherman Lanford, *Essentials of Nutrition*. New York: The Macmillan Company, 1951.

11. *They Never Suspected!* Factual report on a family nutrition study conducted by the Ellen H. Richards Institute, Pennsylvania State College. Mansfield, Ohio: Westinghouse Electric Corporation, Home Economics Institute, 1948.

12. Trulson, Martha D., and others, "New York State Nutrition Survey," *Journal of the American Dietetic Association*, 25:669–676, Aug. 1, 1949.

13. Young, Clara B., and Clara A. Storvick, "Food Habits of Freshmen at Oregon State College," *Journal of the American Dietetic Association*, 25:318–321, April, 1949.

Popular Readings

14. Alvarez, Walter C., *How to Live with Your Ulcer*. Chicago: Wilcox and Follett Company, 1951.

15. Aaron, Harold, "Weight Control," *Consumer Reports,* 17:100–106, February, 1952.

16. Brussel, James A., "What You Should Know about Abdominal Pain," *Today's Health,* 29:16–17, April, 1951.

17. Hagman, Patricia E., *Good Health for You and Your Family.* New York: A. S. Barnes and Company, 1951.

18. Millman, Max, "Exercise and Reducing," *Today's Health,* 29:14–15, May, 1951.

19. U.S. Department of Agriculture, "Family Fare," *Home and Garden Bulletin* 1. Washington: Government Printing Office, 1950.

20. U.S. Department of Agriculture, "Nutritive Content of City Diets," *Special Report* 2. Washington: Government Printing Office, 1950.

21. Wermer, Paul, "Living with Your Ulcer," *Today's Health,* 29:33. June, 1951.

22. Wilkins, Walter E., and Boyd French, *Nutrition for You.* Jacksonville, Fla., 1949.

23. Wilson, Anna May, "Does Fortification Improve the Diet?" *Today's Health,* 29:32–33, March, 1951.

24. Wilson, Anna May, "Is the Basic Seven Out of Date?" *Today's Health,* 29:34–35, February, 1951.

25. Wilson, Anna May, "More Truths about Nutritional Secrets," *Today's Health,* 29:39, December, 1951.

12. Selecting Health Services and Products

The American consumer, including the college student, is confronted with a variety of attractively packaged and highly avertised health products to cure all possible illnesses, as well as to preserve and lengthen life. A multitude of quacks bombard the public with their services, which they guarantee to cure every disease from athlete's foot to cancer. Physical culture specialists, through a mail-order set of prescribed exercises, claim to be able to mold any skeletal frame into a body beautiful. Even more tempting are the aids to beauty, which are supposed to renew, restore, invigorate, and bring to light hidden powers of loveliness for women and manliness, including handsome features, for men.

Endless advertising, designed to ensnare each and every person, fills the daily paper and the weekly and monthly magazines. Advertising of health products and services is broadcast from coast to coast by radio and television stations, supplemented with billboards which decoratively portray a new, healthful, zestful life. Health information with quasi-scientific basis fills the atmosphere through every available medium. The opportunities for filling one's needs for health services and products is greater than ever before. At the same time, the dangers to life and the chance of financial loss, thwarted energy, and wasted time have increased proportionately.

Consumer health is but one aspect, though a significant one, of improving the quality of living. Health consumers are all people who use health products and services. This group includes the well, the sick, the young, the aged, the rich, and the poor. To be an intelligent consumer and to select products and services wisely, it is important for the student to be concerned with answers to the following questions: (1) What are fraudulent health practices? (2) What protection does the consumer have from quacks and nostrums? (3) What are the organizations and agencies protecting the consumer? (4) What are the sources of safe, reliable health information? (5) How can one critically evaluate health information and advertising? (6) How can one select health products and health services wisely? (7) How can one protect himself and others from fraudulent practices undermining the individual and the group? The information in this chapter is presented to assist in answering these questions.

Fraudulent Consumer Health Practices

Definition of "quackery" and "nostrum." Quackery is the practicing of medicine by a faker or an incompetent person. Such an individual claims he has a cure-all or "sure-fire" method of restoring health. The quack preys upon the public, including the so-called "intellectual" class, by his adroit psychological suggestions. The dominating motive of the quack is to make money. It takes no special preparation or education to become a quack.

A nostrum is the product distributed as a cure-all by the quack—legally, a patent or secret remedy sold directly to the public. Proprietaries are chemicals or drugs whose composition or formula is protected by patent or other means against free competition. They are advertised to and used by physicians in the treatment of disease.

Historical examples of quackery. Cure-alls are almost as old as history itself. It has been a weakness of all peoples through the ages to believe in a fountain of youth, an elixir of life which would free them from pain, and restore youth and vigor. Certainly, the quacks prey upon this weakness of mankind as did P. T. Barnum. It is reported that the oldest nostrum, which later developed into a bona fide drug and still is in existence today, is called "hiera picra." This is a powder of aloes and canella, the dried juice of a common oriental plant.[1] Arab doctors, Greek practitioners in Rome, barbers, corn doctors, herbalists, the monastic doctors of the Middle Ages, and early English and American doctors used this drug, and quacks peddled an imitation of it.

One of the most colorful quacks in history was St. John Long of London, a handsome and clever Irishman. He was patronized by many fashionable and noble patrons. He built up a reputation as one who could cure a number of diseases, particularly tuberculosis. His popular treatment consisted of the application of a liniment made up of turpentine, acetic acid, and egg yolk and the inhalation of a vapor. After reap-

[1] John A. Foote, "Medicine Fakes and Fakers of All Ages," *The National Geographic Magazine,* January, 1919, p. 69.

ing a fortune from his so-called tuberculosis "cure," he died at the age of thirty-seven from pulmonary tuberculosis.

The grandfather of American quacks was Elisha Perkins, a physician who became an impostor in 1795 primarily because of the lure of lucrative returns. He discovered that pain was stopped when a metallic instrument was used to separate the gum from a tooth previous to pulling it. He decided that metallic substances influenced nerves and muscles. Therefore, he developed his famous metal tractors to influence the body when applied externally. The tractors consisted of two rods of brass and iron 3 inches long. One side was flat and the other half round. They were called Perkins Patent Tractors, cost 75 cents, and sold for $25 to $30. The purpose of the tractors, according to Perkins, was to draw the disease from the body by starting at the hairline and working back to the neck. He admitted this would not cure a headache caused by excessive drinking. He took his tractors to a session of Congress and sold a number to the distinguished lawmakers. However, he soon was exposed and forced to give up the sale of the tractors. Then he derived Perkins Medical Formula, a combination of vinegar and salt taken in tablespoon doses diluted with three parts of hot water, which was a sure cure for yellow fever according to Perkins. By a strange turn of fate he died of yellow fever in 1799. His work was carried on by his son, who fled to England, where he made a fortune from Perkins Patent Tractors [29]. The cases of Long and Perkins are two selected historical illustrations of quackery indicating fraudulent practices. Many more could be cited.

Present-day pseudoscientific practices. Food, drug, and cosmetic racketeers are not past history but are prevalent in present-day culture. The following examples illustrate this fact:

The market today is deluged with antifat preparations so numerous that there is need to classify them into several categories. There are the laxatives in crystalline salt form whose action rids the body of its food. A second type consists of foods which dull the appetite. The individual using this method of reducing depends upon a restricted diet and a strenuous exercise program. A third variety includes the drug preparations. These are effective but extremely dangerous, since they may contain thyroid preparations or dinitrophenol, which reduces weight by speeding up the bodily processes and literally burning the tissue, including the fat. A fourth type is a product in a class by itself as a weight reducer, and it is hard to believe it could be sold on the open market; government food and drug inspectors have found live tapeworms in this reducing preparation. There is no doubt about the effectiveness of any of the preparations mentioned above. However, the user runs the real risk of gaining a slim figure at the expense of loss of vision, poor health, or even life itself.

Beauty treatments and skin care have provided a fertile field for quacks. Many people forget that health comes from within as well as from without. As the common expression goes, beauty is more than skin deep. Health is not purchased in a jar from the local cosmetic counters. A balanced diet, fresh air and sunshine, proper rest, soap and water, a good cleansing cream, a wholesome environment, and, if necessary, medical treatment will do more for the skin than cosmetic preparations. It is true that cold creams have been used since Roman days. They are valuable for softening the skin, particularly a dry skin, and removing some dirt particles, as well as serving as a lubricant. Special creams claiming to serve other purposes are pure nostrums and a waste of money. Such are the vitamin and hormone creams, which, according to the claims, provide food and nourishment to the skin, or the creams that are supposed to prevent acid skin, remove wrinkles, and restore youthful beauty and loveliness.

One of today's most tragic rackets is conducted by the cancer quacks. Since the causes of cancer or not yet fully known to medical science, many opportunities are open to quacks to advertise their sure cures. These unscrupulous persons take in desperate persons who are grasping at any new hope for a cure. Some types of cancer can be cured when detected early, but surgery, radium, and X ray are the only sure methods of cure. Preventive methods are being used in some industries and occupations where workers are constantly coming in contact with irritants predisposing to cancer. Great strides are being made in cancer research, and cancer clinics and detection centers are increasing in scope and value. The importance of periodical medical examinations as a means of discovering early cancer cannot be overemphasized. Cancer is discussed in further detail in Chapter 14.

In the case of some nostrums, false claims are made by the producers; in others, the wording of the claims is so clever that no one claim can be discounted absolutely. The latter is true in the case of vitamins, especially when they are considered as cure-alls. If a person is in good health and is eating a well-balanced diet, there is no need for additional vitamins. Vitamins prescribed by a physician are a different matter. For example, a doctor prescribes vitamins for patients showing evidence of a minor deficiency condition, to prevent deficiencies in certain wasting diseases, and for pre- and postoperative care. It is the indiscriminate use of vitamins by healthy persons submitting to the wiles of advertisers that is a waste of money.

It was not so many years ago that quacks depended on electricity and electric devices and claimed to bring new health to their gullible patients by means of electric shocks, shining lights, and magnetic fields. Today such instruments are in use, but not as extensively as formerly, for the modern quack has developed new machines to cure all diseases by means of atomic and cosmic waves. Reputable physicians utilize X-ray and therapeutic machines as aids in the treatment of certain diseases. The quack builds machines designed to look like the approved devices and, in addition to treatment in his office with these fake machines, endeavors to sell or lease them for home use. No therapeutic machine today manufactured for home use cures the basic cause of disease [10].

Frauds occur in the sale of medicines today even though drug labels must tell a true story according to law. The smooth talk of salesmen or lecturers promises much more than is claimed on the label. Also, false claims are contained in booklets or brochures accompanying the drugs. The modern quack is still a part of the culture, and he is more subtle and clever than ever before.

Legal Protection for the Consumer

Laws are one means of protection for the consumer. However, the common laws in America provide only slight protection against fraudulent selling of health products. Under the Uniform Sales Act, when there is a breach of warranty or breach of contract, the buyer can proceed as follows: (1) refuse to accept the goods and cancel the contract; (2) keep the goods and sue the dishonest seller for damages; (3) keep the goods and insist on a deduction from the original price [13]. These are not adequate protective procedures because the time and expense involved in suing or showing proof of the seller's fraud make this prohibitive in most cases. Also, consumers are loath to admit that they have been duped, and so they bear the financial loss. Since the common laws give insufficient protection, the consumer looks to statute law for aid. Through the statutes a number of governmental agencies have been established with the expressed purpose of protecting the consumer.

Early food and drug legislation. Congress passed its first legislation exerting control over drugs in 1848. This statute was concerned only with controlling importation of adulterated drugs into the United States. Soon, however, the adulteration of drugs in this country provoked attention to the extent that several states and the District of Columbia passed control measures. In 1906 Congress passed the Federal Food and Drug Act governing the interstate commerce of drugs. The Food and Drug Act made adulteration, which is the addition of inferior substances to products, illegal. It attempted to prevent the inclusion of harmful ingredients in foods and drugs by controlling branding, false statements, omissions of facts concerning the products, and the selling of products under assumed names. This was a serious effort to control quackery and nostrums through interstate commerce. As a part of the functions of the Act, the Bureau of Chemistry, United State Department of Agriculture, made examinations of drugs. In the same year, 1906, the Federal Meat Inspection Act was passed. By this law all meat in interstate or foreign commerce was required to be inspected by the Bureau of Animal Industry, United States Department of Agriculture. By 1927, Congress established a Food and Drug Administration to enforce the 1906 Act. Although the Act was a great step forward, it lacked many enforcement powers and did not apply to many products. Because of the many loopholes in the law the consumer was not adequately protected. Public interest called for better controls.

The Food, Drug, and Cosmetic Act. Congress responded to the public demand with a revision of the Food and Drug Act in 1938. This Act was named the Food, Drug, and Cosmetic Act. It became effective in 1940, providing punitive powers to prevent fraudulent practices.

The Act defined "food" as articles used for food or drink for man or other animals. It included chewing gum and articles used as components of food or drink. Certain health and sanitary safeguards were established to protect the consumer. For example, an illegal food was clearly defined as any food containing a natural or added substance which is injurious to health. The law declared food illegal that is filthy, putrid, or decomposed. Food labels must not be false or misleading and must actually represent the facts concerning the food. The required information must appear in a prominent position on the label. The Act authorized standards of identity, standards of quality, and standards of fill of containers for food [11]. It prohibited traffic in new drugs unless they were tested and approved by the Food and Drug Administration. For example, drugs such as insulin, penicillin, and streptomycin must be from a batch certified by the Food and Drug Administration. Also, drugs must comply with one of three standards, (1) the United States Pharmacopeia (stamped U.S.P.), (2) the Homeopathic Pharmacopoeia (marked H.P.), (3) the National Formulary of the American Pharmaceutical Association (labeled N.F.).

In general, the Act granted power to the Food and Drug Administration to control food, drug, and cosmetic traffic by issuing rules and regulations that have the force and effect of law. For example, criminal penalties for violations were increased; authority was given to establish minimum standards for foods and to prohibit traffic of all food injurious to health. Factory inspection of food, drugs, and cosmetics was authorized for interstate shipments, and truthful labeling of foods, drugs, and cosmetics was required.

Despite the number of provisions covered by the Act, the need for critical evaluation of products is still, to a great degree, left up to the consumer. This is an important reason for consumer health education today.

Other Federal legislation protecting the consumer. Four other acts designed to safeguard the health of consumers are worthy of mention, (1) the Caustic Poison Act, (2) the Tea Act, (3) the Import Milk Act, and (4) the Filled Milk Act.

The Caustic Poison Act became effective in 1927. It requires that certain caustic or corrosive substances must be clearly labeled with the name of the substance, name and place of manufacture, and name of packer and seller or distributor and the word "poison" placed in plain sight in large capital letters. Directions for treatment in case of accidental personal injury must be provided. A few substances covered by the Act include hydrochloric acid, sulfuric acid, nitric acid, carbolic acid, and oxalic acid.

The Tea Act became effective in 1897 and was last amended in 1920. It authorizes the annual establishment of standards of quality, purity, and fitness for consumption of all teas imported into the United States. If a lot, or "chop," of tea imported does not meet these standards, it is rejected.

The Import Milk Act of 1927 was passed to protect the public health and promote the dairy industry of the United States. It prohibits the importing of milk and cream into the country unless the shipper holds a permit from the Administrator of the Federal Security Agency.

The Filled Milk Act of 1923 prohibits the interstate commerce of filled milk if it is adulterated or injurious to health or if its sale constitutes a fraud upon the public. Filled milk is defined as any milk or cream to which has been added, or which has been blended or compounded with, any fat or oil other than milk fat. Such a change in the product makes it an imitation or semblance of milk or cream rather than the true product itself [19].

State, territory, and local laws protecting the consumer. State, territory, and local communities have enacted their own laws to supplement and complement Federal legislation. For example, the California legislature passed its own Pure Foods Act in 1939 patterned after the Federal Act of 1938. The new Act in California added provisions to the Health and Safety Code for control of food, drugs, and cosmetics, giving additional powers to the state department of public health.

The legislature of the Territory of Hawaii likewise responded to the Federal legislation by enacting in 1941 the Hawaii Food, Drug, and Cosmetic Act. This legislation is administered by the Food and Drug Bureau of the Board of Health.

Many county and city health departments, local public health units, and other official agencies at the local level protect the consumer's health every day. A few of the activities which these agencies undertake are inspection of food-dispensing establishments, meat inspection, milk inspection and pasteurization, supervision of the canning of food and the purity of the water supply, and the restriction of sale, possession, distribution, and use of narcotics and poisons.

Much of the effectiveness of the control of food, drug, and cosmetic traffic depends on the working relationships and the cooperation among law-enforcement personnel of the Federal, state, territory, and local agencies and private organizations. More effective control has resulted with improved legislation, similar legislation at each level, better-qualified personnel, and cooperative endeavor through better human relationships at each level. However, there is still room for great improvement in legislation and enforcement. Loopholes in legislation and enforcement make possible intensified activities of the quack and unscrupulous businessman.

Organizations and Agencies Protecting the Consumer

It is reassuring to know that several governmental agencies, professional societies, and private organizations are assuming responsibility for the protection of the consumer. A brief description of some of these organizations and agencies is presented in Table 6. For further information, consult references listed under Suggested Readings.

Table 6. Organizations and Agencies Protecting the Consumer

Organizations and Agencies	*Protective Functions*
Government Agencies	
Department of Health, Education, and Welfare:	
The Food and Drug Administration	Protects consumer from impure or falsely labeled food, drugs, cosmetics, and therapeutic devices in interstate commerce; cooperates with state and local agencies
Public Health Service	Responsible for control and standardization of biological products; enforces Virus, Serum, and Toxin Act of 1944; requires manufacturer of biologicals to hold license
Federal Trade Commission	Prevents price fixing agreements, boycotts, combinations in restraint of trade, and other unfair methods of competition. Maintains jurisdiction over false advertisements of food, drugs, cosmetics, and devices as well as unfair and deceptive acts and practices
The Department of Agriculture	Enforces Federal Insecticide, Fungicide, and Rodenticide Acts. Regulates marketing and labeling of poisons preventing or destroying insects, fungi, rodents, and the like
Post Office Department	Protects consumer by preventing fraudulent schemes, and guards against selling of nostrums by mail
Professional Groups	
American Medical Association	Protects public as well as medical profession against fraud and improper advertising of nostrums and proprietaries. Several councils, bureaus, and committees carry out these functions; for example, Bureau of Investigation checks patent medicines, quacks, medical fads, and other phases of pseudo medicine. Medical schools and hospitals are approved for training of interns. Products meeting requirements are given "Seal of Acceptance"
The American College of Surgeons (a professional society of surgeons in North and South America)	Develops and maintains standards for hospitals, hospital services, and surgical products
American Dental Association	Engages in standardizing materials used in dental practice. Its Council of Dental Therapeutics gives "Seal of Acceptance" to products meeting requirements of Council. Publishes *Accepted Dental Remedies*
Home economics associations	Encourage educational programs in schools and colleges, providing students with understanding of standards, grades of commodities, and services for individuals, families, and communities. American Home Economics Association publishes a monthly *Journal*. Home Economics Education Service of U.S. Office of Education provides numerous materials
Better business bureaus	Protect both businessman and consumer. Some 90 bureaus and a National Better Business Bureau are located in chief business centers throughout United States. These nonprofit organizations educate public to inquire before buying, fight frauds, promote advertising accuracy, reduce unfair competition. Businessmen and business firms support bureaus through an annual subscription. They publish informative literature such as *Facts You Should Know about Health Cures* and *Facts You Should Know about Cosmetics*
National Consumer-Retail Council	Provides a medium for collective bargaining between consumers and sellers. Attempts to accomplish joint planning and action on mutual problems of buyers and sellers. Educational purposes relate to consumers, manufacturers, and distributors
Private Testing and Rating Agencies	
Consumers' Research	Provides unbiased information and counsel for consumer. Established in 1929 at Washington, N.J. Members receive information through *Consumers' Research Bulletins* and an *Annual Cumulative Bulletin*. Ratings of products and services based on judgments from staff, Federal, and state agencies, professional societies, and other research bureaus
Intermountain Consumers' Service, Inc.	Provides its membership with sources of information on products similar to those of Consumers' Research. Publishes *Consumers' Buying Guide*, issued four times a year. A nonprofit research and information agency, located at Denver, Colo. First organized in 1932
Consumers' Union, Inc	Proposes to tell consumers the truth about goods and services, to provide information for making comparison of brands, and to make intelligent selection of commodities. Organized as a nonprofit corporation in 1936. Located in New York, N.Y. Publishes for subscriber-members *Consumer Reports* and an *Annual Buying Guide*. Ratings of products are made by staff of Consumers' Union, by consultants employed by commercial research concerns, by government, and by other technical research agencies. Products approved only after laboratory tests, controlled-use tests, expert opinion, or experience tests
Magazine Testing and Rating Services	
Good Housekeeping	Issues a "Seal of Approval" guaranteeing that merchandise advertised does what it says it will do. Replacement or refund of money is made by *Good Housekeeping* if product is not as advertised
Parents' Magazine	Issues two seals: (1) a guaranteed Seal in which the magazine stands behind product for refund or replacement; (2) "Studied and Commended Seal" which provides a guarantee to consumer and denotes a recommendation for product and manufacturer

Evaluating Health Information

Selection of reliable sources of health information and advice about health products and services is vital to consumer health and merits attention. With the advent of television, added to such media as the radio, magazines, newspapers, and billboards, the constant stream of health information reaching the average citizen is attaining flood-tide proportions. Health information should be appraised by scientific guides; that is, reliable and unreliable sources of health information should be differentiated by applying sound scientific criteria. Then a selection of the products and services needed should be made on the basis of the findings.

Unreliable sources of health information. Unsafe sources are (1) the customs and superstitions of the culture which do not withstand the test of the scientific method; (2) information based on ignorance and prejudice; (3) the expoundings of the quack or information devised by him for the consumption of the uneducated and gullible; and (4) the commercialized health information advanced for the sole purpose of selling a product regardless of its effect on the individual.

Customs and superstitions. Many of the customs of our ancestors have helped materially in protecting, saving, and improving human health. The utilization by our forefathers of natural forces such as sunshine, sleep, rest, and invigorating work are good examples. On the other hand, many customs from early days are built on beliefs in magic or spirits or are based entirely on superstitions. Fortunately, with the progress of science and the increase of knowledge throughout the land, mythical customs and superstitions have waned, particularly the more serious ones. A belief in witchcraft, for instance, has disappeared from civilized society. No longer are the following beliefs held as they were at one time:

A baby will not grow if a hat is placed on his head before he is a year old.
Illness of a child may be prevented by bathing him in greasy dishwater.
A sore throat is cured by drinking water out of a stranger's shoe.
You will not be sick the following year if you dip your head in the ocean on January 1.
Sleeping with a dog prevents rheumatism.

Despite the great advance of scientific knowledge, however, customs and superstitions continue to exert an influence on the conduct of many. There is still belief in signs and omens. Charms are worn upon the person or affixed to the automobile to bring good luck and ward off disaster. The belief in lucky or unlucky circumstances is prevalent. The reading or telling of fortunes continues to be a profitable business and an expensive pastime. An interesting superstition pertains to the sneeze. In the early days of Greece and Rome the sneeze was an ominous sign and had to be counteracted by a protective saying. Today one frequently hears someone say after a person sneezes, "God bless you!" or the German version, "*Gesundheit!*" meaning "good health" [25].

Many such beliefs are trivial or minor. However, accepting superstitions and beliefs without critically appraising them can lead to poor health practices and needless expense. Since all untested beliefs are likely to be dangerous to health, every intelligent person should subject his health beliefs to the scientific method.

Ignorance and prejudice. Ignorance and prejudice are other unreliable bases for health information. It should be remembered that an adviser can be highly educated in the arts, languages, or history and at the same time be thoroughly misinformed and highly prejudiced in matters pertaining to health.

Health cults are frequently the result of ignorance or of narrow, one-sided education. The cultist is one who, regardless of education, training, and experience, claims to cure all disease. Also, he believes in but one dogma or particular belief. He exhibits a "closed-mindedness" indicating extreme prejudice. His stock in trade consists of superstitions and a belief in magic and miracle cures.

Another example of blindness, of ignorance and prejudice, is the individual who insists on self-diagnosis and self-treatment. The old adage, "He who hath himself for a doctor hath a fool for a patient," is more true today than ever before. Yet many are willing to stake their health and their very life on self-diagnosis and self-treatment. Many of the 5,000 yearly deaths in the United States from appendicitis are due to faulty self-diagnosis and self-treatment. Serious dangers threaten when persons making their own diagnosis purchase patent medicines and treat themselves. They are relying upon guesswork for diagnosis and upon possibly harmful, expensive products for cure of conditions which, for the most part, demand immediate expert medical attention. The gullible and ignorant every day are influenced by high-powered advertising and dramatic testimonials.

The quack as an unreliable source. Although the quack previously has been referred to, he must be included as an unreliable source of health information. The quack is the medical pretender whose silver tongue boasts of his achievements, who advertises in the daily papers or periodicals, who cites the testimonials of cured patients, who promises miracle cures of heart disease, cancer, arthritis, kidney disorders, and the like. Quacks flourish for a number of reasons. Many diseases cure themselves after running their course, and the quack takes the credit for the work nature has performed. A large percentage of the population's ills are minor disorders due to nervous or emotional causes. The quack's fanfare, glib talk, soothing ways, mystic powers, sure-cure elixirs provide needed confidence, sympathy, and a form of psychotherapy. Always, it is well to remember that the dominating motive of the quack is money, not the welfare of the individual.

Testimonials. Testimonials are the backbone of nostrum advertising. They have an important commercial value due to the supposed experience of the testimonial writer. They serve as one of the best baits for prospective customers of the quack. There is no scientific value to the testimonial; it may have been purchased outright by the quack, written by him or his agent, or written in good faith by those who believe they have been or will be cured. In one investigation by the Post Office Department, 75 per cent of the testimonials came from deceased persons [3].

Bona fide medical testimonials are impossible to obtain, since it is unethical for any member of the American Medical Association to give a testimonial. The testimonial, then, is an unreliable guide for health information or products.

Commercialized health information. The health appeal in commercial advertising has developed tremendously within the last decade. This rise has been so marked that it is a definite part of the culture and has grown to big-business proportions. Appraisal of this type of health information is important because some commercial health information is desirable, while much is undesirable and unreliable. The reliable kind is that furnished by organizations whose prime purpose is to keep people alive and well. A good example of this type of organization is the life insurance companies, which are developing excellent health education materials for their policyholders, for school children, and for the general public.

A second type of commercial health information relates to health products such as household staples, clothing, foods, beverages, and the like. Such health information is furnished by advertising designed to sell a product, in which the health motive is used as the selling power. Breakfast cereals, milk, fruits and vegetables, enriched bread, and health shoes are illustrations of the products sold through an appeal to the health motive. The dangers from such advertising lie in the possibility of overemphasis, of distortion of the truth, of misinterpretation by the public.

A third type of commercial health information concerns the hygienic products, such as cosmetics and soaps with germicidal virtues and medicinal qualities, dentifrices, deodorants, feminine-hygiene products, hair tonics, pimple creams, and the like. The greatest danger from information exploiting these products, and also from using them, is the encouraging of harmful health practices. Furthermore, false health values are built up. Also of real consequence is the fact that purchasing such products relieves consumers of large sums of money annually.

A fourth type of information is furnished by the quack selling his nostrums. These hazards have been discussed previously [12].

The common method of communicating health information. John Peterson,[2] in talks to civic groups, has repeatedly stated: "The most common method of communicating health information is over the backyard fence." There is a great deal of truth in this statement. Time and time again the average American needing health information contacts a friend or neighbor for advice. At the college level, the friend or neighbor is a roommate, a fraternity brother, a sorority sister, a fellow club member, or a study partner.

The accuracy of the friend's recommendation will depend upon his preparation and experience and also on whether or not he has appraised critically the situation, the person, or the product he is recommending. Possibly he will operate entirely on ignorance, bias, prejudice, misinformation, or superstition. Possibly he will recommend another friend, a relative, or a product simply on an emotional basis.

Most well-meaning American citizens are eager to diagnose, prescribe, and even treat a friend or neighbor on the basis of their own past ills, and it is true that the intelligent quick thinking of friends has saved many lives. A sound procedure for the individual seeking the advice of a friend is to listen to his information, appraise it in the light of scientific criteria for evaluating health information, and check it with at least one other unquestionably reliable source.

Criteria for evaluating health information. It is evident from the foregoing discussion that some guide lines for judging health information are needed. The following are suggested criteria to assist the student in using judgment.

Before accepting health information or following health advice one should ask:

1. Who is the person or organization presenting the information?
2. What are the educational background and professional experience in the health sciences of those providing the information?

[2] Director of the Health Division, Welfare Council, Philadelphia, Pa.

3. What reputation does the person or organization have in the community?

4. What are their motives? To improve health and prolong life? Are they using the health motive as a sales appeal? Is the primary purpose to make money? Is there a subtle but consistent reference to money?

5. How is the information presented? In an educational, scientific manner? Or are the propaganda devices utilized, such as name calling, glittering generalities, transfer, testimonials, plain-folks appeal, card stacking, and bandwagon technique?

(The foregoing marks of propaganda were developed by the Institute of Propaganda Analysis.)

Reliable sources of health information. Sources that meet the criteria for evaluating health information are as follows: (1) recognized authorities in the health sciences who are competent to present scientific facts; (2) men and women educated and experienced in health sciences and education; (3) religious counselors who operate on a basis of ethics and scientific fact; (4) health organizations and agencies administered and staffed by experienced and scientifically educated personnel; (5) public and private agencies operated by scientifically educated personnel for the protection of the consumer.[3]

Recognized authorities educated in the health sciences. These include physicians, surgeons, and dentists, graduates of approved professional schools, particularly those who: (1) have passed their speciality board examinations in a specialized field, such as pediatrics, psychiatry, ophthalmology, preventive medicine, orthodontia, pedodontia, and the like; (2) have been awarded the professional title of "Fellow" for distinguished professional service; (3) have gained experience through years of service and are rewarded with an impeccable reputation in the medical or dental profession and in the community; (4) have conducted research projects in the medical and dental science fields, contributing new knowledge or techniques for improving healthful living; (5) have won distinction through their teaching ability in the health sciences; (6) have written extensively for the professional publications and lay periodicals, such as *Today's Health,* communicating scientific information to the profession and the general public.

Men and women educated and experienced in the health sciences. These comprise such persons as health educators, both school health educators and public health educators, who have special preparation in methods of health education and are equipped to interpret scientific

[3] Walter H. Brown and Oliver E. Byrd, *Evaluation of Health Information.* Unpublished syllabus, Stanford University, 1942.

health information to children, youth, and adults; who are concerned that people received prompt and adequate medical and dental care; who are engaged in activities that assist in solving both individual and community health problems; and whose primary purpose is to help individuals and groups to learn how to live healthfully. Science and social science professors, teachers, research workers, public health nurses, medical social workers, and others who have had basic preparation and experience in the science fields of chemistry, physics, physiology, anatomy, bacteriology, zoology, biology, anthropology, sociology, and psychology are examples of persons who can be relied upon for sound, scientific health information.

Religious counselors. Doctors of divinity, ministers, rabbis, priests, and other religious counselors who are well-trained in spiritual guidance and human relationships, whose faith and worship are founded on ethics and not mere secularism, are reliable sources.

Health organizations and agencies. Health organizations and agencies are discussed in Chapter 17 (see pages 424 to 442).

Public and private consumer agencies. Public and private agencies operated by scientifically educated personnel for the protection of the consumer are of special importance to consumer health education. This group is considered in a preceding section of this chapter.

Selecting Health Products

The process of selecting health products. Every consumer at some time or other buys a simple drug, cosmetic, or therapeutic device. Selecting the right health product appears to be a simple process until one discovers the numbers of brands, the varieties of sizes and shapes, the variations in weight, and the numerous price levels for each single item. Consumer confusion is the natural result. The easy way out is to take the clerk's advice, regardless of whether he has had thirty years' experience or whether it is his first day on the job. The person with discriminating judgment is not satisfied by this method. He wants to ask some questions, and he is willing to consider some guide lines to assist him in the selection process, for two reasons: (1) to protect his health; (2) to protect his pocketbook.

Guide lines for selecting products to protect and maintain health. The intelligent consumer:

1. Follows the advice of his physician. Buys products prescribed by him, realizing that his supervision and recommendations are for the individual's best interests.

2. Does not permit pharmacists, druggists, or store clerks to prescribe health products.

3. Reads the label on products. Remembers that the Food, Drug, and Cosmetic Act requires the producer to tell the consumer the contents of the product, what it will do, how to use it, and when and when not to take it.

4. Buys products bearing a seal of acceptance or a seal indicating a high-quality standard. Remembers that the American Medical Association and the American Dental Association, through their special committees, "accept" products meeting their standards. Recalls that the letters U.S.P., N.F., and H.P. mean that drugs meet the standards of the United States Pharmacopeia, the National Formulary, and the Homeopathic Pharmacopoeia.

5. Is critical of and does not buy drugs or devices offered as cure-alls or curatives for serious diseases, such as heart disease, cancer, tuberculosis, and kidney diseases.

6. Is skeptical of products advertised under propaganda techniques.

7. Is skeptical of and refuses to purchase devices or machines to cure disease offered for sale or lease for use in the home.

8. Reports frauds and suspected frauds in writing to the nearest bureau of the Food and Drug Administration or the better business bureau.

Guide lines for making the most of the health dollar. The intelligent consumer:

1. Knows what is needed before buying. This means buying on the basis of need, not to "keep up with the Joneses," to satisfy his vanity, or merely to take advantage of a bargain.

2. Compares values. Checks the quality and purpose of the product and its design. "Shop and save" is a good motto, since prices may vary for the same item from store to store. The one-store buyer pays more.

3. Buys on the basis of standards in grade labels, in weights, in measures, and other standards of quality. Utilizes the standards of the Department of Agriculture for qualities of canned fruits, vegetables, meats, butter, and eggs. Buys the cheapest brand meeting the grade A standard when there are several grade A products.

4. Buys on the basis of intended use. When standards are shown on grade levels, grades A, B, or C can be purchased wisely on the basis of intended use. For example, canned tomatoes, grade A, can be reserved for special occasions, since they are slightly higher priced. Grade B is of the same nutritional value but less perfect in size or appearance and is suitable for general use.

5. Buys from private brands. This is a particularly wise procedure in purchasing cosmetics and toiletries. Such products sold by a reputable dealer with U.S.P. or N.F. marked on the label can mean substantial savings over nationally advertised brands.

6. Buys the larger quantity. Larger sizes and quantities result in savings. Checks the cost per ounce of drugs and toiletries. Notes the savings in the long run.

7. Watches for buying opportunities. Appraising needs in advance and watching for regular and special sales saves money.

8. Pays cash from cash-and-carry stores. Such firms operate for less and sell for less. However, paying cash at a credit firm does not result in savings.

9. Subscribes to a commodity testing service. Membership in one of the testing services, such as Consumers' Research, Intermountain Consumers' Service, Inc., or Consumers' Union, Inc., provides information about the quality and price of products which can result in substantial savings over a period of time [16, 26].

Selecting Health Services

The importance of selecting a competent health adviser. One of the most vital factors in promoting and maintaining healthful living is choosing the proper health advisers. It is to these professional persons—the medical doctor (general practitioner, surgeon, medical specialist), doctor of dental surgery (the dentist, the dental specialist)—that one entrusts his life and certainly the quality of his living. In discussing the student health service as a part of the college health program in Chapter 3 of this book, it was pointed out that the majority of colleges and universities throughout the country do not provide complete medical and dental services for the college group. As a result, many college students, on their own for the first time, are faced with the problem of selecting competent health advisers. If college students do have complete health service coverage during college, the problem is merely delayed until they establish their own homes after acquiring a college education.

The task of selecting the right health adviser is important because the human organism is the most delicate and highly interrelated and integrated of all mechanisms. Anyone who even superficially has studied the human body—its structure and function—cannot help being awed by its delicate functions. When this complex organism is out of adjustment, for whatever cause, the most competent health adviser is needed to assist in regaining a healthy state. Preventive service to keep one healthy is equally important to living a full life, or even more so.

Types of doctors and health specialists. Because of the multiple use of the term "doctor," it is necessary to distinguish between those using this title. Originally, the term meant "teacher," and that meaning remains today when the title of doctor of philosophy or doctor of education is assigned to one awarded an advanced academic degree. From the medical point of view it denotes a person licensed to practice medicine. The osteopath, the chiropractor, the naturopath, and the Christian Science practitioner are representatives of other healing arts and may in some instances use the title "doctor." In selecting a health adviser, it is necessary to understand the various types of medical practice and their theory and required training.

Medical doctor. The medical doctor serves as a counselor, one to whom the individual can confide personal problems of adjustment as well as conditions pertaining to his physical well-being. However, the medical adviser is more than a counselor; he provides preventive services to protect one's total health. He gives continuous supervision to health needs, based on his findings in periodical health examinations, laboratory tests, and many subjective evaluations, which altogether give him a complete health history. When illness comes, he is able to stop pain, to alleviate suffering. He offers medical care, including surgery, sufficient to rehabilitate the individual to a healthy state.

The medical adviser today realizes that he alone cannot furnish this complicated service of providing adequate preventive and sickness care. The task requires a team of well-trained personnel. The center on this team is a cooperative patient who works with, rather than against, the doctor's advice. The medical adviser, the quarterback, calls upon the specialist from the various medical specialties when the condition warrants it. He arranges for hospitalization and nursing service. He is constantly in touch with consultants, technical assistants, and research workers. Also, he is working at all times with the public health officials in protecting and improving the health of the total community group.

The healing art of medicine is based on scientifically proved principles of preventing, curing, and alleviating disease. The medical doctor is carefully selected from among many students on the basis of scholarship, personality, character, and professional aptitude. He spends nine years in training under the careful supervision of leading scientists. The highest type of code of ethics governs his practice. Medical organizations at the local, state, and national level promote professional standards and offer opportunities for advanced study and continuous medical education.

Doctor of osteopathy (D.O.). Osteopathy was originally based on the theory that disease is caused by structural maladjustment and that body manipulation rather than drugs is the therapeutic medium. It has advanced from the point where it was a cure-all theory to the stage where body manipulation is but one therapeutic agent among many. At present, osteopathic physicians are striving to approach medical physicians in training and professional standards.

The osteopaths, through their professional organizations, particularly the American Osteopathic Association, are continually raising their professional standards. They require scientific training in the chemical, physical, and biological sciences as foundation for their practice. The subject matter of their curriculum resembles the medical curriculum. In eleven or more states they take the same examinations as the medical doctor in order to be licensed to practice. Staff members of some county hospitals now include osteopathic physicians and surgeons. Despite the rise in standards, the osteopaths are not yet as well trained in their schools as are the medical doctors. Schools of osteopathy do not have the financial support, the high-grade faculty, or the equipment and facilities that are characteristic of the modern medical school.

Doctor of chiropractic (*D.C.*). The chiropractic theory is based on the belief that the nervous system controls all other systems and all physiological functions of the human body and that interference with the nerve control of the systems impairs their functions and induces disease. According to this theory, all diseases and illnesses are caused by slight dislocation, or subluxation, of one or more of the spinal vertebrae, which results in pressure upon the nerves. Hence cure of all diseases takes place through the adjusting of the dislocated vertebrae.

The doctor of chiropractic obtains his degree from one of five accredited colleges in 30 per cent less time than it takes the average medical student in medical school. The difference in length of training is even greater for chiropractic graduates from unaccredited colleges, of which there are a number throughout the country. Some schools require a high school education; others do not. Several of the colleges offer a four-year course. Usually a student can be admitted on the first day of any month. Faculty members are holders of doctor's degrees other than the medical doctor's degree; so the quality of instruction also does not compare with that of the medical doctor. A third difference between the two professions is the lack of training afforded chiropractic students in the study of disease in man [24].

The doctor of chiropractic is well trained in the art of adjusting the vertebrae. He is not trained to cure diseases caused by microorganisms or degenerative diseases such as heart diseases, cancer, and nephritis.

Doctor of naturopathy (*N.D.*). Naturopaths are drugless healers similar to the chiropractors. These practitioners depend upon nature's forces, such as water, air, sunlight, electricity, exercise, rest, diet, and mental and moral science for the cure of disease. Naturopaths believe that no one natural force can cure all diseases, and so the practitioner works out the best combination of these forces to suit the individual's case. A dozen or so naturopathic colleges award diplomas. Some of these schools award the doctor of naturopathy and the doctor of chiropractic degree, as well. A high school education is required in some of the colleges and merely recommended in others. As in the case of the chiropractic schools, a student is admitted on the first day of any month. The faculty is similar in make-up to the faculty of chiropractic schools.

In recent years naturopaths have drifted from their dependence on nature's remedies to pursue the more lucrative therapeutic methods utilizing electrical treatment, violet ray, X ray, spectrochromes, colonic irrigations, and the like. In certain conditions, such treatments are of some therapeutic value and can be compared with physiotherapy conducted by trained physiotherapists who are under the direction of medical doctors. Other methods are sheer quackery and are expensive and time-consuming when competent medical care is needed.

Criteria for selecting health advisers. If it is an important task to select health advisers, then it is necessary to establish a set of criteria to aid the college student in the selection process. The following are suggested criteria which are suitable for both medical and dental advisers: (1) Are they licensed to practice within the state in which they reside? (2) Are they graduates of approved medical schools or dental schools? (3) Are they members in good standing of local, state, and national professional societies? (4) Are they members of staffs of approved hospitals and clinics in the community? (5) Do they periodically increase their skill and extend their knowledge through professional conferences, meetings, and postgraduate studies? (6) Do they possess a type of wholesome personality that inspires confidence and interest in the individual and people in general? (7) Have they established a reputation for professional ethics, character, integrity, and dependable service? (8) Have they had a variety of professional experience to develop skills in providing medical or dental care?

Procedures for selecting health advisers. To apply the criteria suggested for selecting health advisers requires some time, thought, and effort. Yet all such time and trouble is well spent if competent advisers are selected. If the student is away from home, it is a wise procedure to obtain references from the family physician and dentist with whom he has been associated. Former advisers are always glad to recommend competent physicians and surgeons and dentists in a new locality. The following suggestions are made for those who are not able to contact their former advisers or who are living under different circumstances:

1. Secure the names of competent medical and dental practitioners from two or more sources:
   a. The county medical and dental societies.
   b. The student health service.
   c. Approved hospitals in the community.
   d. The local health department.
   e. The nearest class A medical school or approved dental school.
   f. Educated, well-informed friends at the college or university or in the community.
2. Check professional membership by contacting the professional societies or their directories (found in most public libraries).
3. Check standing and reputation in the community by consulting educated, well-informed friends or acquaintances at the college or university or in the community.
4. Make an appointment with the doctor or dentist, and personally find out whether or not he inspires confidence and meets the established qualifications.

Medical care. A variety of health services are necessary to promote and protect the health of the individual and group. In addition, when illness or defects cannot be prevented, competent health services are essential for diagnosis, treatment, care, and rehabilitation. All these personal services are classed under a broad interpretation of the term "medical care" [14]. Such medical care is furnished by the members of the medical profession who use clinics, hospitals, and other health facilities.

One of the hotly contested and debated questions in present-day society is, Should medical care be provided on a compulsory or a voluntary basis? For many years there has been more heat than light in the controversy. If the issue is closely examined, it is evident that there has been more progress than appears on the surface and that there are many points of agreement on both sides in the contest. Both sides agree that every individual has the right to adequate medical care, regardless of race, creed, or economic status. There is real agreement that a prepayment plan of paying for medical care is wise and desirable. Also, there is agreement among most parties that an insurance plan is the best type of prepayment plan. The basic point of disagreement is over the type and kind of insurance plan. One group led by organized labor, particularly the CIO and AFL, contends that a compulsory health insurance plan is the best means of providing medical care for all persons. On the other hand, the American Medical Association is the proponent of a voluntary system of health insurance sponsored and operated by them and by the American Hospital Association. An intelligent approach to the issue calls for a further examination of the pros and cons of both plans.

Compulsory health insurance. The supporters of compulsory health insurance believe that voluntary insurance for medical care, including hospitalization, does not meet the health needs of the citizens of the United States. It is argued by this group that a substantial portion of the population in the United States cannot afford medical care. Some 6 million persons receive public assistance and cannot pay the costs of adequate medical care. Slightly higher in the financial scale but little better off from the standpoint of ability to pay for medical care are millions who are close to the level of public aid but who do not receive it. An estimated 100 million persons can meet the costs of minor illnesses and inexpensive care but cannot afford large or continuing medical costs [14].

Furthermore, advocates of compulsory health insurance believe their plan of paying for medical care works if it is coordinated with services already provided through public health programs. This includes the administration of insurance benefits by state and local public health agencies. Also, this plan including disability insurance would be coordinated with the present system of old-age and survivor's insurance. State and local health agencies would organize health services with physicians and hospitals. Negotiations and administering of the agreements for payments would take place with representatives of insured persons and health personnel, all of whom are involved in the plan.

The plan for compulsory health insurance is based on the principle of the individual's ability to pay a percentage of his income, such as 3 to 4 per cent, for comprehensive health care. All the people of the nation would be covered, and comprehensive medical care would be available.

Those in opposition to compulsory health insurance argue that the quality of medical service would be seriously affected under a compulsory system. They believe that organized medicine would be controlled by government agencies and that the professional standards of the private practice of medicine would be lowered.

Voluntary health insurance. A recent survey of health insurance coverage in the United States shows that 66 million persons, or approximately 44 per cent, are insured against hospital expense; 41 million, or 27 per cent of the total population, are protected to some degree against surgical costs; and 17 million, or 11 per cent, are insured against the cost of nonsurgical services [14].

There are three prepayment voluntary insurance programs operating throughout the country, which illustrate the types of voluntary plan. One is the prepayment plan administered on a nonprofit basis, such as Blue Cross and Blue Shield; the second is health insurance offered by commercial insurance companies; and the third is the comprehensive local health insurance plan illustrated by the Health Insurance Plan of Greater New York.

The Blue Cross and Blue Shield plans constitute the predominant type of voluntary health insurance throughout the nation. Blue Cross provides for hospitalization in a contracting hospital for each period of disability. It covers all conditions requiring hospital care, with the exception of rest cures, workmen's compensation cases, and service-connected disabilities. Blue Shield is the medical-care counterpart of Blue Cross. Each can be utilized separately or together as the individual chooses. Blue Shield for some income groups covers the complete medical-care needs; in other instances, depending upon the income of members, the physicians are permitted to charge additional fees over and above the insurance payment. In general, Blue Cross and Blue Shield plans provide protection for the individual against costs of catastrophic illnesses and maternity care. Under recent negotiations of labor and management with Blue Cross, national and uniform coverage for large groups of workers and their families has been arranged. For example, the entire hospital bill is covered under automobile-industry contracts.

The health insurance plans of insurance companies also protect the individual for hospital, surgical, and nonsurgical expenses, according to a schedule of fees. They, too, protect against costs of catastrophic illnesses. The major insurance companies offer sound plans, but one must exercise care not to be taken in by current health insurance rackets. Many "fly-by-night" companies are now operating so-called "health insurance plans." Regardless of the plan, one needs to investigate carefully before joining.

Several local-area comprehensive medical-care plans are in operation. Examples are (1) the Health Insurance Plan of Greater New York, (2) the Permanent Health Plan on the West coast, (3) the labor Health Institute of St. Louis, and (4) the Ross-Loos Clinic in Los Angeles. These plans include wider benefits for subscribers, such as preventive and diagnostic services and complete care at home, at the office, and in the clinic and hospital. This is a type of group practice in which the principle of free choice of physician is limited to the members of one group. However, a member is free to change his group if there is more than one group belonging to the plan. This is contrasted with the complete free choice of physician under the first voluntary health plans described above. Comprehensive coverage is the advantage of the local-plan type.

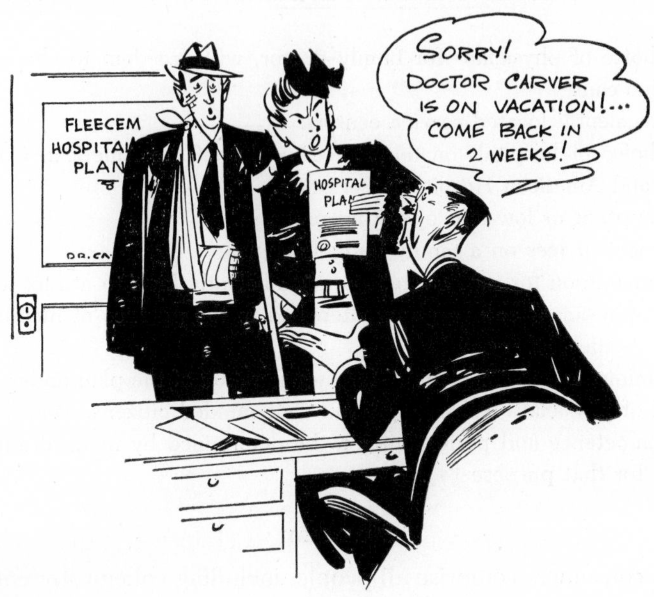

Fig. 12.1. Before you invest—investigate! (*Los Angeles Better Business Bureau.*)

Such plans are limited to the membership in the local area; yet they provide complete care for their members in that area.

Voluntary health insurance plans can meet the needs of the people of the United States if in the future more complete coverage and more comprehensive benefits are provided the individual and his family.

Criteria for selecting a medical-care plan. It is evident that many health insurance prepayment plans are in operation. The majority of these are attempting to meet the medical-care problems of the public; however, as in other fields, there are some plans that are not serving the best interests of the consumer. It is a wise consumer health practice to find out the details of a plan before one becomes a member, as has been pointed out. The following are suggestive criteria which serve as a guide in selecting a plan. These are high standards that are incorporated in present-day plans or are in the process of becoming operative.

An excellent prepayment medical-care plan provides:

1. High-quality medical care by a family physician and coordinated services with specialists. Both family physician and specialists are affiliated with an approved hospital where there is competent nursing service.
2. Adequate medical care covering both acute and chronic diseases for dependents as well as the wage earner.
3. Membership for the subscriber as an individual as well as through a group affiliation.
4. A choice of physicians for family doctor, with freedom to change when there is due cause.
5. Conveniently located service centers.
6. A choice of hospitals on the accredited list of the American College of Surgeons and American Hospital Association.
7. A nonprofit or low-cost operating program.
8. Payment of fees on a family budgeting plan.
9. Remuneration for medical personnel sufficiently high to attract and hold competent physicians and surgeons interested in the practice of medicine and continued medical education.
10. Administrative responsibility for the operation of the plan under a group composed of physicians, subscribers, and civic-minded citizens. Medical standards of competence and performance to be determined by medical authorities organized for that purpose [4].

Summary

Health consumers comprise all people, including college students, who use health products and services. The main problem of consumer health is how to get maximum protection, value, and satisfaction from health information, products, and services. The intelligent consumer utilizes sound criteria based on scientific facts to evaluate health information and select health products and services for the purposes of protecting his health and getting his money's worth.

The consumer receives protection through Federal, state, and local laws and regulations and through the activities of professional and private consumer organizations.

The individual consumer cannot completely solve the problem himself, but he can make significant contributions. He can:

1. Make sure he understands consumer health education as an integral part of the over-all consumer education movement.
2. Inform others about their rights and privileges as consumers and the type of protection and safeguards presently available, as well as those needed in the near future.

3. Use judgment in purchasing products and services, since manufacturers are influenced by the actions of consumers. Each purchase counts in this respect.

4. Report frauds and suspected frauds to the proper authorities.

5. Support and work for improved legislation affecting the consumer at the local, state, and Federal levels.

6. Support and work for better producer-consumer relations, particularly better medical-care plans.

Suggested Activities

1. Trace the development of quackery through the ages to the present day. Present findings to the class.

2. List health superstitions obtaining today. Use the scientific method to check their validity. Why are these prevalent?

3. Study testimonials found in newspapers and periodicals. Analyze them on the basis of the suggested criteria for evaluating health information. Select one or two choice testimonials, and follow up their source. Report on findings.

4. Analyze the propaganda of quacks. What loopholes can you find in their sales talk?

5. Secure copies of the Food, Drug, and Cosmetic Act from the Government Printing Office, Washington, D.C., and of the food and drug legislation in your state. How do they compare? How do Federal, state, and local agents work together? Formulate suggestions for additional legislation to protect the health consumer.

6. Visit the nearest bureau of the Food and Drug Administration. Investigate the workings of this organization, and report to the class.

7. Visit the nearest better business bureau, or write for its material. How does it protect the consumer against fraud? How does it deal with individuals violating business ethics? How is it working to improve business practices?

8. Bring various products or wrappers from products to class. Appraise these on the basis of criteria for selecting health poducts.

9. Appraise advertising over radio and television or in magazines and newspapers, using the identifying marks developed by the Institute of Propaganda Analysis. Identify the types of technique used in each advertisement.

10. Organize a panel discussion on compulsory versus voluntary health insurance.

11. Organize and present a sociodrama on the activities of the modern quack.

12. Invite a physician and a dentist to discuss their ideas on choosing health advisers.

13. Analyze the various types of commercial health information. Make a list of the commercial concerns you find are safe, reliable sources of health information.

14. Appraise the commodity-testing services. Prepare a statement on their

usefulness to the consumer and the consumer movement. How should they be improved in the near future?

15. Develop a list of the medical specialities, and present it to the class.

16. Study and compare the various healing arts on the basis of training, experience, professional activities, professional ethics, contributions to science and human welfare, and the theory of healing.

Suggested Readings

1. Axelrod, S. J., "The Medical Care Bookshelf," *American Journal of Public Health and the Nation's Health,* 43:381–398, April, 1953.

2. Better Business Bureaus, *The Public Interest, The Better Business Bureau Movement.* New York: The Association of Better Business Bureaus, 1950.

3. Bureau of Investigation, *Testimonials.* Chicago: American Medical Association, 1940.

4. Campbell, Persia, *The Consumer Interest: A Study in Consumer Economics.* New York: Harper & Brothers, 1949.

5. Coles, Jessie V., *Standards and Labels for Consumer's Goods.* New York: The Ronald Press Company, 1949.

6. Committee on Cost of Medical Care, "The Healing Cults," *Publication* 16. Chicago: University of Chicago Press, 1932.

7. Consumer Education Study Staff, "Using Standards and Labels," *Consumer Education Series, Unit* 5. Washington: National Education Association, 1945.

8. Consumers' Union, "To Tell the Truth," *Consumer Reports,* 17:44–63, January, 1952.

9. Food and Drug Administration, *Federal Food, Drug and Cosmetic Act and General Regulations for Its Enforcement, Revision* 4. Washington: U.S. Department of Health, Education, and Welfare, 1953.

10. Food and Drug Administration, "Read the Label on Food, Drugs, Devices, Cosmetics," *Miscellaneous Pamphlet* 3. Washington: U.S. Department of Health, Education, and Welfare, 1951.

11. Food and Drug Administration, "Import Requirements of the U.S. Food, Drug and Cosmetic Act," *Publication* 2. Washington: U.S. Department of Health, Education, and Welfare, 1947.

12. Galston, Iago, "Hazards of Commercial Health Advertisement," *American Journal of Public Health,* 21:242–248, March, 1931.

13. Getz, S. George, *The Consumer and the Law,* Consumer Education Series. Washington: National Education Association, 1947.

14. Goldman, Franz, and Hugh Leavell, "Medical Care for Americans," *The Annals of the American Academy of Political and Social Science,* 273:1–192, January, 1951.

15. Huntington, Emily H., *Cost of Medical Care.* Berkeley: University of California Press, 1951.

16. Margolius, Sidney, *The Consumer's Guide to Better Buying.* New York: New American Library of World Literature, Inc., 1951.

17. Report of the Committee on Labor and Public Welfare, U.S. Senate, *Health Insurance Plans in the United States,* Appendixes, Part II. Washington: Government Printing Office, 1951.

18. Sorenson, Helen, *The Consumer Movement.* New York: Harper & Brothers, 1941.

19. Temporary National Economic Committee, "Investigation of Concentration of Economic Power," *Consumer Standards Monograph* 24. Washington: Government Printing Office, 1941.

20. Williams, J. F., *Investing in Your Health,* Consumer Education Study, National Association of Secondary-school Principals. Washington: National Education Association, 1946.

Popular Readings

21. Aaron, Harold, *Good Health and Bad Medicine.* New York: Robert M. McBride & Company, 1940.

22. California Chiropractic Association, *This Is Your Doctor of Chiropractic.* Los Angeles, 1953. (Pamphlet.)

23. *Consumer Reports,* 1953 *Buying Guide Issue.* New York: Consumers' Union, Inc., 1952.

24. Doyle, Kathleen C., "Science vs Chiropractic," *Public Affairs Pamphlet* 191. New York: Public Affairs Committee, 1953.

25. Fielding, W. J., *Strange Superstitions and Magical Practices.* Philadelphia: The Blakiston Company, 1945.

26. Gaer, Joseph, *Consumers All,* National Problems Series. New York: Harcourt, Brace and Company, Inc., 1940.

27. Fishbein, Morris, *Shattering Health Superstitions.* New York: Liveright Publishing Corp., 1930.

28. Fishbein, Morris, *New Medical Follies.* New York: Boni & Liveright, 1927.

29. Lamb, Ruth, *American Chamber of Horrors.* New York: Farrar & Rinehart, Inc., 1936.

30. Livingston, Helen E., "National Health Insurance," *Public Affairs Pamphlet* 85. New York: Public Affairs Committee, 1950.

31. "Medical Men or Quacks," *Today's Health,* 31:40–41, May, 1953.

32. Smith, Austin, *The Drugs You Use.* New York: Revere Publishing Company, 1948.

33. Solomon, Charles, *The Traffic in Health.* New York: Navarre Publishing Co., 1937.

34. "Voluntary Health Insurance for the Individual Subscriber—Its Problems, Progress and Promise," *Progress in Health Services,* 4:1–4, March, 1953. (Health Information Foundation, New York.)

PART FIVE

Building Defenses for Effective Living

13. Preventing and Controlling Communicable Disease

Greater progress has been made in recent years in preventing and controlling communicable disease than in any other area affecting the health and welfare of man. This contribution to mankind has alleviated much suffering, prevented the loss of countless working hours, saved many persons from untimely deaths, and increased the span of life. Despite this record, no single scourge caused by microorganisms has been wiped out completely. Much remains to be learned about how to prevent and control disease before actual freedom from the ill effects of disease for individuals and communities is possible. Regardless of the great advances in disease prevention, there is much yet to be accomplished to solve the residual problem of communicable disease.

College students are still affected much too often by the insidious or unsuspected occurrence of disease, usually at the most inopportune time. Communicable diseases such as tuberculosis are responsible for students dropping out of college, postponing temporarily, and in some cases permanently, a planned college education. Each term, students are absent from important class activities and examinations because of illness. From a social point of view, illness upsets the best plans for the crowning social events and outstanding athletic contests, not to mention an occasional much-looked-forward-to vacation period. Also, communicable diseases cut down the ability to produce and to attain established goals. Another important fact is that communicable diseases not properly cared for may lead to unnecessary complications or to more serious chronic and degenerative diseases. It must be admitted, too, that some college students do not develop an appreciation for effective living, free from disease, until they have experienced an illness. Other students, owing to lack of scientific knowledge, worry unnecessarily about disease, the possibility of contracting disease, or how disease might affect them personally. Actually, students are confronted with a great challenge. They are afforded opportunities for education and research in later years as never before in history. It is the young scientists of today who, more than likely, will provide the missing information about these unknown disease-prevention and -control factors.

These concerns of students about disease, logical or illogical, right or wrong, can best be dealt with by providing scientific information about disease and its prevention and control. The following discussion answers several pertinent questions: (1) What is the meaning of infection and disease? (2) What are the principles and methods of disease prevention and control? (3) What are the common communicable diseases of the college age group? (4) What is one's role as a citizen in preventing and controlling disease for himself, his family, and his community? Specific and implied suggestions are made in relation to the latter question.

The Modern Concept of Disease

In Chapter 1, health is defined as a positive quality of life enabling the individual to make successful personal and social adjustments. This quality results from the biological equilibrium existing between the person and his environment. Also, health is viewed as a positive condition of the organism, disease being the negative. The word "disease," is a combination of "dis" and "ease," meaning "not at ease."

Definition of disease. The individual with disease, then, is not at ease. He is unable to function according to his capabilities. A modern definition of infectious or communicable disease is as follows: Disease is an unfavorable resultant of the nature of the biologic equilibrium existing between the human host and an infectious agent in a particular environment [7, 23]. More simply stated, disease is the visible reaction of the individual, the human host, to a parasite, an infectious agent.

Epidemiology. A brief explanation of the science of epidemiology and its functions aids in an understanding of the modern concept of disease. Epidemiology is a discipline concerned with the occurrence of disease as it affects groups of people. Many of the solutions to problems pertaining to communicable disease are made through this field of endeavor. It pertains to all diseases, although its chief efforts are directed toward the communicable disease.

Epidemiology is the study of the occurrence of disease through: (1) first-hand information from the bedside of the sick individual, the clinical approach; (2) controlled conditions in the laboratory, the experimental approach; and (3) observation of disease under natural conditions of the population within the environment, the detectivelike or true epidemiological method [23].

Epidemiology today views disease as a total process. The cause of disease involves more than a disease organism. The characteristics of the individual or the population attacked and the particular environment are

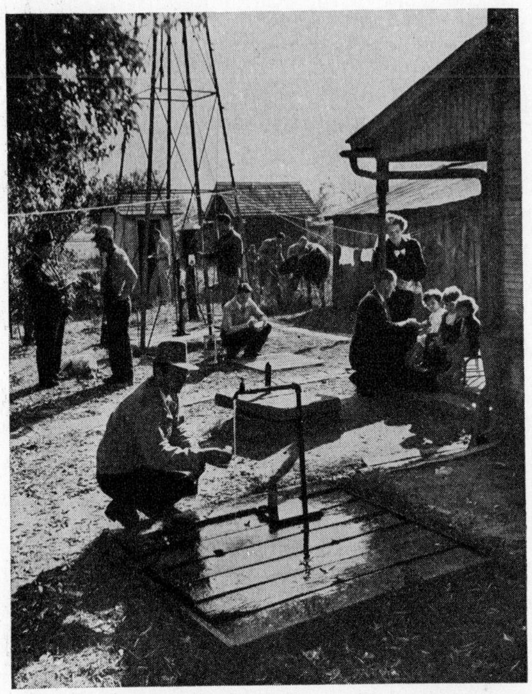

Fig. 13.1. Field epidemiology of poliomyelitis. (*Life magazine and U.S. Public Health Service. Photo by Life photographer Francis Miller, copyright Time, Inc.*)

important factors in the process. Therefore, in the prevention and control of disease all factors must be brought into focus. This is the basic point of view of present-day epidemiology.

Principles of Disease Prevention and Control

The keynote of disease prevention is the science of epidemiology. Therefore, the principles of disease prevention and control are observable in the actions of the epidemiologist and his associates. The epidemiologist is concerned with the series of events that makes disease possible, the disease process, and ways and means of controlling disease. He is especially concerned with the individual who is host for the disease, the disease-producing organism or agent, and the related environment. Even today it is not always possible to know all the factors about a disease. The epidemiologist by necessity is forced to determine the factors that are known about a particular disease. Armed with the available information, he looks for weaknesses in the disease-producing process where one or more procedures may be applied to prevent or control the disease.

An example of the work of the epidemiologist is shown in a venereal-disease-control program. A case of venereal disease is reported to the health department. Immediately, the job of the epidemiologist is to determine the identity and the descriptions of the persons with whom the patient had contact. He also attempts to find out the circumstances involving the contact. Such information includes the place, the date of exposure, and the relationship of the contact to the patient. While obtaining the information, the epidemiologist also tries to reeducate and reorient the patient. A third function of the epidemiologist is the following up of the contacts to find the source of infection. When found, this person is treated, and a source of infection is eliminated. During all steps or stages of the epidemiological study, reeducation and reorientation of patients and contacts are carried on as an important aspect of control and prevention.

The epidemiologist may discover the weak link in the disease-producing chain; however, he is not the only person involved in ultimate control. Prevention and control depend upon a team of individuals working together to guard the health of the community. These team members include the private physician, the health officer and his staff (epidemiologist or communicable-disease-control officer, sanitarian, public health nurse, and public health educator), research workers, and members of voluntary health agencies interested in the eradication of special diseases, as well as Mr. and Mrs. Average Citizen.

The infectious-disease process. *Infection* is the result of the invasion of the body by pathogenic, or disease-producing, organisms. As soon as pathogenic organisms come in contact with the body tissues, an interaction takes place between them and the body processes. The invading organisms, in varying numbers and with their own particular virulence, grow, multiply, and attempt to overcome the body's defensive mechanism. If the struggle results in a supremacy of the microorganisms, then *infection* occurs. When infection produces overt evidence in the body, the condition is called disease. Such signs and symptoms of disease are chills, fever, rash, lesions, nausea, headache, diarrhea, and the like. Disease, then, is the visible aspect of the infectious process [2].

If a stalemate is reached between the two opposing forces, a symbiotic relationship exists. This means a living together, or close association, of two different organisms—the infectious agent and the host. It is a situation in which an individual harbors pathogenic organisms without apparent ill effect to himself. Nevertheless, in this state as a carrier, the individual is capable of transmitting disease-producing organisms to others. If, on the other hand, the forces of the body overpower the microorganisms in the struggle between the individual and disease-producing organisms, no infection or disease takes place. Furthermore, no other persons are infected.

When infectious disease occurs, it develops through several stages as follows: (1) an incubation period, in which the organism is growing, multiplying, and overcoming the body processes; (2) the onset, the stage in which signs and symptoms of the disease appear; (3) a progressive stage, in which the disease develops fully. The outcome will be that (4) the disease agents are victorious, resulting in the death of the individual and suicide for the invading organisms; or (5) the individual overcomes the disease and proceeds through a stage of convalescence and recovery.

An anonymous poem humorously pictures the interaction process between the host and the pathogenic organism:

What a Chance!

Cheer up!
You have two chances—
One of getting the germ
And one of Not

And if you get the germ
You have two chances—
One of getting the disease
And one of Not

And if you get the disease
You have two chances—
One of dying
And one of Not

And if you die,—Well
You still have two chances

The range between the extremes of no infection and severe infection is described in what is called an infectious-disease spectrum. The spectrum is comparable to the color spectrum showing the intensities and variations in colors. Actually, there are two spectra. The first is the spectrum of infection, which provides the over-all picture. The second is a disease spectrum, which is included within the broader spectrum of infection.

In the broader spectrum the range of infection is charted from no detectable effects (subclinical) as extremely mild and mild infections to moderate and severe infections. The second spectrum, the disease spectrum, also has its range from extremely mild and mild to severe or fatal diseases.

Often the mild cases are the unrecognized infections in carriers or missed cases. These cases are more responsible for the spread of infection because they go unnoticed. The infectious-disease spectrum provides valuable information for the authorities concerned with prevention and control methods.

The infectious process leading to the development of an infectious disease progresses through a series of events as follows: (1) there is a specific causative, or etiological, agent; (2) the agent is found in a suitable reservoir (man or animal), the source of infection; (3) the agent escapes from the source; (4) it is transmitted to a susceptible host; (5) it gains entrance into the new host; (6) after entering the host it develops sufficient numbers or virulence or both to overcome the resistance of the host [2]. A breakdown at any one point in the series or chain of events means that the infection or disease does not develop. Information relative to these six factors is essential in the prevention and control of disease. Therefore, each factor is discussed briefly for the purpose of developing understanding of the total process.

Causative, or etiological, agents. The agents producing infectious or communicable disease are minute micro-organisms. For purposes of the discussion in this chapter they are classified as bacteria, fungi, rickettsiae, viruses, protozoa, and metazoa.

Bacteria. Bacteria are one-celled plant forms belonging to the Schizomycetes class of organisms. They range in size from ultramicroscopic to those which are almost visible to the naked eye. However, none can be seen clearly without the aid of a microscope. Bacteria are found everywhere in nature. Most bacteria are nonpathogenic and do not cause disease; they play vital roles in the carbon and nitrogen cycles, particularly in the decomposition of waste materials. A relatively small number of bacteria are pathogenic, or disease-producing, microorganisms.

Bacteria exhibit one of three shapes. The rod-shaped bacteria are called bacilli; the round, spherical forms are cocci; and the spiral forms

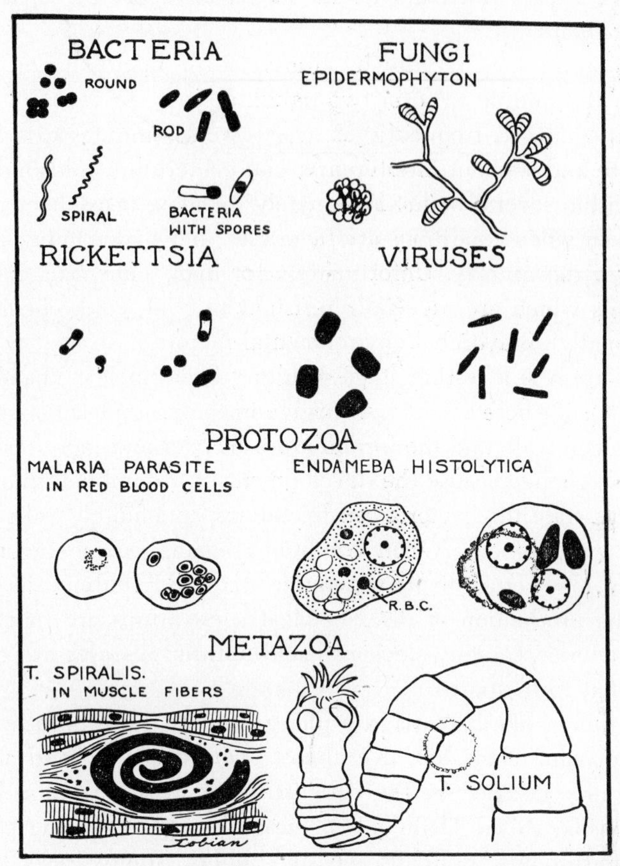

Fig. 13.2. Causative agents producing communicable diseases (greatly enlarged). (*Drawing by Jacqueline Tobian.*) *Bacteria:* the three usual shapes of bacteria—round, rodlike, and spiral, also spore forms. *Fungi:* illustrated by Epidermophyton, one type of fungus causing athlete's foot. *Rickettsiae:* some characteristic shapes (note the similarity to bacteria). *Viruses:* two forms of viruses drawn from photographs taken with an electron microscope. *Protozoa:* the protozoon causing malaria, a parasite in red blood cells; and *Endamoeba histolytica,* the causative organism of amebic dysentery. *Metazoa:* a roundworm, *Trichinella spiralis,* the causative agent of trichinosis, encysted in muscle fibers; and *Taenia solium,* the pork tapeworm.

are spirilla, resembling a comma or corkscrew. The bacilli are the causative organisms of diphtheria, typhoid fever, tuberculosis, and anthrax, to name several examples. The cocci cause pneumonia, gonorrhea, scarlet fever, and boils. The less coiled variety of the spiral forms (spirilla) are the causative organisms of cholera. The closer-coiled type are the spirochetes causing syphilis. The classification of spirochetes is a disputed point. They are classified as bacteria, as protozoa, or in a separate classification of their own.

Bacteria reproduce rapidly by transverse or binary fission. One cell divides in the middle to form two daughter cells. In favorable environments this occurs as frequently as every twenty minutes to a half hour. At this rate and without interference, one bacterium could multiply into 500,000 within several hours. Fortunately for man, many bacteria do not survive even when conditions are favorable, and under unfavorable conditions they die quickly. Unfortunately for man, some bacteria produce spore forms which are especially resistant to heat, cold, chemicals, and other normally unfavorable environmental factors.

A spore form is a resting stage resulting from nuclear changes in the vegetative cell. There occurs a shrinkage in the protoplasm, a contracting within the cell wall, and the forming of a heavier and more resistant cell wall. These changes cause the development of a dumbbell-shaped structure. In this state the bacteria can live almost indefinitely even in an unfavorable environment. When conditions again become favorable, the spore form may return to its vegetative state and continue its cycle, including the production of disease. Most spore forms are found in rod-shaped bacteria. Tetanus (lockjaw) and anthrax diseases are caused by bacteria that form spores.

Fungi. Fungi, like bacteria, are plant forms that are both helpful and harmful to man. They, too, live almost everywhere on land and in the sea. They are classified by the botanist along with algae and lichens in the subdivision called Thallophyta. Fungi are spore-forming plants that include mushrooms, puffballs, yeasts, blights, smuts, rusts, rots, and molds. Pathogenic fungi attacking man are microscopic in size. Fungus infections of the skin, discussed more in detail later in the chapter, are prevalent and widespread. For example, athlete's foot and ringworm are two common and troublesome fungus infections. Two more serious diseases caused by fungi are coccidioidomycosis, commonly called "valley fever" or "desert fever," and histoplasmosis. Both diseases are often fatal in their acute forms. The spores of the fungus that causes coccidioidomycosis are found in the soil. People are infected when they breathe the spores into their bodies with dust.

Fungi have a useful as well as a harmful side. On the positive side is the fungus penicillium, the genus of molds from which the drug penicillin is extracted. Molds and their relatives constitute the greatest source of present-day antibiotics. In the future, fungi may be more helpful than destructive to man as their activities are better controlled.

Rickettsiae. Rickettsiae are disease organisms named after their discoverer, Howard Ricketts. Ricketts described these organisms as the causative agents of two characteristic rickettsial diseases, typhus fever and Rocky Mountain spotted fever. He died of typhus during his studies. Rickettsiae are spherical or rod-shaped, resembling bacteria. In size they are between bacteria and viruses and are barely visible under the microscope. They are found in the tissues of man, other animals, and insects and are transmitted by insects such as lice and ticks. Like viruses they are difficult to grow in laboratory media, although some strains have been cultivated in special tissue media.

Viruses. The virus is the smallest of all the causative agents and for this reason has been referred to as "the little bug that wasn't there." Viruses are not visible by means of the ordinary microscope. However, they can be seen with the electron microscope, or their presence may be determined in the laboratory by injecting material suspected of virus infection into a susceptible animal. Many viruses are so small that they pass through the smallest-pored porcelain filters used to retain bacteria. On the other hand, some viruses can be filtered out by small, dense filters which allow only a few kinds of bacteria to pass through. Some research workers believe viruses are autocatalytic bodies which injure a cell, with the result that the cell itself is stimulated to produce additional viruses of the same type. It is the general belief today that animal viruses are living, while some plant viruses may not be. It is safe to say that much is yet unknown about the nature of viruses. It is known, however, that viruses reproduce or are reproduced only within living cells. The cells of the chick embryo are a common virus medium used in experimental study in the laboratory. A characteristic of many virus diseases is the producing of a lasting immunity. Diseases in which an attack confers an immunity of comparatively long duration or a lasting immunity are smallpox, mumps, measles, poliomyelitis, and yellow fever. However, the common cold, influenza, fever blisters, and warts are virus diseases in which little or no immunity is produced.

Protozoa. Protozoa are one-celled animal organisms, the lowest of animal life, found in many thousands of forms. Only a few, twenty-five or so, are human parasites causing infectious diseases. Protozoa vary greatly in size; the smallest are comparable to the most minute bacteria, and the largest exceed the largest bacteria by many times. Like bacteria they reproduce rapidly in a variety of ways, including both asexual and sexual reproduction. Usually, protozoa depend on an intermediate host for transmission. Strangely enough, an attack of a protozoan disease produces little, if any, immunity. Some protozoa develop a spore stage in which they form cysts. In this stage, similar to bacteria spores, they are capable of living for long periods of time. Three common human diseases caused by protozoa are malaria, African sleeping sickness, and amebic dysentery.

Metazoa. The metazoa fall in a broad, general classification of many-celled animals of higher organization. Metazoa include flukes, tapeworms, hookworms, trichinae, and insects such as the itch mite.

Flukes cause dysentery and other infections. Tapeworms, so named because they resemble a measuring tape, include pork, beef, fish, dog, rat, and monkey tapeworms. The adult tapeworm fastens itself by hooks in its head to the wall of the host's intestine, where it obtains its food from the host. While in the intestine, it lays eggs, which pass out of the body with the feces. The eggs are eaten by an intermediate host, such as a cow or hog. Larvae develop in the new host, bore through the wall of the intestine, and enter the blood stream. The blood stream carries them to the muscles where they develop cysts. Human beings become infected when they eat the flesh of the infested cow, hog, or fish not sufficiently cooked to kill the cysts.

Hookworm is a disease caused by a parasite which is capable of piercing the skin. It is common in tropical countries where frost does not cover the ground. The hookworm attaches itself to the intestinal wall. There it injures the host by sucking blood, eating the epithelial tissues, and producing a toxin.

Trichinosis is the disease caused by trichinae, which are small, round worms. Man acquires the disease by eating infested pork not cooked sufficiently to kill the trichinae. The worms enter the small intestine. After a few days when the female eggs have been fertilized by the male sperm, the larvae pass into the blood stream and are carried to the muscles, where they become encysted. These cysts cause extreme muscular pain. While in the intestines the worms cause gastrointestinal disturbances which also can be severe.

Three bloodsucking lice cause disease in man, (1) the head louse, (2) the body louse, and (3) the pubic, or crab, louse. Lice lay eggs, or nits, on clothing or at the base of body hair. The eggs hatch in about seven to ten days. Lice begin to suck blood from the host immediately after developing from the egg. They feed a number of times a day and more often at night when the host is quiet. They spread by direct contact, person to person, or by contact with infested personal belongings, including clothing.

The itch mite is an insect which burrows into the skin. It lays its eggs under the superficial layer and produces intense itching. Scabies, another insect disease, is also caused by mites. The female mite burrows into the horny layer of skin, remaining in her burrow until removed. Eggs are laid from which larvae hatch. They leave the burrow and enter the hair follicles. Here a nymph stage develops, and the nymph becomes an adult, either a male or an immature female. The entire cycle takes place in ten to fourteen days. Scabies is highly contagious, being transmitted by personal contact.

The effect of microorganisms on the body. Much is yet to be learned about the struggle between the causative agents of disease and the body processes. It is known that these microorganisms affect the body in the following ways: (1) they destroy body cells and tissues; (2) they cause mechanical injury; and (3) they secrete toxins, or poisons.

Destruction of body cells and tissues. Many forms of bacteria, most of the viruses, the rickettsiae, and some protozoa and metazoa invade the tissues directly. For example, the hemolytic streptococci dissolve red blood corpuscles, and the staphylococci in boils injure the white blood cells. The tuberculosis bacilli destroy tissues extensively, gas bacilli in wound infections destroy muscle tissue, viruses kill cells, especially nerve cells, malaria parasites invade the body cells, and tapeworms and hookworms damage tissue and rob the host of food and blood.

Production of mechanical injury. Because of the rapid multiplication of microorganisms from a few to billions in a few hours, the tissues of the body are affected by a material burden in some diseases. For example, the blood flow is altered, vessels are blocked, and the function of cells, tissues, and organs is interfered with and interrupted.

Secretions of toxins or poisons. Bacteria, particularly, secrete poisons, although other microorganisms such as some viruses, rickettsiae, and metazoa may also give them off. Bacteria release two types of toxin, (1) exotoxins and (2) endotoxins. Exotoxins are liberated poisons excreted freely by living bacteria and occur in most bacterial diseases. The bacilli causing diphtheria have a local effect, producing a sore throat as well as symptoms throughout the body by the freeing of toxins. In tetanus the toxin formed by the bacteria is liberated and carried by the blood stream to the nerve cells of the central nervous system.

The second type of toxin produced by bacteria, the endotoxins, are the result of the dead or killed bacteria themselves. This is sometimes referred to as the effect of split proteins. The toxin within the bacteria bodies, which are protein material, is released when the bacteria are split, or disintegrated. The bacillus causing typhoid fever is an example of this type.

Source of infection. Since the word "source" means "origin" or "ultimate cause," "source of infection" refers to the place, called "reservoir of infection," where the causative organisms live, grow, and multiply. There are two sources of infection: man and animals. Of the two, man is the most significant because human tissues are excellent media for the growth and development of microorganisms. Man then serves as a reservoir during an attack of a disease. Also, he may be a carrier during convalescence, that is, a temporary carrier, or a healthy carrier in a chronic state. Man may present an atypical case; examples are a walking case of typhoid fever, an abortive case of infantile paralysis. In such situations the individual goes about his normal daily business but at the same time may spread disease. Most diseases are spread by personal contact with an individual serving as the reservoir of the infectious agent.

Animals, likewise, are a source of infectious disease. A number of diseases are acquired by man from animals. Bovine tuberculosis is an example. Man is infected with this disease when the bacilli are transmitted from the cow through milk. Brucellosis, or undulant fever, is acquired by man from drinking the raw milk of infected cows or by handling the diseased animals. Rodents serve as a reservoir for plague, and dogs are the principal source of infection for rabies.

The natural environment, to a limited degree, also serves as a reservoir for infection. The soil and dust contain many pathogenic organisms, particularly spore forms. Soil and dust constitute the source of infection in coccidioidomycosis (valley fever) and in tetanus.

Mode of parasite escape. As long as man or animals serve only as reservoirs, harboring disease-producing organisms, new infections do not take place. Other factors are necessary for the transmission of disease. The next step in the infectious process is the liberation of microorganisms from the source. The escape of organisms from the body depends upon (1) their location in the body, (2) the tissue in which the organisms are reproducing, and (3) available exits. The mouth and nose are exits through which infectious agents are expelled in sneezing, coughing, and expectorating. These exits expel infectious materials from tissues, for example, in the respiratory tract in which microorganisms readily grow and multiply. The intestinal tract serves as an exit through which feces, intestinal discharges, liberate disease-producing organisms, particularly bacteria. The urinary tract is comparable with the intestinal tract as a means of escape for disease-producing microorganisms. Surface lesions, open sores, likewise, are means of exit. Since the latter are readily visible, they are more likely to receive attention than are the normal body processes expelling causative organisms.

Mode of transmission. The means by which microorganisms are spread from the source of infection to the susceptible host furnish invaluable information for controlling communicable disease. Methods of transmission are related directly to the previously discussed channels of exits from the body. Microorganisms may escape from the sources; however, unless they are transmitted to a new host, infection does not spread. It is for this reason that knowledge of the mode of transmission is often the vital point of attack for those attempting to control disease.

There are two common means of transmitting infection: (1) by direct contact, person to person; (2) by indirect contact, by means of inanimate objects, by insects or other animal vectors, and through the air.

Infection spread by direct contact is the most frequent method by which one individual infects another. Direct contact means actually touching the infected person or the source of infection or coming in close enough contact for transfer of the agent. Microorganisms expelled from the mouth and respiratory tract are transmitted through close contact, that is, by transmission of droplets containing disease-producing microorganisms through the air for a distance of 3 feet or less [1]. Colds, influenza, pneumonia, diphtheria, mumps, measles, chickenpox, smallpox, and tuberculosis are a few of the diseases transmitted by this means. A few diseases are transmitted by direct physical contact, such as the prevalent venereal diseases, syphilis, gonorrhea, and chancroid.

Several ways of transmitting infectious agents illustrate indirect contact. Microorganisms are transmitted indirectly by vehicles of infection, such as milk, water, other food, and inanimate objects, including articles of clothing and eating utensils. Typhoid fever, undulant fever, and tuberculosis and diphtheria are examples of diseases in which the disease-producing organism may be transmitted through milk. Typhoid fever, dysentery, and cholera organisms are spread through water. Trichinosis, typhoid fever, dysentery, and streptococcal infections are spread through food. The most dangerous inanimate objects are those which a number of persons handle frequently. The common drinking cup, public roller towels, and improperly washed eating utensils are classic examples.

Insects and other arthropods transfer microorganisms both mechanically and biologically. Flies and cockroaches may transfer disease-producing microorganisms on their feet, appendages, or bodies as a mechanical means. The transfer is biological when the microorganisms undergo changes within the insect conveyers. Such a process occurs in the female Anopheles mosquito carrying the protozoa causing malaria, or in the *Aedes aegypti* mosquito in which the development of virus takes place, or in ticks harboring the rickettsia organism.

Entry of organisms into the new host. Transmission of microorganisms to the new host is in itself not sufficient to produce infection. The microorganisms must gain entrance to the body before they can grow, multiply, and produce infection. The natural openings of the body, the mouth, nose, throat, urinary tract, and intestinal tract, are the main portals of entry. Any break in the skin also opens the way for infectious agents. A cut, an abrasion, an open wound, a scratch, a bite are all means of breaking through the protective mechanism of the skin. The individual himself causes some of these breaks. Another person, animals, or insects are responsible for others. Insect diseases are the result of the insect bites which make possible the entrance of the infectious agents. Fortunately, most infectious agents cannot penetrate the regular surface of the skin. One exception is the hookworm, which is able to pierce the soft skin between the toes or the back of the hand. The mucous membranes may be directly infected by the gonococcus causing gonorrhea. This is discussed further in the section on The Venereal Diseases.

In some instances the portal of entry determines whether or not infection takes place. Some microorganisms are not carried to the tissues where they grow and multiply unless they enter the right portal of entry for them. A dog bite which breaks the skin and deposits the rabies virus starts the infectious process, but the rabies virus in other portals of entry, the mouth, for example, does not lead to infection. The specific organisms are highly selective in reference to portals of entry. They must use a portal of entry in the body that leads to a site in the body favorable to growth. Another example is the infectious agent causing dysentery. If deposited in an open break in the skin, it does not produce disease. But if the agent gains entrance through the mouth, is swallowed, and enters the intestinal tract, infection may result.

Susceptibility of the host. When microorganisms enter the new host, the struggle between the host and the microorganisms is set in motion in a similar manner to the contest that took place in the original host. The agents of infection may live, multiply, and produce infection or disease, in which condition the host is a susceptible person lacking resistance, the ability to ward off disease. Or the agents may live and multiply without producing disease; in this condition a state of symbiosis is reached, with the host becoming a carrier. Or the body defenses may overcome the infectious agents, in which condition the microorganisms are killed and the body develops its power of resistance.

Important to the epidemiologist and the physician is knowledge of the incubation period. This is the time during which the infectious agent is growing, multiplying, and producing disease, or, more accurately, it is the period of time from the entrance of the infectious agents into the body until the development of signs and symptoms. The incubation period varies according to the specific disease. In some diseases, for instance, syphilis, the disease is communicable during the incubation period. The period of communicability is that time during which the etiologic agent can be transferred from an infected person to another host or to another source of infection.

Resistance and immunity. Resistance consists in the body mechanisms of defense warding off the invasion of infectious agents. It is the power of the individual to prevent the growth and multiplication of infectious agents after they have entered the body. Immunity is a high degree of resistance and is the ability to ward off disease because of inherited, acquired, or conferred powers [21]. The body defensive measures form the barriers against the infectious agents attempting to gain entrance into the body.

The first line of body defense. The skin, the protective covering of the body, plays a major role in the first line of defense. Although many kinds and varieties of infectious agent are found on the skin, it prevents their spread to the inner tissues where they can grow and develop readily. In general, microorganisms are unable to penetrate the skin unless there is a break in its surface, such as a cut or wound, which forms an unnatural opening. Hookworms already have been cited as an exception to this statement. Logically, then, most microorganisms gain entrance to the body through the natural openings.

Other defensive measures in the first line of body defense operate at these points. Each portal of entry is protected from the attack of infectious agents by mechanical protective means. For example, the mucus, a sticky, thick secretion of the mucous membranes, lines the nose, the lungs, and the digestive tract. Mucus traps microorganisms when they come in contact with its sticky solution, much like flypaper catching flies [5]. Ciliated cells in the upper passages in the lungs and nasal passages move microorganisms to areas where other defensive measures can act upon them. For illustration, the cilia in the lungs push disease-producing microorganisms upward to the pharynx, where they are swallowed and destroyed in the digestive tract. Another accessory defensive measure is the filtering out of foreign materials in the nasal cavity by hairs. These hairs, by mechanical means, keep infectious agents from penetrating into the deeper tissues of the body.

Many microorganisms are destroyed in the stomach if they have passed through the mechanical barriers. The high acid content of the gastric juice serves as a chemical means of destroying or retarding the growth of infectious agents and thus keeps large numbers of microorganisms from entering the intestinal tract. The intestinal tract in turn rids itself of microorganisms through its discharge of waste materials. Reflexes also are accessory aids to body defense. Coughing expels microorganisms from the respiratory tract, vomiting removes infectious material from the digestive tract, and the blinking of the eyes and eye secretions protect the eyes from bacterial growth.

The second line of body defense. If microorganisms evade the mechanisms of defense constituting the first line, then other measures are called upon to prevent the development of infection. The white blood corpuscles and antibodies together constitute the second line of body defense.

White blood corpuscles, also called leukocytes or phagocytes, are amebalike cells which surround and engulf microorganisms, digesting and killing them. This process is called phagocytosis. The term "phagocyte" comes from the Greek words meaning "to eat" and "hollow vessel," or "cell." Phagocytes have the ability to change their shape and move about freely in the tissues. The leukocytes and lymphocytes are but types of white cell. Leukocytes are the largest of the white blood corpuscles and the most numerous, composing about 70 per cent of the white cells [5]. The lymphocytes, located in the lymph nodes, are smaller types of white cell. Fixed phagocytes are cells that line the capillaries in the liver and spleen. They are larger in size than the leukocytes.

Antibodies are chemical substances found in the blood which combat microorganisms. The exact chemical nature and the method of production of antibodies are not known. It is believed, however, that an antigen is usually a foreign protein substance. When this substance is introduced into the body, it causes the body to develop its own antibodies. There are several kinds of antibody which have specific functions. The lysins, or bacteriolysins, act directly on bacteria, dissolving them. Antitoxins are antibodies that neutralize the toxin produced by bacteria, such as the diphtheria bacillus. The precipitins precipitate the toxin or foreign protein, thus taking it out of solution. The agglutinins cause bacteria to clump together, aiding the white blood corpuscles in surrounding and engulfing them. The opsonins prepare bacteria for ingestion by the white blood cells.

In some diseases the white blood corpuscles play a greater role than do the antibodies, and vice versa. These defensive mechanisms may also play a reciprocal role. Both are vital in the defense against disease. Recent experiments indicate that, in acute bacterial infections in which the struggle between the host and the bacteria is waged in an extracellular environment, phagocytosis is highly important. Phagocytes destroy bacteria by themselves when inflammation occurs; in this instance, the strands of fibrin formed in the clotting blood plasma aid the phagocytes, and the white blood cells use these strands to trap bacteria and engulf them. When viruses, some bacteria, and a few protozoa develop within cells, in intracellular infections, phagocytes are less effective. An example of the cooperation of white blood cells and antibodies is the host's fight against pneumonia. Two species of microorganisms causing acute pneumonia are the pneumococcus and Friedländer's bacillus. These agents possess capsules which serve as an armor against phagocytes. When the capsules are removed, the microorganism is susceptible to white blood corpuscles. Strangely enough, an antigen in the microorganism's capsule stimulates the formation of antibodies. These antibodies coat the microbes, which become opsonized, or more desirable for the phagocytes. When they are so prepared, the phagocytes are able to engulf and kill them. These antibodies are specific and react only to these types of antigen [24]. The defense in intracellular infections and chronic infections presumably is carried out by antibodies or processes at present unknown.

Defenses outside the body. Microorganisms are killed by natural forces existing outside the body as well as through the ingenious defensive mechanisms of the body. Drying kills pathogenic organisms except spores. Sunlight is effective in killing bacteria and their spores. Ultraviolet rays are used in some controlled areas as a means of killing microorganisms. High temperatures kill pathogens, as in the pasteurization of milk. Disease-producing organisms may be killed by other organisms, for example, bacteriophages. Bacteriophages are bacterial parasites which also kill bacteria. However, they have not proved successful as therapeutic measures for combating disease. An unfavorable environment which lacks food, warmth, or moisture causes bacteria to die readily. Chemical products such as the antibiotics—penicillin, streptomycin, Aureomycin, bacitracin, Chloromycetin, gramicidin, neomycin, and tyrothricin—inhibit multiplication of or kill pathogenic organisms. Carbolic acid, creosote, and Lysol are effective chemical disinfectants.

Natural immunity. Natural immunity is the inherited power of species, races, and individuals to resist infection. Species immunity means that a species has natural power to resist disease to which another species is susceptible. Man has a natural immunity against many animal diseases, while animals are immune to many of man's diseases. Races within a species also possess natural immunity to disease. For example, some authorities believe that American Indians and Negroes are more susceptible to tuberculosis than are white men. At the same time, the Negro is immune to malaria and yellow fever to a greater degree than is true of members of the white race [21]. This fact may be due to natural selection, by which the susceptible die off in each generation while the immune survive and reproduce. Natural racial immunity is believed to be established in this manner. Natural individual immunity depends upon one's personal inheritance. It is the immunity with which one is born.

Acquired immunity. Acquired immunity is developed by active or passive means. Active immunity is a specific resistance developed through the body's own efforts. The individual develops his own antibodies in relation to a particular disease, and these antibodies last for a period of time depending upon the disease. *Active immunity* is acquired in the following ways: (1) By infection with or an attack of a disease. In the process of infection or disease, the body develops sufficient antibodies to resist other attacks. Typhoid fever, scarlet fever, whooping cough, plague, smallpox, chickenpox, measles, German measles, mumps, and yellow fever are examples of diseases producing an active immunity. (2) By artificial means. A virus is weakened or attenuated by injecting it into an animal that has greater resistance than man. For example, smallpox virus from the cow introduced into man produces a mild form of cowpox. A virus may be attenuated by drying as in the case of rabies vaccine. Dead organisms, killed infectious agents, are used for vaccines in a number of diseases. Weakened toxins are developed by combining formalin with the toxin of diphtheria to form a toxoid. The toxoid is injected into the body to produce antibodies. In each of these ways the disease-producing organism is weakened artificially. It is then administered in the body and acts as an antigen, and the body develops its own antibodies. An active immunity is the result.

Passive immunity is produced in the individual by injecting into his body antibodies obtained from another person or from an animal. The tissues of the person receiving the immunity play no part in producing the immunity. Diphtheria antitoxin obtained in the blood serum of the horse and then injected into a susceptible person produces a passive immunity of temporary duration.

Methods of Prevention and Control

Charles E. Smith, Dean of the School of Public Health, University of California, describes the control measures of disease in terms of "the

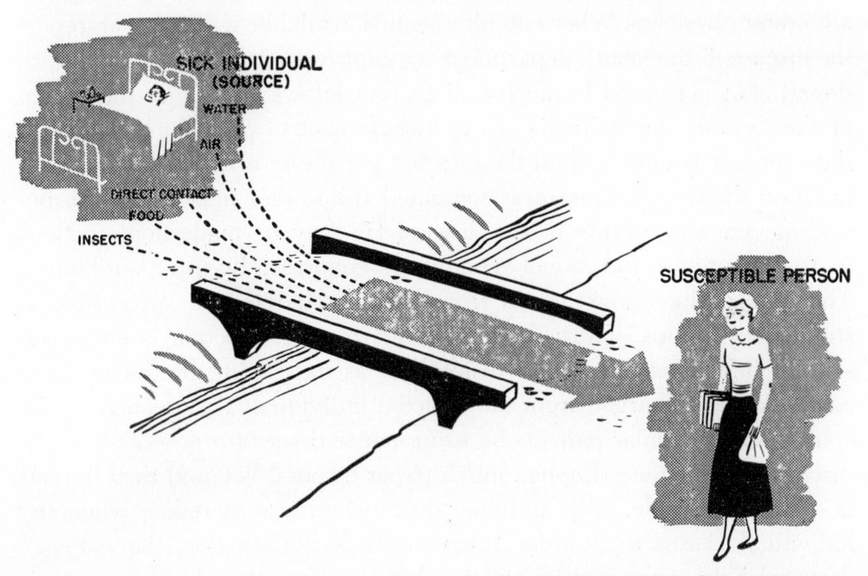

Fig. 13.3. The bridge between source and susceptible individual. For disease to occur, infectious agents must escape from the source, make their way across the bridge, and enter and become established in the susceptible person. (*Drawing by Al Dunkel.*)

Bridge between Source and Susceptible." In his discussion, he cites an epidemiological analogy used by Neil McKinnon of the Toronto School of Hygiene. In this analogy the infectious process is compared to two people on opposite sides of a stream with a bridge between them. The person on one side of the stream represents the source of infection. The person on the other side is the susceptible person. For disease to occur, infectious agents must escape from the source, make their way across the bridge, and enter and become established in the susceptible person [18]. Successful control comes from finding the weakest link in the infectious cycle and applying effective measures. With this principle in mind, prevention and control measures can be directed at three points:

(1) eliminating the source of infection; (2) breaking the lines of communication across the bridge; (3) protecting the susceptible, and developing immunity if possible.

Eliminating the source of infection. If the source of infection for a communicable disease is known, the source may be destroyed or made noninfectious. Only in a few diseases can the source be destroyed completely. Bovine tuberculosis and rabies are examples [18]. The next alternative, applying to human sources, requires less drastic steps. In the first place, the disease must be reported to the health officer by the attending physician. Where no physician is available, a citizen can report the disease to the health department. Prompt reporting enables the health department personnel to muster all current knowledge about the source of the disease and immediately to initiate control procedures. Quickly, then, a fence is built around the infected person by isolating him. During isolation the infected person is separated from other persons for the period of communicability of the disease. He may be made noninfectious by treatment as in the case of syphilis and gonorrhea by using antibiotics. The flow of infectious agents from the infected to the susceptible is stopped by means of disinfection. Concurrent disinfection is employed so that infectious material is disinfected as it is being produced or as soon as it is discharged from the infected individual. Disinfection of the sputum of tubercular patients by using paper tissues for nose and mouth discharges which are dropped into a paper disposal bag and then burned is such an example. Also, terminal disinfection is undertaken when the individual ceases to produce tuberculosis bacilli, that is, the patient's personal belongings and inanimate objects within the physical environment are disinfected [1]. Burning, boiling, heating to a high temperature, scrubbing with hot, soapy water, sunning or exposing to light rays, and using chemicals are appropriate means of disinfection.

Quarantine means the limiting of freedom of movement of persons exposed or suspected of exposure to communicable disease for the period of communicability. This includes any known contacts, members of the family, and any other exposed people. The health department has its specific rules for the length of the quarantine period depending upon the particular disease. Recently, some health departments have liberalized quarantine regulations for contacts. Quarantine has been dropped in the case of whooping cough, with greater emphasis on isolation of the patient. Quarantine of poliomyelitis contacts has been modified from strict regulation to one left up to the judgment of the local health officer [15]. A periodically revised guide for health departments in developing their regulations is the American Public Health Association publication, *The Control of Communicable Diseases in Man* (see reference 1).

New medical discoveries have added to the effectiveness of controlling sources of infection. Owing to contagious atypical cases, missed cases, and various carrier states, source control alone is not enough. Attack on disease must be taken from other points as well.

Breaking the lines of communication. Cutting the lines of communication from the source of infection to the host is an effective means of controlling the spread of disease. Such control is comparable to destroying the bridge crossing the stream between the source of infection and the susceptible person. Measures for cutting communication include purifying the water supply, sanitation of sewage and wastes, protection of food and milk supplies, and the destruction of intermediate hosts.

A general control measure is purifying the water supply. This procedure protects against the infectious agents carried by water that cause the water-borne diseases. Typhoid, paratyphoid, Asiatic cholera, and dysentery are examples. Water is purified slowly through plain sedimentation, an effect of the rate of flow by which many suspended materials settle to the bottom. Chemicals may be added to the water to coagulate the solid materials and speed sedimentation. Lake and reservoir waters are filtered as a means of removing bacteria. Small amounts of water can be disinfected by boiling for ten minutes or can be sterilized in thirty minutes [18]. The use of chlorine in the water is a standard means of disinfecting water for large-scale use.

Proper sewage disposal is an important means of controlling the spread of intestinal diseases. In rural areas sanitary excreta disposal consists in emptying wastes into a pit privy of 6-foot depth or in employing a septic tank which is buried underground and has an adequate water supply under pressure [18]. Local and state health departments and the United States Public Health Service provide detailed plans for the construction of these sewage-disposal units. Urban communities use modern sewage-disposal plants employing physical, chemical, and natural devices for treating waste materials.

Means of breaking the line of communication for rat-borne diseases consist in ratproofing buildings, eliminating food and trash, placing circular metal disks on ropes mooring ships to docks, and destroying rats by poisoning, trapping, and fumigation [18].

The line of communication for diseases caused by metazoa is broken comparatively easily: thus trichinae are killed in pork when it is thoroughly cooked, and hookworm cannot penetrate the feet if shoes are worn.

Protecting the susceptible. Destroying the bridge between the infected person and the susceptible host is only a partial answer, as was the case in source, or reservoir, control. Unfortunately, it is not always possible to control communicable diseases by cutting lines of communication. Therefore attention must be given to the third aspect of prevention and control, protecting the susceptible. The susceptible person can isolate himself, change his environment by leaving the area, use available protective devices, and increase his resistance.

The susceptible person can build a screen around himself to keep out flies, mosquitoes, and other insects, but this, too, is only a temporary, partially successful protective measure. He can run away from communicable diseases by traveling to other parts of the country or the world. However, disease-producing organisms know no boundary lines. With present-day means of transportation, no part of the world can be isolated completely, free from invasion by microorganisms. Quarantine at seaports and airports does aid in limiting the spread of infection since it serves as a protective line of defense around geographical areas. In actuality, quarantine is more of a filter than an impregnable protective covering for the susceptible.

The most effective protective measure for the susceptible host is increasing resistance through the body's defensive mechanism. This process changes a susceptible into an immune person. Though it is not possible to immunize against all communicable diseases, the list of diseases for which immunization can be obtained is steadily growing in number. Diseases against which the individual can be protected by either passive or active immunity are given in Table 7.

Effective control through immunization is possible for diphtheria, influenza (specific for epidemic strain), whooping cough, plague, rabies, Rocky Mountain spotted fever, smallpox, tetanus, typhoid, typhus, and yellow fever. New immunizing methods now in experimental form are soon to be employed to increase the effectiveness of control through immunization.

The susceptible individual may be protected from developing a disease or the severity of attack lessened by prompt prophylactic measures after the organisms have invaded the body. The use of chemicals to prevent disease is a chemoprophylactic method of prevention. Atabrine taken by the susceptible individual protects against the malaria protozoon. Silver nitrate solution applied to the eyes of the newborn baby serves as a highly effective preventive measure against the gonococcus. The sulfonamides are a chemotherapeutic preventive and control measure against some diseases. Although their use is not so widespread now, with the new antibiotics they are effective against the pneumococci and

Table 7. Immunizations *

Disease	*Type of immunity*	*Effectiveness*
Cholera	Active (killed spirilla)	Of value, not absolute protection; temporary protection
Diphtheria	Active (toxoid)	Most effective preventive measure
	Passive (antitoxin)	
Infectious hepatitis	Passive (human immune globulin)	Of value in epidemics
Influenza	Active (weakened virus from chick embryos)	Valuable against specific strain of virus. Temporary protection—1 year. New vaccines reported to produce lasting immunity of 2 years or more
Measles (rubeola)	Passive (convalescence serum; human immune globulin)	Temporary protection
German measles (rubella)	Passive (human immune globulin)	Doubtful and unpredictable, primarily prophylactic
Mumps	Active (attenuated virus)	Not widely used
Pertussis (whooping cough)	Active (separately or mixed with diphtheria toxoid)	Most effective preventive measure
	Passive hypertussis (Immune serum)	
Q fever	Active	For laboratory workers
Plague	Active (attenuated virus)	Temporary protection—reimmunize every 6 months or in presence of disease
	Passive (antiplague serum)	Temporary (3 weeks)
Poliomyelitis	Active (attenuated virus)	In experimental stage
	Passive (gamma-globulin)	Temporary protection in some cases
Rabies	Active (killed or attenuated virus)	Effective measure if bitten or contaminated with rabid virus
	Pasteur (Semple) chick embryo fixed virus	Most effective for animals
Rocky Mountain spotted fever	Active (killed rickettsiae)	Most effective protection. In infected area repeat series annually
Smallpox	Active (attenuated virus, cowpox virus)	Most effective protection; stimulating doses every 3 years and in presence of disease
Tetanus	Active (toxoid)	Most effective protection; booster shots required 1 year after initial series and when wounded or burned
	Passive (antitoxin)	
Tuberculosis	Active (*Bacillus Calmette-Guerin,* BCG) (attenuated bacilli)	Present experimentation shows some important protective effect
Typhoid and paratyphoid	Active (killed bacilli)	Effective measure. Revaccinate every 2–3 years. Used in conjunction with sanitary measures; does not replace them
Typhus	Active (killed rickettsiae)	Effective though not absolute. Prevalence reduced, severity of attack lessened. Seasonal immunization and in presence of disease
Yellow fever	Active (attenuated virus)	Very effective measure. Duration 4–6 years

* Based on data from:
"Immunization against Disease," *Consumer Reports*, 17:32–33, January, 1952.
Roscoe L. Pullen, *Communicable Diseases*. Philadelphia: Lea and Febiger, 1950.
William P. Shepard, Charles E. Smith, Rodney R. Beard, and Leon B. Reynolds, *Essentials of Public Health*. Philadelphia: J. B. Lippincott Company, 1948.
William W. Stiles, *Individual and Community Health*. Philadelphia: The Blakiston Company, 1953.

the streptococci of meningitis. Specific serums are another prophylactic measure. For example, antitoxin may be given soon after exposure to diphtheria. Gamma-globulin administered after the fifth day of exposure to measles provides an effective protection. Gamma-globulin administered before exposure offers a short-time passive immunization against poliomyelitis.

Comparatively few antibiotics are effective in controlling disease, although the number is growing rapidly. Even the medical profession has difficulty keeping up with the new antibiotics, and for this reason only a few examples are given here. Penicillin is one of the least toxic and the most useful antibiotics. It is administered to combat pneumococci, streptococci, staphylococci, gonococci, and the spirochete of syphilis. Streptomycin is successful against tularemia and against secondary bacterial infections occurring with influenza and pneumonia. It is most widely used against tuberculosis bacilli, although it is not absolutely effective against tuberculosis and it does produce a toxic effect on the nervous system. Less toxic is a variety identified as dihydrostreptomycin.

Chloromycetin is preferred to overcome the typhoid bacillus and the rickettsial infections, such as Q fever and Rocky Mountain spotted fever. Aureomycin with its great penetrating power is applied against rickettsial diseases, coccal bacterial diseases, and spirochetes that are resistant to penicillin. Terramycin, another drug produced from the Streptomyces earth molds, is proving effective against syphilis, amebiasis, brucellosis, and some rheumatic diseases. Two useful antibiotics made from bacteria are tyrothricin, used as an antiseptic in bandages and dressings and for upper-respiratory-tract infections, and bacitracin, for wound infections and upper-respiratory-tract infections.

The susceptible individual can contribute to his powers of resistance by promoting and maintaining his general health. Proper diet, adequate sleep and rest, appropriate exercise, fresh air, and sunshine aid in developing general resistance to disease. Such resistance is of considerable importance against disease-producing agents causing tuberculosis, some streptococci infections, and the common cold [13]. The utilization of immunizations for specific diseases is paramount for increasing one's individual resistance.

Health education of children, youth, and adults through educational experiences in schools, colleges, and universities and in the community contributes to the prevention and control of communicable diseases. Scientific knowledge of control measures, together with positive attitudes and practices, is necessary for intelligent action. Cooperative action on the part of the individual citizen, the private physician, and the personnel of the official and voluntary health agencies makes successful prevention and control programs possible.

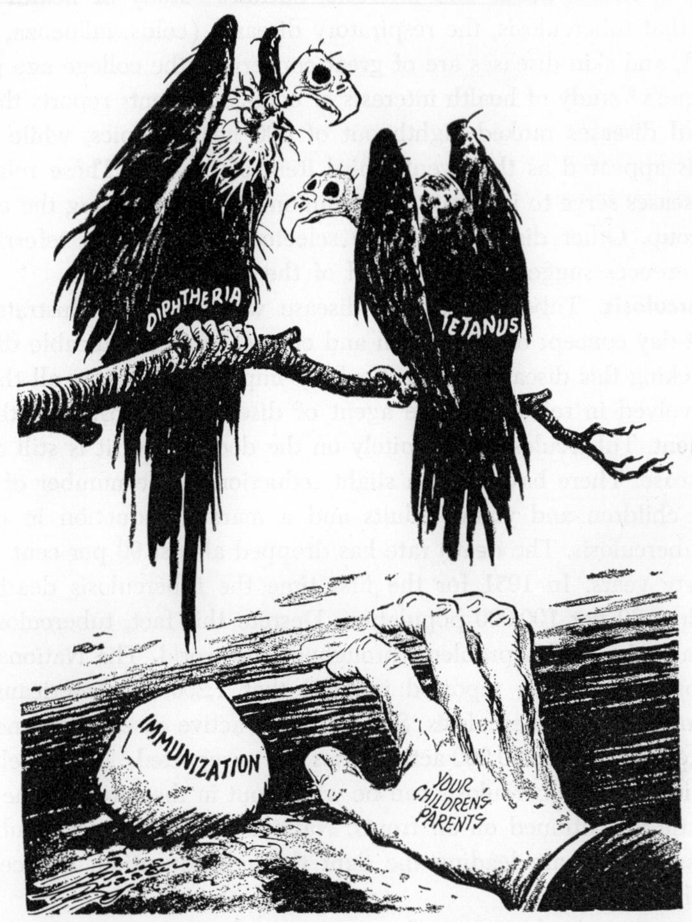

Fig. 13.4. "Two birds with one stone." (Courtesy of Bruce Russell, Los Angeles Times, and Los Angeles City Health Department.)

Some Diseases Pertinent to the College Group

Essential information pertaining to the reportable communicable diseases is presented in the report of a committee of the American Public Health Association, *The Control of Communicable Diseases in Man* [1]. Each disease is discussed in terms of means of identification, etiologic agent, source of infection, mode of transmission, incubation period,

period of communicability, susceptibility and resistance to it, prevalence, and methods of control. This source serves as an informative handbook on communicable diseases.

A few diseases are selected for discussion in this chapter based on studies of health needs and interests. Sutton's [1] study of health needs shows that tuberculosis, the respiratory diseases (colds, influenza, pneumonia), and skin diseases are of great concern to the college age group. Lantagne's [2] study of health interests of college students reports that the venereal diseases ranked eighth out of 300 health topics, while poliomyelitis appeared as the twenty-third item of interest. These relatively few diseases serve to illustrate the common diseases affecting the college age group. Other diseases may be selected for study by referring to the references suggested at the end of the chapter.

Tuberculosis. Tuberculosis is a disease which clearly illustrates the present-day concept of prevention and control of communicable disease. In attacking this disease it is particularly important to know all the factors involved in relation to the agent of disease, the host, and the environment. Tuberculosis is definitely on the decline; yet it is still a serious disease. There have been a slight reduction in the number of cases among children and young adults and a marked reduction in deaths from tuberculosis. The death rate has dropped almost 90 per cent in the last forty years. In 1951 for the first time the tuberculosis death rate fell below 20 per 100,000 population. Despite this fact, tuberculosis remains a major health problem throughout the world. The National Tuberculosis Association reported in 1952 that 1,200,000 Americans had active or inactive tuberculosis. Some 400,000 active cases exist, and it is estimated that some 150,000 active cases are unreported.[3] Nevertheless, it is predicted that tuberculosis can be wiped out in the future if the present battle is continued on all fronts. National, state, and local tuberculosis associations are leading the fight through education, service, and research.

Recognition of tuberculosis. In primary, or first-infection, tuberculosis, the tuberculosis bacillus, the infectious agent, causes a small lesion, or "spot," in the lung tissue after an incubation period of a month or more. The organism spreads to the lymph glands, causing them to enlarge and

[1] Wilfred C. Sutton, *Determining the Health Needs of College Students.* Unpublished doctoral dissertation, University of California, Los Angeles, 1954.

[2] Joseph Lantagne, "An Analysis of Health Interests of 1,000 Junior College Students in California," *Junior College Journal,* 21:429–433, April, 1951.

[3] Mary Demsey, "The T.B. Picture Today," *National Tuberculosis Association Bulletin,* 38:86, June, 1952.

become inflamed. Often the infection is stopped at this point as the host's resistance establishes an equilibrium with the tuberculosis bacilli.

In some cases resistance is not sufficient even early in the disease to bring about an equilibrium with the agent, and the bacilli then may travel in the blood or lymph stream to other parts of the body. Tubercles develop at these points. This traveling, or galloping, type of tuberculosis is called miliary tuberculosis, meaning that milletlike seeds are established throughout the body. Generally, this primary type of tuberculosis heals itself without treatment. However, when resistance is low, the invader may overcome the body defenses and the disease progresses to destructive pulmonary tuberculosis, and possibly death.

Reinfection tuberculosis, or the adult type, varies from insignificant tubercles which do not progress to a severe disease with great destruction of the lungs that frequently results in fatality. Reinfection occurs when infected sputum is inhaled into the lungs, or the bacilli from an infected gland invade a bronchial tube, or bacilli from a lesion proceed into a blood vessel. In such instances, this spread of the infective agent results in complications such as pleurisy and laryngitis. Also, a chronic state may develop in which the disease is active for many years. The person with such a chronic case belongs in a hospital or a sanatorium where he receives the best care and cannot spread the infection to others.

Tuberculosis is a disease capable of infecting all the tissues and organs of the body. The most common site of infection is the lungs, which is characteristic of pulmonary tuberculosis. Other forms include tuberculosis of the bones and joints, and of the intestines, kidneys, and the meninges. Tuberculosis also attacks animals, as in bovine tuberculosis. Bovine tuberculosis is well controlled now in the United States by means of tuberculin testing of cattle, destruction of infected animals, and sanitary handling and pasteurization of milk.

Control of tuberculosis is aimed at three vital points previously developed under Methods of Prevention and Control. These are discussed below.

Eliminating the source of infection. The source, or reservoir, of infection is both human and animal, the human source being by far the greater. The attack on the source is threefold: (1) discovering patients as soon as possible after they become infectious by means of tuberculin testing, X-ray examinations, and routine examinations of contacts; (2) prompt placement of patients in institutions that provide isolation facilities available for as long a period as an individual remains infectious; (3) prompt and adequate treatment to make patients noninfectious. Improved medical and surgical methods of treatment are important. Treatment cannot replace case finding and isolation; all three measures must be utilized.

Cutting lines of communication. Transmission of tuberculosis occurs largely through continuous and intimate direct contact such as is characteristic of family relationships. Droplet infection through the air by means of coughing, sneezing, talking, and the like, is considered a common method of transmission. Lines of communication can be cut by (1) isolating tuberculosis patients from susceptibles; (2) using good personal health practices, such as covering the mouth and nose with a handkerchief when sneezing or coughing and refraining from spitting in public places; (3) rinsing and scalding with hot water dishes and other utensils handled by the infected person; (4) eliminating silica dust in quantities in industrial plants; and (5) pasteurizing milk and milk products.

Protecting the susceptible. The susceptible can be protected through specific measures as well. It is essential to provide healthy environmental conditions, such as good housing, adequate nutrition, suitable occupations, and freedom from physical and mental strain, and to furnish health education to children, youth, and adults. Another factor is the use of BCG to immunize the especially susceptible groups, such as doctors, medical students, nurses, hospital and laboratory personnel, and individuals in the family who are naturally exposed, as well as persons in communities where tuberculosis is especially prevalent. An important need is for an improved vaccine which produces a greater immunity than BCG. Therefore, continued research is vital if the susceptible are to be fully protected.

If control measures are ineffective and tuberculosis does develop, it is now possible to attack the tuberculosis bacilli directly with chemotherapy. Streptomycin by itself or in combination with sulfadiazine is one example of chemotherapy that has proved partially successful. Many new drugs, too new and too numerous to list, are being used to arrest the course of the disease. Although there is great promise for control through chemotherapy, this measure still remains in the experimental stage. Standard treatment includes bed rest, collapse of the lung, and surgery, often in combination with chemotherapy. All treatment procedures must be undertaken by competent physicians and surgeons. Adequate nursing care is essential for effective recovery from tuberculosis.

The common cold. Man's most prevalent disease is the common cold. It is the number one disease in the college population as it is in the general population. The common cold is responsible for more loss of time from school, work, and recreation than all other diseases combined. Most people have at least one cold a year. A majority of the population suffer from three or more yearly.

A cold is characterized as a self-limited, acute disease of the upper respiratory tract. Some colds affect the whole respiratory tract, producing some bodily discomfort, such as a headache and slight rise in temperature. Inflammation frequently is localized in the mucous membranes of the nose, sinuses, and throat. Signs and symptoms include congestion of the nose and throat, dryness, hoarseness, coughing, and occasionally loss of voice. The nasal congestion is followed by a watery flow from the nose accompanied by sniffles and sneezes.

The common cold is mild in effect, but it is also serious because it may be the forerunner of secondary infections such as pneumonia, influenza, laryngitis, bronchitis, and sinusitis. As a self-limited infection the duration of a cold usually varies from two to seven days.

A cold is caused by one or more viruses. An accepted theory exists that a lowering of the tissue resistance enables viruses to overcome the body's defensive mechanism and inflammation of the mucous membranes results. The complications are caused by streptococci, staphylococci, pneumococci, and influenza bacilli.

Colds are spread by direct contact from person to person. Coughing, sneezing, and even talking expel droplets into the air, and the virus is thus transferred to susceptible persons. Droplets may be carried through the air for short distances, as far as 12 feet, and may remain suspended in the air for as long as three hours.

The incubation period is twelve to seventy-two hours. Colds may be transmitted to others before the symptoms develop fully. The period of communicability is in the early stages of the disease, usually one to four days.

Colds show a seasonal rise in prevalence beginning in October, followed by a depression, then an upswing, with the highest incidence occurring from December to April. Naturally, the lowest period is during the summer months.

Only a temporary immunity follows the attack of the common cold, which accounts for repeated colds during a year. No artificial immunity is effective against a cold. Vaccines made from bacteria, commonly referred to as "cold shots," have not proved successful. The preparation of an immunizing procedure made from viruses is still in the experimental stage. The effect of antihistamines in controlling colds is known to have been exaggerated in popular articles. Cowan and Diehl, in an experiment on university students, found that antihistamines had no important effect in preventing or diminishing the severity of colds.[4] Other authorities believe that colds may be effectively controlled if antihistamines are taken within an hour or two after the appearance of the first symptoms. Since antihistamines produce ill effects in some people, it is wise to take them only on the advice of a physician.

The individual can protect himself from becoming infected with a cold by (1) avoiding as much as possible people with colds who are coughing, sneezing, or blowing their noses; (2) keeping up his resistance by sufficient sleep, rest, recreation, and proper diet; (3) washing his hands with soap and water before eating or handling food; (4) not employing towels, eating and drinking utensils, toilet articles, etc., used by others; (5) keeping the head, back of the neck, and feet warm and dry; (6) avoiding drafts and sudden temperature changes; and (7) scheduling a regular medical examination for general physical checkup.

It is important to take precautions in the early stages of a cold for one's own protection as well as for others'. Intelligent health practices include (1) getting as much rest as possible after one is exposed to a cold or feels a cold developing (going to bed during the first stages of a cold is an excellent practice, particularly if one has a fever); (2) keeping warm and dry, avoiding undue exposure or indiscretion (one does not throw off a cold by strenuous exercise, or "working it out"); (3) eating light meals with nourishing food; (4) increasing the fluid intake by drinking plenty of water, fruit juices, soups, and the like; (5) protecting other people by staying away from them and by covering the nose and mouth with a handkerchief when coughing or sneezing; (6) blowing the nose carefully to avoid forcing infection into sinuses, eustachian tube, and middle ear; and (7) calling a physician if a cold is severe, with chills, fever, aches, and pains throughout the body, or if it persists for a longer period of time than usual.

Poliomyelitis (infantile paralysis). Poliomyelitis is an acute, infectious, crippling disease caused by a virus organism. It affects persons of all ages, although approximately 80 per cent of the reported cases occur in children under fifteen years of age. Unlike the diseases previously discussed, poliomyelitis is most prevalent during the summer months, March and April being the months with the lowest incidence. About half of the cases cause paralysis. There have been a marked increase in cases

[4] D. W. Cowan and H. S. Diehl, "Antihistamic Agents and Ascorbic Acid in the Early Treatment of the Common Cold," *Journal of the American Medical Association,* 143:421–424, June 3, 1950.

during the last ten years and a slight but definite increase in the death rate during this period.

The virus is found principally in the nervous tissues of the spinal cord and central nervous system. Occasionally it is found in the blood stream, in lymph glands, and in the intestinal tract. Three types of the poliomyelitis virus are isolated, referred to as types 1 (Brunhilde), 2 (Lansing), and 3 (Leon). The virus causes lesions in the nervous system, destroying neurons in the motor areas of the brain and spinal cord. Bulbar poliomyelitis is the most serious type, occurring when the virus attacks the base of the brain.

Early symptoms of the disease are headache, sore throat, fever, nausea, constipation, fatigue, listlessness, and pains or stiffness in the muscles. A spinal tap is helpful in determining whether the symptoms are due to polio or to some other infection producing similar symptoms.

The incubation period is seven to fourteen days but in some cases ranges from five to thirty-three days. The method of transmission is not absolutely known. It is known that human beings are the reservoir of the virus. It is believed that direct contact is the common method of transmitting the disease. Individuals who have light or abortive cases may be carriers of the disease. Flies are suspected as carriers since they have been found to be contaminated with virus material during epidemics. There is no reliable evidence that other insects, food, or water are media for transmitting the virus [1].

There appears to be a relationship between tonsillectomies, operations on sinuses, mouth, and nose, and the like, and the development of poliomyelitis. These operations are not recommended by many medical authorities during epidemic periods and months of high incidence.

There are no absolute preventive measures available at this time. Gamma-globulin gives a valuable passive immunity for a period of a few weeks. State health departments are being supplied with gamma-globulin to service each state in polio epidemics and during the polio season. Usually, an attack of the disease produces a permanent immunity; however, repeated attacks do occur. Active immunization against poliomyelitis is now in the experimental stage. To date a small number of human beings have been successfully immunized with weakened polio virus, although it is not yet known whether those immunized can resist an epidemic. An active immunization, if it continues to prove successful, is a great step forward in the prevention and control of this scourge.

The antibiotics are not yet a specific control measure for poliomyelitis. Quarantine is not recommended because of the many normal individuals harboring the virus. Early detection of the disease, isolation of the infected person during the fever stage, concurrent disinfection of discharges of the patient as well as articles used, and immediate bed rest are effective control measures. Competent medical and nursing care, physical therapy, and rehabilitation of patients with disabilities are all important aspects of the care and treatment of poliomyelitis patients. Hot packs for early muscle soreness and spasm, followed by reeducation of muscles as practiced by Sister Elizabeth Kenny and others, are successful methods of treating symptoms. Respirators, or "iron lungs," are used in respiratory paralysis.

Until there is an effective preventive for poliomyelitis, the individual and family group need to be aware of and practice known precautions for avoiding or lessening the effect of the disease. Such precautions, especially important when polio is present in the community, include the following: (1) keeping the resistance high and maintaining as good health as possible; (2) avoiding crowds, particularly during epidemic and seasonal periods; (3) watching for signs and symptoms such as a fever with headache, sore throat, muscle pains or weakness, or stiff neck or back; (4) going to bed immediately when signs and symptoms appear and calling a doctor; (5) insisting on prompt diagnosis and treatment of suspected polio; (6) avoiding overfatigue and chilling as well as other means of lowering resistance; (7) avoiding swimming in polluted waters or waters not known to be safe; (8) keeping clean and redoubling sanitary precautions, such as hand washing before eating; (9) protecting against flies by screening, use of chlordane and Dieldrin, covering garbage, and the like [32].

The National Foundation for Infantile Paralysis, supported by the March of Dimes fund, is a voluntary health agency leading the fight for the eradication of poliomyelitis. The Sister Elizabeth Kenny Foundation is engaged in improving the treatment of the disease. Health departments, hospitals, and research centers also are assisting in efforts to conquer poliomyelitis.

The venereal diseases. There are some eight diseases classified as venereal diseases, three of which are important in the United States: syphilis, gonorrhea, and chancroid. Venereal diseases are so named because their common means of transmission is sexual intercourse. Specifically, they are diseases spread by mucous-membrane contact. The venereal diseases rank as one of the major social problems because of the resultant physical and mental suffering, sterility, destruction of life, cost to the public, decrease in production of goods and services from loss of time and inefficiency, and general effect on men, women, and children living in an environment where such diseases are present.

Syphilis. Syphilis rightfully is called the "killer" among venereal diseases. The exact mortality rate is unknown owing to many unreported cases. Syphilis is a direct or contributory cause of other diseases which result in death. It is a major cause of death in paresis, locomotor ataxia, apoplexy, and heart diseases. In 1951 there were 198,640 cases of syphilis reported by state health departments despite a 49 per cent reduction in number of cases [8].

Syphilis is caused by a spirochete, *Treponema pallidum.* This is a spiral organism which lives only a short period of time outside of the body. It is easily killed by heat, drying, sunlight, and disinfectants. The spirochete is capable of entering the body through the normal ports of entry, through minute breaks in the skin, and directly through mucous membranes. It is not able to pierce the skin.

Sexual intercourse is the chief means of transmission, although direct contact with infected persons through kissing or a break in the skin may also transmit the spirochete. Indirect contact, as with toilet seats, hotel beds, library books, restaurant silverware, and the like, is rarely a means of transmission, since the organism lives only a short time in a dry environment.

The average incubation period is approximately three weeks, though it may last ninety days. The first sign or symptom characterizing the first stage of the disease is the development of a chancre at the point of entry into the body. Usually, this is a hard lump of tissue with firm edges. However, it may appear as an ulcerated sore with a thin secretion that becomes hardened after a few days. Both types are painless, with no general bodily symptoms. The chancre disappears of its own accord whether treated or not. This gives the false impression that the disease is cured by the body defenses. The first stage is the most infectious stage.

The second stage of the disease develops some three to eight weeks after the disappearance of the chancre. In this stage bodily symptoms appear. There are possible fever, headache, swollen lymph nodes, small pink or white sores in the mouth and about the genital organs and anus, sore throat, loss of appetite, patch loss of hair, and a copper rash. Even these signs and symptoms may be extremely mild and so may be overlooked. This stage, too, is an infectious one, with the disease spreading through direct contact, including kissing.

Between the second and third stage a latent period occurs which may last for several months or years. The spirochete is proceeding into the deep tissues of the body.

The third, or tertiary, stage is characterized by the development of gummas—firm, nodulelike tissue formed in practically any part of the body. The gummas often break down into destructive ulcers. Also, in the third stage the disease grows progressively worse. For example, there is involvement of the brain, resulting in paresis, a destruction of brain tissue; infection of the spinal cord, causing locomotor ataxia (tabes dorsalis); an attack on the heart and blood vessels, causing inflammation of the aorta and weakening of the blood vessel walls resulting in aneurysms. In this stage the disease is least communicable.

Syphilis is not hereditary, but it is congenital. The spirochete may be transmitted by an expectant mother to her unborn child during pregnancy if she is not treated and rendered noninfectious.

Control measures for syphilis include the following: (1) case finding by competent personnel to discover the source and each contact; (2) prompt recognition of the disease by identifying the spirochete under a dark-field microscope in the first and early second stages of the disease, by blood tests [Wassermann, Kahn, Kline, VDRL (Venereal Disease Research Laboratory), and Hinton tests] in the second stage, and by competent clinical diagnosis in any stage; (3) prompt treatment with penicillin to effect cure in the early stages, administered by private physicians or free clinics in health departments; (4) health education of the public as a means of prevention and control of early infections through scientific information and intelligent practices [8].

Gonorrhea. Gonorrhea is the commonest of the venereal diseases. Its frequency is two or three times that of syphilis. As with syphilis the exact number of cases throughout the country is not known. During 1951, 270,459 cases of gonorrhea were reported by state health departments. Many additional cases occur that are not reported, since persons infected with the disease are likely to be secretive about it, and others do not know that they are harboring it. Medical authorities state that no other disease known to medical science has caused so much suffering and sorrow as gonorrhea.

Gonorrhea is caused by the gonococcus, a coffee-bean-shaped form of bacteria. The gonococcus is easily distinguished with the aid of the dark-field microscope. The organism grows and multiplies on mucous membranes. It affects the mucous membranes of the urethra (the urine duct or tube), the vagina in the female, the rectum, and the conjunctiva—the delicate mucous membrane lining the eyelid and eyeball. Usually the gonococcus is contained in pus, a creamy-yellow discharge from the infected parts. It is important that this pus should not come in contact with other mucous membranes.

The most common form of transmission is sexual intercourse. By this means the genital organs are contaminated. It is possible to contaminate the eyes when soiled fingers or soiled materials transfer pus containing the gonococcus to the mucous membranes of the eyes. Also, the vaginal secretions from an infected mother may cause infection in the conjunctiva of the eye of a newborn baby. This is the reason for applying the 1 per cent solution of silver nitrate to the eyes of every newborn baby as a routine procedure. Towels or other articles contaminated with pus may be a means of transmitting the infection. As with syphilis, the organism dies quickly outside the body.

The incubation period is one to fourteen days, usually three to five. In men, the urethra quickly becomes inflamed. There is a burning or stinging sensation at the time of urination, though it is well to note that this symptom may be due to causes other than gonorrhea. Pus is discharged from the urethra, and there is general discomfort such as fever, fatigue, and depression.

As a result of the inflammation, scar tissue forms in the urethra, distorting and constricting the passage and interfering with the flow of urine. If untreated, the gonococcus spreads to other genital parts, including the prostate, seminal vesicle, and epididymis. Sterility is a common result of infection of these organs. The urethra is often the first site of gonorrheal infection in women. The vagina and cervical canal of the uterus are next involved, and the infection, if untreated, may progress to the fallopian tubes, causing intense pain. Inflammation of the tubes may lead to sterility.

Greater complications arise when the organism finds its way into the blood stream and to the heart. The valves of the heart may be damaged. Gonorrheal arthritis with high fever and intense pain results when the organism attacks the joints.

Measures for controlling gonorrhea are similar to those for syphilis. Avoiding contacts with the infected and prompt medical treatment with antibiotics are successful preventive and control measures.

Chancroid. Chancroid is a venereal disease associated with filth and poor hygienic practices. It is less prevalent and less serious than either syphilis or gonorrhea. The rod-shaped Ducrey's bacillus does not live where soap and water are used plentifully. Chancroid is characterized by the appearance of one or more soft chancres, or ulcers, on or near the genitals or elsewhere on the body, whence it may be transferred to other parts if the discharge is spread by the hands or by soiled clothing. The disease sometimes resembles syphilis but has a short incubation period of three to five days. Both diseases may occur, with syphilis symptoms developing later. Chancroid is transmitted generally by sexual contact. As in syphilis, a break in the skin is necessary before the bacillus penetrates and sets up an inflammation. The first sign is a small sore on the affected part, which increases in size and ruptures through the skin, forming an ulcer. The sore is soft, spongy, and painful compared with the hard chancre of syphilis. Usually the penis in the male or the labia or vagina in the female is infected. The ulcers may damage these genital organs. Prevention and control measures are similar to those for syphilis and gonorrhea.

Skin diseases. The role of the skin as the first line of body defense already has been established. Because the skin is in contact with many disease-producing organisms and environmental irritants, it, too, is subject to a number of diseases. Diseases affecting the skin include: erysipelas, scabies, pediculosis, cold sores, shingles, ringworm, impetigo, and others.

Tinea, or ringworm, is an example of a skin disease prevalent among college students. It is caused by a variety of fungus infections affecting the body in general, the scalp, and the feet.

Tinea pedis. Tinea pedis, or ringworm of the foot (epidermophytosis: athlete's foot), is discussed here because it is the most common of all fungus infections. Men are affected more often than women, undoubtedly owing to more profuse perspiration and more direct contact with infected persons. The causative organisms are three fungi, Microsporon, Trichophyton, and Epidermophyton. After an undetermined incubation period, a lesion with a vesicle or vesicles appears on the soles of the feet, between the toes, and in some cases on the hands. The vesicle may break, discharging a watery fluid. Some forms are characterized by fissures in the skin followed by scaling. Once a fungus becomes established, it may become a stubborn chronic disease. Secondary eruptions similar to eczema also may occur along with the primary fungus infection. Such conditions are called "ids" and are believed to result from sensitive reactions to the fungi or the products of the fungi. Each type of fungus forms its own id.

Prevention of athlete's foot requires special care in keeping the feet clean and dry, particularly between the toes. Dusting with talcum between the toes aids in drying. Wearing sandals, wooden clogs, or protective slippers in possibly contaminated areas is a wise procedure.

Prompt medical attention is important in effecting a cure. Competent medical care provided early is less expensive and prevents secondary complications frequently occurring with self-treatment or no treatment at all. There is no scientific evidence that foot baths placed at shower or swiming-pool entrances and exits assist in the prevention of fungus infections.

Summary

Communicable diseases are those diseases transmitted from person to person either directly or indirectly. The modern concept of disease is expressed through the science of epidemiology. This science shows the necessity of bringing all factors relating to prevention and control of disease into focus, including what is known about the host, the disease-producing organism or agent, and the related environment.

For the individual a knowledge of the principles of the prevention and control of disease is essential in order to understand disease and to enable him to assume his responsibility as a citizen. These principles are based on such items as (1) the factors involved in the infectious process, (2) the factors involved in the body's defensive mechanism, and (3) methods of preventing and controlling disease.

Several communicable diseases selected on the basis of the needs and interests of college students have been discussed briefly. They include tuberculosis, the common cold, poliomyelitis, three venereal disases, and one fungus skin disease, athlete's foot.

Suggested Activities

1. Trace the course of man's fight against communicable diseases during the last fifty years. What factors have accounted for the rapid advance and the marked decline in incidence and death?

2. Select one of the popular or historical references, and study the major epidemics that have wrought havoc with mankind.

3. Investigate the new immunization procedures now in the experimental stage. Report on those which give promise of contributing to the prevention and control of disease.

4. Investigate the new drugs now in the experimental stage which may prove to be specifics for controlling disease.

5. How can the individual contribute to the prevention and control of communicable disease in the college environment? As a citizen in the community? Suggest a plan for a coordinated community attack against disease.

6. Select one or more diseases from the following list: influenza, pneumonia, septic sore throat, mumps, amebic dysentery, food poisoning, undulant fever, impetigo, scabies, tularemia, malaria, rabies. Organize information regarding

prevention and control measures with reference to (*a*) the source of infection, (*b*) the means of transmission, and (*c*) the measures for protecting the susceptible.

7. Select diseases not described in the chapter that are major problems in your community. Develop a report on one or more of these diseases, using the following as outline headings: identification, the etiologic agent, the source of infection, the mode of transmission, the incubation period, the period of communicability, susceptibility and resistance, prevalence, and methods of control.

8. Preview, show, and discuss the following films: (*a*) *How to Catch a Cold* (sound, color, 10 minutes), International Cellucotton Products Company, Walt Disney Production; (*b*) *Antibiotics* (sound, 14 minutes), Encyclopaedia Britannica; (*c*) *The Body Fights Bacteria* (sound, 17 minutes), McGraw-Hill Text-Film, 1948; (*d*) *Rodney* (sound, 15 minutes), National Tuberculosis Association.

Suggested Readings

1. American Public Health Association, *The Control of Communicable Diseases in Man.* New York, 1950.

2. Anderson, Gaylord W., and Margaret G. Arnstein, *Communicable Disease Control,* 3d ed. New York: The Macmillan Company, 1953.

3. Bloomfield, A. L., "Some Problems of the Common Cold," *Journal of the American Medical Association,* 144:287–292, Sept. 23, 1950.

4. Burnet, Sir Macfarlane, "The Influenza Virus," *Scientific American,* 188; 27–31, April, 1953.

5. Carlson, Anton, and Victor Johnson, *The Machinery of the Body,* 3d ed. Chicago: University of Chicago Press, 1948.

6. Cooley, C. H., *Social Aspects of Illness.* Philadelphia: W. B. Saunders Company, 1951.

7. Gadston, Iago, *The Epidemiology of Health.* New York: Health Education Council, 1953.

8. Greenberg, Morris, and Anna V. Maltz, *Modern Concepts of Communicable Disease.* New York: G. P. Putnam's Sons, 1953.

9. "Immunization against Disease," *Consumer Reports,* 17:32–33, January, 1952.

10. Maxcy, K. F., revision of M. J. Rosenau, *Hygiene and Preventive Medicine.* New York: Appleton-Century-Crofts, Inc., 1951.

11. Perkins, James E., "The Shape of Things to Come in TB Control," *National Tuberculosis Association Bulletin,* 39:57–58, 66–67, April, 1953.

12. Raper, Kenneth B., "The Progress of Antibiotics," *Scientific American,* 186:49–57, April, 1952.

13. Hanlon, John, *Principles of Public Health Administration.* St. Louis: The C. V. Mosby Company, Medical Publishers, 1950.

14. Leavell, Hugh Rodman, and E. Gurney Clark, *Textbook of Preventive Medicine.* New York: McGraw-Hill Book Company, Inc., 1953.

15. National Foundation for Infantile Paralysis, "Recommended Practices for the Control of Poliomyelitis," *California's Health,* 7:25–28, Aug. 31, 1949.

16. Pullen, Roscoe L., *Communicable Diseases.* Philadelphia: Lea & Febiger, 1950.

17. Salle, A. J., *Fundamental Principles of Bacteriology,* 4th ed. New York: McGraw-Hill Book Company, Inc., 1954.

18. Shepard, William P., Charles E. Smith, Rodney R. Beard, and Leon B. Reynolds, *Essentials of Public Health.* Philadelphia: J. B. Lippincott Company, 1948.

19. Smillie, Wilson G., *Preventive Medicine and Public Health,* 2d ed. New York: The Macmillan Company, 1952.

20. Stiles, William W., *Individual and Community Health.* Philadelphia: The Blakiston Company, 1953.

21. Top, Franklin, *Handbook of Communicable Diseases,* 2d ed. St. Louis: The C. V. Mosby Company, Medical Publishers, 1947.

22. Winslow, C. E. A., *Man and Epidemics.* Princeton, N.J.: Princeton University Press, 1952.

23. Winslow, C. E. A., Wilson G. Smillie, James A. Doull, and John E. Gordon, *The History of American Epidemiology.* St. Louis: The C. V. Mosby Company, Medical Publishers, 1952.

24. Wood, Barry, Jr., "White Blood Cells v. Bacteria," *Scientific American,* 184:48–52, February, 1951.

Popular Readings

25. Fishbein, Morris, *1953 Medical Progress.* Philadelphia: The Blakiston Company, 1953.

26. Hagman, E. Patricia, *Good Health for You and Your Family.* New York: A. S. Barnes and Company, 1951.

27. Heiser, Victor, *An American Doctor's Odyssey.* New York: W. W. Norton & Company, 1936.

28. Pomeranz, Herman, and Irvin S. Koll, *The Family Physician.* New York: The Greystone Press, 1951.

29. Schifferes, Justice J., *How to Live Longer.* New York: E. P. Dutton & Co., Inc., 1949.

30. Smith, Geddes, *Plague on Us.* New York: Commonwealth Fund, Division of Publication, 1941.

31. Tobey, James A., *Riders of the Plague.* New York: Charles Scribner's Sons, 1930.

32. U.S. Department of Health, Education, and Welfare, Public Health Service, "Poliomyelitis," *Health Information Series,* No. 8. Washington: Government Printing Office, 1953.

33. Zinsser, Hans, *Rats, Lice and History.* Boston: Little, Brown & Company, 1935.

14. Understanding Chronic and Degenerative Diseases

Advances in the control and prevention of communicable diseases have increased the average life span of Americans. As a result, more persons are surviving to the age when they are afflicted with the so-called "chronic" or "degenerative" diseases. Deaths resulting from "heart failure" are to be expected among seventy- and eighty-year-old men and women. However, the fact is that chronic diseases disable or kill many individuals at all ages, from infancy on. The college-age student is likely to be aware of problems associated with such diseases as cancer, heart diseases, diabetes, kidney diseases, or allergies because many persons in his age group are victims of such diseases. In addition, he is quite likely to have a father or mother affected by one or more of these or other chronic diseases.

To comprehend the significance of the chronic-disease problem, one should be able to answer the following questions: What are the diseases or disorders which are considered to be chronic or degenerative? To what extent do the various chronic diseases affect the different age groups? What are the factors which contribute to the onset of chronic diseases? What can the individual do to assist his physician in the early detection and effective treatment of chronic or degenerative disease? What can he do to support medical research, which is so vital to understanding and improving the means of controlling chronic diseases? All these questions cannot as yet be answered completely, but additional information is coming in every day.

The Chronic-disease Problem

The diseases which spread or are communicated from person to person are discussed in the preceding chapter. If one considers the meaning of "chronic" literally, some of the communicable diseases which persist for

Table 8. Leading Causes of Death in the United States, 1900, in Descending Order *

Cause of Death	*Death Rate per 100,000 Population*
All causes	1,719
1. Pneumonia and influenza	202
2. Tuberculosis	194
3. Diarrhea and enteritis	143
4. Diseases of heart	137
5. Cerebral hemorrhage	107
6. Nephritis	89
7. Accidents	72
8. Cancer	64
9. Diphtheria	40
10. Meningitis	34
First ten causes	1,082

* Louis I. Dublin, *The Facts of Life from Birth to Death*, p. 105. New York: The Macmillan Company, 1951.

a long period of time are chronic in nature. Tuberculosis is an example of a communicable disease which, on the basis of long duration, may be considered as chronic. The diseases discussed in this chapter, however, have a persisting or long-lasting quality but are not transmitted from person to person. Chronic or degenerative diseases cannot be attributed to a specific organism such as the bacillus which causes tuberculosis. For the most part, the causes of chronic diseases are complex in nature and in many instances are not understood completely.

Chronic diseases as a cause of death. Mortality statistics provide evidence of the significance of the chronic diseases as a health problem. Data in Table 9 show that six of the ten leading causes of death in the United States in 1950 were chronic diseases. These six chronic diseases killed more than five times as many persons as did the other four leading causes of death. Compare with data for 1900, shown in Table 8.

As an individual ages, his tissues undergo changes which increase his chances of becoming a victim of one or more of the chronic diseases. However, chronic diseases are not, as commonly believed, a problem confined to the older segment of the population. The fallacy of such a belief is shown, at least partially, by the fact that chronic or degenerative conditions of cardiovascular disease and cancer cause more deaths among school-age children in the United States than do all the infectious and parasitic diseases combined [7]. Table 10 lists leading causes of death in

Table 9. Leading Causes of Death in the United States, 1950, in Descending Order *

Cause of Death	*Number of Deaths*	*Death Rate per 100,000 Population*
All causes	1,456,000	962.7
1. Diseases of heart	535,889	354.3
2. Malignant neoplasms	211,090	139.6
3. Vascular lesions affecting central nervous system	156,513	103.5
4. Accidents	90,620	59.9
5. Influenza and pneumonia	47,093	31.1
6. Tuberculosis (all forms)	35,633	22.2
7. General arteriosclerosis	30,490	20.2
8. Chronic and unspecified nephritis and other renal sclerosis	25,567	16.9
9. Diabetes mellitus	25,076	16.6
10. Congenital malformations	18,450	12.2

* Data from National Office of Vital Statistics, "Estimated Numbers of Deaths and Death Rates for Specified Causes: United States, 1950," *Current Mortality Analysis*, 8:12–15, May 9, 1952.

the fifteen- to twenty-four-year age group. The inclusion of eight chronic diseases suggests their importance to individuals of college age.

Chronic diseases as a cause of disability. Deaths alone do not show the extent of the chronic-disease problem. The disability which results is of equal or greater importance. Some of the consequences of prolonged disability from chronic diseases are the cost of medical expenses, the loss in man-hours from work, the suffering of the patient, and the disruption of normal family living.

The degree to which individuals in the various age groups are affected by disability is illustrated partially by the following statement: [1]

> It is true that the highest rate of prevalence of chronic disease and disability occurs among the older persons in the population, but, as the National Health Survey discovered, more than three-quarters of those with chronic illness and two-thirds of the invalids are between the ages of fifteen and sixty-four and more than half the chronic invalids are under the age of forty-five.

On the basis of such factors as days lost, number of invalids, number of cases, and number of deaths the chronic diseases are listed in the following order of social importance: (1) heart diseases, (2) arteriosclerosis and high blood pressure, (3) nervous and mental diseases, (4)

[1] National Health Assembly, *America's Health: A Report to the Nation*, p. 85. New York: Harper & Brothers, 1949.

Table 10. Leading Causes of Death in the 15–24-year Age Group in the United States, 1950, in Descending Order *

Cause of Death	*Number of Deaths*	*Death Rate per 100,000 Population*
All causes	27,996	126.1
1. Accidents	11,875	53.6
2. Tuberculosis	2,554	11.5
3. Malignant neoplasms	1,960	8.8
4. Diseases of heart	1,362	6.1
5. Homicide	1,238	5.6
6. Suicide	884	4.0
7. Deliveries and complications of pregnancy, childbirth, and the puerperium	762	3.4
8. Influenza and pneumonia	672	3.0
9. Chronic and unspecified nephritis and other renal sclerosis	645	2.9
10. Congenital malformations	421	1.9
11. Vascular lesions affecting central nervous system	380	1.7
12. Acute poliomyelitis	310	1.4
13. Rheumatic fever	280	1.3
14. Benign neoplasms of unspecified nature	270	1.2
15. Acute nephritis and nephritis with edema, including nephrosis	240	1.1
16. Diabetes mellitus	220	1.0
17. Appendicitis	200	0.9

* Data from National Office of Vital Statistics, "Estimated Numbers of Deaths and Death Rates for Specified Causes: United States, 1950," *Current Mortality Analysis*, 8:12–15, May 9, 1952.

rheumatism, (5) nephritis and other kidney diseases, (6) tuberculosis, (7) cancer and other tumors, (8) diabetes mellitus, (9) asthma and hay fever, and (10) diseases of the gallbladder and liver [13].

Although chronic diseases are an important health problem at all ages, it is apparent that, the longer persons live, the more likely they are to develop one of the chronic diseases.

THE AGING POPULATION

A thorough discussion of the problem of chronic disease invariably includes a consideration of the age of afflicted persons and the change taking place in age composition of the population of the United States.

Age composition of the population. Pronounced changes in the age composition of the population of the United States have occurred during the last century. These changes are illustrated graphically in Figure 14.1. The increase in the age groups from forty-five and older has been steady.

Estimates for the future indicate that about 36 per cent of the population will be forty-five or older by 1975 [8].

Among the factors producing the change in age composition are (1) the decline in fertility or reduction in the size of families, (2) a decline in immigration to a point where it has almost negligible effect, and (3)

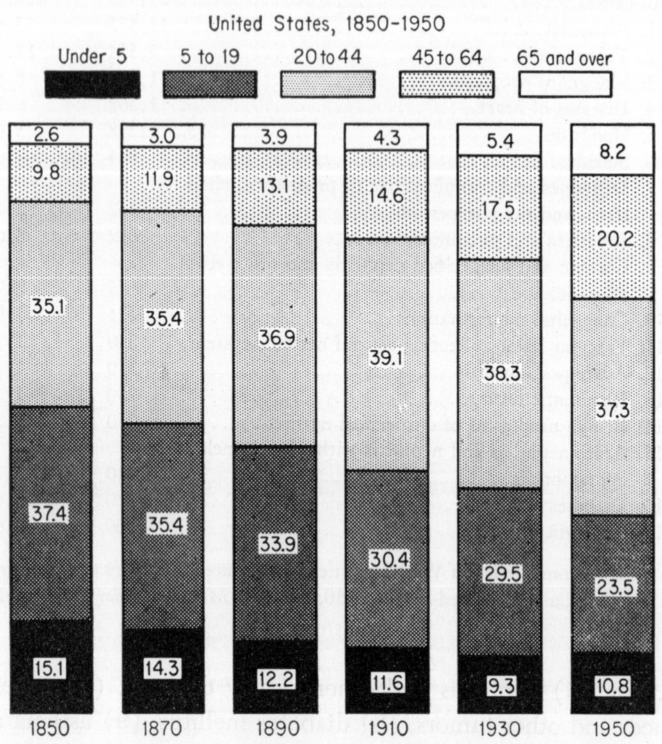

Fig. 14.1. Per cent distribution of total population by age. *(By permission from Louis I. Dublin, The Facts of Life from Birth to Death, copyright 1951, The Macmillan Company.)*

declines in mortality rates in the younger age groups [8]. The decrease from an average of 8 children for each woman of childbearing age in 1800 to an average of 2.2 children per woman who had passed childbearing age in 1950 illustrates the extent of the reduction in size of families.

Gerontology and geriatrics. Gerontology is the science of old age. The gerontologist is concerned with all aspects of the aging process of all materials. Geriatrics is one branch of the science of gerontology. The geriatric specialist is a physician who is concerned with preventing disease, prolonging life, and promoting health for persons past middle life. The geriatrician is to the older person what the pediatrician is to children.

With the cooperation of the patient the geriatric specialist is able to accomplish the important objective of adding vigor to the later years. If the beginning symptoms of a chronic or degenerative disease are detected and the patient takes advantage of what is known about the disease, he has an excellent chance of avoiding its disabling effects. The physician prefers to have his patients come to him while they are in good health instead of waiting until aging and disease produce conditions for which treatment is relatively ineffective.

Diseases of the Heart and Circulatory System

Deaths due to diseases of the cardiovascular system, the heart and the blood vessels, increase in proportion to the effectiveness with which medical science is able to prevent deaths due to other causes. Evaluation of the progress in controlling cardiovascular diseases on the basis of mortality rates alone is inaccurate. Death from heart disease is almost certain if one lives long enough.

The age at which cardiovascular disease causes death and disability is an important criterion for evaluating the extent of the problem. White [2] indicates the significance of this criterion:

> Unfortunately, however, at present, the increase in mortality from cardiovascular-renal disease does not occur only in old persons. There has been a great increase of the disease in young adults and those of middle age within the last half generation. There is actually a greater increase in these middle years between thirty and sixty than in the later years. Here lies the challenge, presented mostly by such conditions as hypertension and coronary atherosclerosis.

Cardiology, the medical speciality dealing with detection and treatment of the cardiovascular diseases, is relatively new. The effectiveness of present-day treatment is remarkable if one considers that most of the progress in the control of heart disease has been made during the last quarter century.

Solution of the problem of heart disease is dependent upon the physician, the cardiac patient, the potential cardiac patient, and the medical research worker. Early recognition of symptoms, regular visits to a phy-

[2] Paul D. White, "Heart Disease Forty Years Ago and Now," *Journal of the American Medical Association,* 149:799–801, June, 1952.

sician, and cooperation in carrying out his prescription for prevention and treatment are the patient's responsibilities. The patient is assisted in doing his part by understanding the nature of cardiovascular diseases and the factors which contribute to their onset.

Heart disease means many things. Heart disease is not a single disease. A reference to heart disease without a more specific definition of the nature of the condition is somewhat like saying that an individual is ill. Many diseases involve the heart and blood vessels directly, while others exert a secondary effect on these organs. The classification of heart diseases into various types and kinds is recognized by authorities as one of the great medical advances. The identification of different diseases makes it possible for the physician to provide specific treatment for each, and more effective control is the result.

Different types of heart disease are more prevalent or more likely to cause difficulty at different ages. During infancy congenital defects are the most frequent cause of death due to heart disease. Congenital defects are imperfections in structure of the heart or blood vessels at the time of birth. Infections provide the primary cause of heart disease during school age and early adult life. Rheumatic fever is the most common specific cause of heart disorders during this period of life. Hypertension, or high blood pressure, is the cause of the greatest difficulty during the middle years of life, and coronary disease takes the heaviest toll during the later years. Arteriosclerosis (hardening of the arteries) and stroke (apoplexy) are common in the older age groups and frequently are associated with hypertension or coronary disease as cause of death or disability.

The suggestion that specific types of heart disease produce greater effects at different ages does not mean that they are not felt at other ages. Hypertension is not limited to the middle-aged, nor is coronary disease limited to the elderly.

Cardiovascular system. The heart and the blood vessels which make up the cardiovascular system provide the "pump" and the "pipes" for circulating blood to the cells in all parts of the body.

The heart. The force which moves the blood throughout the body is provided primarily by a muscular organ approximately the size of a fist. Figure 14.2 illustrates the structure of the heart and the pathway of the blood as it flows through the heart. The three layers of heart tissue (endocardium, myocardium, and pericardium) receive their own blood supply through a system of blood vessels, the coronary vessels, and not by absorption through the wall of the heart. Damage to any of the three layers of tissue or to the coronary blood vessels as a result of infection, injury, or aging may result in disruption of normal circulation.

Contraction of the walls of the left ventricle forces blood into the large arteries. This contraction, called systole, forces the walls of the

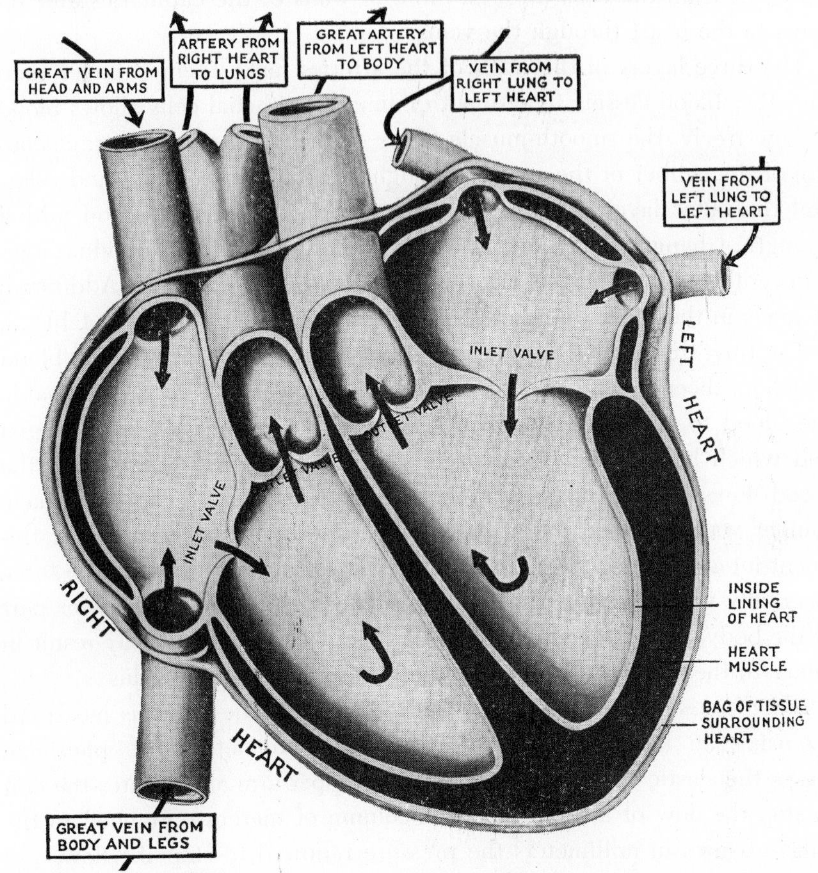

Fig. 14.2. Diagram of the heart. (By permission from *Your Heart,* p. 1, Metropolitan Life Insurance Co., 1951.)

arteries to expand. Relaxation of the ventricle walls, called diastole, relieves the pressure on the blood in the arteries and allows the walls of the arteries to contract and assist in the forward movement of the blood. The alternate expansion and contraction of the arteries with each "beat" of the heart causes the pulse. The average pulse rate of an adult male at rest is approximately seventy-two beats per minute, of an adult female approximately eighty, but considerable variation from this may be normal for a given individual. Some outstanding distance runners have had a pulse rate in the fifties or lower. The pulse rate is increased by such factors as physical activity and nervous tension.

The blood vessels. The blood is carried to the various parts of the body by the arteries. It exchanges its food and oxygen supply for waste materials from the cells through the thin walls of the capillaries and returns to the heart through the veins.

The three layers in the walls of the arteries make them stronger than the other blood vessels. The smooth lining of epithelial cells allows blood to flow freely, the smooth-muscle fibers of the middle layer permit control of the caliber of the vessels through its ability to contract and relax, and the outer layer of connective tissue provides elasticity and added strength. Changes which take place in the arteries as an individual ages reduce the ability of the arteries to expand and contract. Additional changes in the inner lining of the arteries slow down the flow of blood.

The tiny, thin-walled capillaries are the "end of the line" for the blood which has been moving away from the heart. These minute vessels enable the blood to reach all the living cells which require food and oxygen and which have waste materials to eliminate. From the capillaries the blood flows into the veins and then back to the heart. The veins have thinner walls than do the arteries and, in addition, have valves at frequent intervals along their course. The valves help to overcome the force of gravity which inhibits the return of venous blood from the lower part of the body. Interference with normal venous flow of blood may result in injury to the valves and may eventually result in varicose veins.

Blood pressure. The pressure required to move the blood is measured by using an instrument called a sphygmomanometer. The physician wraps the elastic cuff around the patient's upper arm and inflates the cuff to stop the flow of arterial blood. A column of mercury attached to the cuff measures in millimeters the pressure required to stop the flow.

The pressure at its highest point is called systolic pressure. The low-pressure reading is the diastolic pressure. A reading of 120/80 means a systolic pressure of 120 and a diastolic pressure of 80. The normal range in systolic pressure is about 110 to 140 for the average person, and the diastolic range is 70 to 90 [21]. The difference between systolic and diastolic is the pulse pressure.

Blood. Blood makes up about one-thirteenth of the body weight and is composed of formed elements, the red blood cells, the white blood cells, and platelets, suspended in a fluid called plasma. An individual weighing 150 pounds has approximately 5 to 6 quarts of blood.

The plasma portion of the blood is largely water. Organic salts and other substances are suspended or dissolved in the water. The red blood cells, erythrocytes, contain hemoglobin, which is responsible for the oxygen-carrying ability of the blood. An insufficiency of these cells or of hemoglobin in the cells results in a condition known as anemia. New blood cells are produced continuously in the red marrow of the bones,

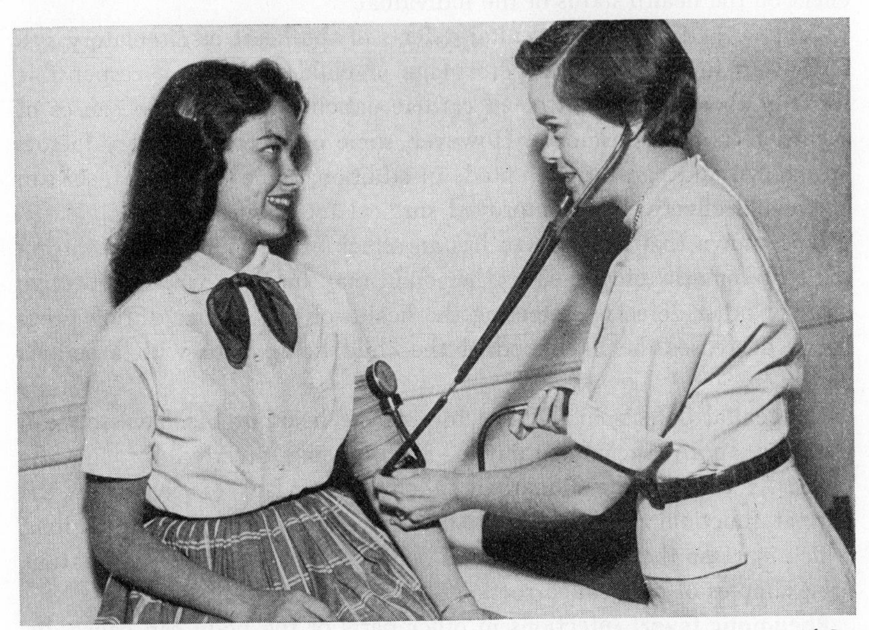

Fig. 14.3. A sphygmomanometer is used in recording blood pressure. (*Courtesy of Dr. Paul Kinney and Pasadena City College.*)

and old red cells are destroyed by the liver and spleen. The number of red cells, approximately 5 million per cubic centimeter for males and 4½ million for females, remains relatively constant under normal conditions. Determination of the red cell count and measurement of hemoglobin content of the red cells provides the physician with information relative to the nature of one's illness.

The white blood cells are of different types. Leukocytes and lymphocytes are the two most common types. Leukocytes are formed in the same area of the bone marrow as are the red blood cells. The lymphocytes are formed in lymphatic tissue. The white blood cells are less abundant than are the red blood cells; the normal range is between 5,000 and 10,000 per cubic centimeter. The functions of white blood cells are not understood as clearly as are those of red blood cells. However, the function of the leukocytes in combating infection is extremely important to the survival of the individual, as was indicated in Chapter 13.

The primary function of platelets is in clotting of the blood. The clotting process is essential in controlling loss of blood. Diseases or disorders which inhibit or interfere with the normal function of any of the constituents of the heart, blood vessels, or blood have a corresponding effect on the health status of the individual.

Congenital defects. Congenital defects of the heart or circulatory system occur in only a small percentage of children and are responsible for only about 2 per cent of all cardiac patients. Some of the causes of such defects are not known. However, some of the contributory factors are known and can be prevented. In addition, some of the defects can be treated effectively by improved surgical techniques.

It is known that if a woman has an attack of German measles during the early months of pregnancy her child may be born with a defective heart or other defects. Protecting the health of the mother during pregnancy decreases the likelihood of the child being born with a serious defect.

Congenital defects in the structure of the heart or blood vessels can result in an insufficient supply of blood being diverted through the lungs. As a result, the individual suffers from a lack of oxygen for the normal functioning of his body tissues. The "blue baby" operations, which increase the amount of blood being sent to the lungs for aeration, are examples of surgical correction of such defects.

Rheumatic fever. Infections in other parts of the body can cause disturbances in the function of the heart. At the present time, rheumatic fever and syphilis are the most frequent causes of heart disease which are infectious in nature. As a result of improved treatment for syphilis, damage from this disease is expected to decrease considerably. Rheumatic fever remains as the greatest danger to the heart of the school-age person and the young adult. Rheumatic fever and chronic rheumatic heart disease are a major cause of death in the fifteen- to twenty-four-year-old age group. Tuberculosis and cancer are the only diseases which cause more deaths in this age group.

Cause of rheumatic fever. Although the exact cause of rheumatic fever is not known, the disease is associated closely with streptococcus infections of the throat. The symptoms of rheumatic fever frequently are observed after a "strep" infection. The part that hereditary susceptibility and environmental factors play in the onset of rheumatic fever is not known definitely but is being explored by research workers.

Unfortunately for the individual, one attack of rheumatic fever does not protect him from future attacks. The danger of recurrences makes it essential that the first attack be recognized and the damage minimized. Steps should be taken to prevent additional attacks by controlling streptococcus infections.

Detecting rheumatic fever. Rheumatic fever is a general systemic disease which may or may not cause damage to the heart. Frequently the symptoms of rheumatic fever are mild, and damage to the heart is slow in appearing. Some of the symptoms which indicate the presence of rheumatic fever are nosebleeds, loss of appetite, fatigue or weakness, slight persistent fever, and pain in the muscles or joints. Appearance of such symptoms in a young person, especially following throat infections or colds, should be brought to the attention of a physician.

Rheumatic heart disease, which results from rheumatic fever, generally consists in damage to the endocardium and scarring of the valves of the heart. Damage to the valves permits blood to leak back into the auricles from the ventricles. The leaking of blood during contraction of the ventricle can be heard by the physician through his stethoscope. The sound is called a murmur. All murmurs do not indicate a serious malfunction of the heart, however.

In addition to listening to heart sounds, the physician makes use of the X ray and the fluoroscope to determine the size, shape, and relative position of the heart. The electrocardiogram records the electrical impulses associated with contractions and relaxation of the heart muscles, and the tracings provide evidence of any malfunction.

Even the blood provides information for the physician. A blood sedimentation test—measurement of the rate and extent to which red cells settle to the bottom of a blood sample—is of value in diagnosis.

Preventing rheumatic heart disease. Although rheumatic fever does not always result in damage to the heart, prevention and effective treatment of rheumatic fever are the basis for preventing rheumatic heart disease. Preventing infections due to hemolytic streptococcus is a fundamental step in the control of rheumatic fever and rheumatic heart disease.

Medical care in the early stages of rheumatic fever is essential in preventing serious complications. Treatment of infections is carried on by the physician, and complete rest and proper diet are prescribed for the patient. Complete rest during the acute stages of the disease lessens the burden on the heart and decreases the likelihood of permanent damage.

The use by physicians of cortisone and ACTH to prevent heart damage from rheumatic fever offers hope in controlling this menace to the hearts of children and young adults [20, 24].

Those who have recovered from an attack of rheumatic fever are advised to maintain their physical vigor through a balanced program of rest and activity and by eating proper foods. In addition, they are advised to avoid exposure to respiratory infections and to seek medical attention in case of exposure. Prevention and control of streptococcus infections are more readily accomplished since the discovery of penicillin and other similar drugs.

Hypertension—high blood pressure. Of the conditions affecting the cardiovascular system, hypertension is one of those most talked about and least understood by lay persons. Hypertension means high blood pressure, or pressure which is above average. It is important to note that blood pressure varies with individuals and with the same individual at different times. Emotions such as fear, anger, and worry cause blood vessels to constrict, and the blood pressure is thus increased. Many individuals have high blood pressure for most of their life and seem to suffer little or no ill effects. Others have blood pressure above normal, associated with serious complications. Worrying about blood pressure adds to the difficulties by increasing the pressure.

Blood-pressure problems are an individual matter. Actually, high blood pressure is a sign or symptom rather than a disease. The associated conditions, as in the arteries or kidneys, determine the seriousness of the hypertensive condition.

Causes of hypertension. Secondary hypertension may be caused by malfunction of the adrenal or pituitary glands or by disorders in other parts of the body. Renal hypertension is an example of a secondary hypertension associated with kidney disease.

High blood pressure which occurs without apparent organic cause is called essential hypertension. The emotionally tense and highly irritable person is more likely to develop essential hypertension than is the relaxed person. Although the exact cause of essential hypertension is not known, a hereditary factor apparently is a contributing cause in many cases [21, 26]. The increase in occurrence of hypertension among older persons is an indication that age is another factor in the onset of high blood pressure. However, hypertension may be found at any age, even in babies. The average age of onset is about thirty-two years.

The overweight person and the individual with a short, stocky build have a higher incidence of essential hypertension than does the person of average weight and tall, slender, narrow-chested build [11, 21].

Effects of hypertension. High blood pressure indicates that the heart is required to exert greater effort in order to circulate the blood. The amount of resistance determines the size of "pump" which is needed. The increased resistance for the heart to overcome may result in an enlargement of the heart muscle. It is possible for a strong heart to become enlarged and be uninjured by increased pressure over a period of years. A weak heart is unable to cope with the additional demands with which it is confronted.

The increase in pressure not only adds to the burden on the "pump" but also places extra strain on the "pipes," or blood vessels. Strong, elastic arteries can withstand the added strain for many years. Weakened or non-elastic arteries are less able to withstand the pressure. Changes in the structure of blood vessels associated with hypertension may result in an insufficient supply of blood to organs. The organs most frequently and most seriously affected by hypertension are the heart, the brain, and the kidneys.

High blood pressure does not always cause symptoms which can be detected by the individual. There may be general symptoms, such as headache, dizziness, lightheadedness, and vertigo, which can be due to some other condition. The cause should be determined by a physician. High blood pressure can be diagnosed accurately only by measurement with an instrument such as the sphygmomanometer. Regular medical examinations enable the physician to detect changes in blood pressure and other signs which indicate the onset of hypertension.

In preventing complications from high blood pressure it is important to follow the advice of the physician regarding kind and amount of physical activity, diet, use of tobacco and coffee, rest, control of weight, and control of emotions.

Arteriosclerosis. Arteriosclerosis, hardening of the arteries, is closely associated with high blood pressure, coronary diseases, and apoplexy, which are common among the older members of the population.

Arteriosclerosis occurs to some extent in everyone who survives for a long enough period of time. However, it is more common in men than in women, it affects men approximately ten years earlier than it affects women, and it tends to occur earlier in persons with diabetes [21, 17].

The importance of arteriosclerosis is suggested by Wright: [3]

The significance of this single process may be realized when it is understood that according to actuarial predictions, of the 25 million persons in this coun-

[3] Irving S. Wright, *Diseases of the Heart,* pp. 4–5. New York: American Heart Association, 1950.

try over 50 years of age, 15 million (60%) will die of some involvement of the heart, kidneys, or brain, and in a vast majority of persons this involvement will be on the basis of arteriosclerosis.

Arteriosclerosis is the result of a series of changes in the wall of the artery. Some of the changes are not understood, but it is known that the fibers in the middle, or muscle, layer deteriorate and that fatty materials are deposited in the inner lining of the artery. The final result of the changes is calcification of the artery. Instead of being flexible vessels, the arteries become rigid tubes.

Weakness in the artery walls which causes hemorrhage, or a change in the inner lining which causes partial or complete stoppage of the flow of blood may be the end result of the arteriosclerosis.

Coronary heart disease. Coronary heart disease is a result of changes in the arteries supplying the heart and a subsequent interference with the flow of blood. The heart muscle needs a supply of food and oxygen and must eliminate waste products the same as any other muscle of the body. Failure of the heart muscle to be supplied adequately produces more dramatic and severe results than does the same insufficiency in other muscles.

Some persons, the minority, die quickly as a result of the first attack of coronary disease. Fortunately, many survive the first attack and are able to enjoy many useful and happy years. The chance for recovery depends upon the extent of the damage, the ability of the body to repair or compensate for the damage, and the maintaining of a sensible program of healthful living.

Angina pectoris. Angina pectoris is a symptom of disturbance in the coronary circulation. Pain results because the heart muscle is deprived of its normal supply of oxygen. The pain of angina pectoris has characteristics which aid in its identification. The term "strangling in the chest" is a description applied frequently. The pain occurs under the breast bone and may radiate out to either arm, although the left arm is affected more frequently. Pain from angina pectoris may be mild or severe, depending somewhat upon the extent of the interference with the coronary blood supply.

Coronary thrombosis. A blood clot which remains stationary is called a thrombus. Coronary thrombosis is a closing or blocking of a coronary artery by a blood clot. If the stoppage involves a large branch of the artery, the individual is likely to die quickly. If the stoppage involves a small branch of the artery, the circulatory system sometimes is able to overcome the difficulty by means of collateral circulation, making use of other blood vessels. This ability of other blood vessels to compensate for a blockage of one vessel is a fine example of the adaptability of the human organism.

The heart muscle fibers whose blood supply is cut off undergo changes. Some of the fibers die. Over a period of time the damaged fibers are replaced by scar tissue, and the wound is healed. Until the healing process is completed, there is danger of hemorrhage in the area. Resting the whole body decreases the amount of work required of the heart and, in turn, reduces the strain on the injured area. By avoiding excessive strain during the healing process, an individual increases his chances of living a comparatively normal life thereafter.

Stroke, or apoplexy. Stroke, or apoplexy, means the same thing as cerebral hemorrhage. Strokes may cause death immediately, or they may be so mild as to escape detection. The extent of the damage depends upon the area of the brain involved and the amount of bleeding which occurs. Blood may simply leak through the walls of the capillaries or may escape owing to a break in the blood vessel wall. Individuals with arteriosclerosis and hypertension are more susceptible to a breakdown in the blood vessels. They may suffer a series of strokes over a period of years.

The paralysis of facial, arm, or leg muscles on one side of the body is a frequent result of a stroke. Pressure on the brain due to the hemorrhage causes the paralysis. If the injury to brain tissue is slight and the blood is gradually reabsorbed, permanent damage may be slight. When brain cells are killed, they do not regenerate and paralysis is permanent. In addition, personality changes sometimes result from pressure in an area of the brain.

Kidney Diseases

"Nephritis" and "Bright's disease" are terms commonly used to designate kidney disease. The name Bright's disease refers to Richard Bright, an English physician, who demonstrated in 1827 that albumin in the urine indicated the possible presence of kidney disease.

Nephritis means an inflammation of the nephrons, or filtering units of the kidneys. Chronic and acute nephritis cause the death of over 25,000 persons each year in the United States. Nephritis is eighth among the leading causes of death and is a problem for both young and old. In the one to fourteen age group, it is eighth among the leading causes of death; in the fifteen to twenty-four age group, chronic and acute nephritis combined rank sixth [14].

Kidneys. Two bean-shaped organs each weighing about ⅓ pound and each containing upward of 1 million filtering units are responsible for removing the end products of protein digestion and other waste products from the body. Complete failure of this filtering system causes death. Partial failure results in an impairment of function which sometimes makes itself known by changes in the amount of urine one passed, changes in the composition of the urine, edema (excess accumulation of fluid in body tissues), backache, or general fatigue.

The filtering units in the kidneys are called nephrons. Each nephron consists of a minute, cuplike chamber called Bowman's capsule and a tubule. The tubule follows a winding pathway ending in the collecting chamber of the kidney, where the urine accumulates and then passes through the ureters to the bladder. Blood comes into the nephrons under high pressure as it passes rapidly from the aorta into the renal artery and thence to the filtering chamber, or capsule. In these chambers the renal artery divides into a network of capillaries, the glomeruli. The surface provided by the many small blood vessels allows fluid to pass into the chamber surrounding the blood vessels and thence into the tubule. It is estimated that at least 600 quarts of blood passes through the kidneys each day and that about 60 or more quarts of fluid is removed and passes into the tubules [5]. As the fluid passes down the 2-inch length of the tubule, reabsorption of useful materials takes place and the waste materials continue through the tubule into the collecting area of the kidney. From the 600 quarts of blood which passes through the kidneys each day only about 1½ quarts of fluid is removed and eliminated as urine.

Urine normally contains urea, uric acid, and creatinine, which are end products of protein metabolism in the body. In addition, sodium chloride, potassium, calcium, and magnesium salts and phosphoric and hydrochloric acid are found in varying amounts. Urine normally is slightly acid in reaction although the effect of diet may cause it to become slightly alkaline. The bulk of the urine is water, which carries the solid waste materials.

The selectivity of the nephron in reabsorbing substances needed by the body and eliminating harmful substances can be disturbed by various types of disorder which affect the kidney. Failure of the kidney to eliminate harmful substances produces the symptoms mentioned earlier.

Causes of kidney diseases. Hench and Odel suggest the following grouping of causes of kidney diseases: (1) germs which cause a local infection; (2) bacterial poisons produced by germs or formed in infected areas of the body; (3) toxins which do not arise from bacterial sources (mercury, lead, poisons arising in burns); (4) infections and intoxications resulting from mechanical interference to the normal passage of urine (stones or enlarged prostate); (5) abnormalities of growth which interfere with normal function (cysts and benign or malignant tumors) [5]. In addition, renal sclerosis, or hardening of the renal arteries, affects kidney function by disturbing the normal supply of blood to these organs.

The burden placed upon the kidneys by infection in other parts of the body is not inconsiderable. Infected teeth and tonsils and other infections, seemingly remote, mean additional work for the kidneys, which must eliminate toxins produced as a result of such conditions. However, the normal kidney is able to carry an extra burden in most circumstances because of the abundance of filtering units. This abundance of nephrons is demonstrated by the fact that an individual is able to live and remain in good health with only one kidney.

Occasionally, poisons or toxins accumulate too rapidly, and the nephrons are unable to perform their function as rapidly as they should. The accumulation of waste material in the blood stream as a result of kidney insufficiency produces general systemic poisoning called uremia.

Detection of kidney diseases. Some symptoms of kidney malfunction can be detected by the individual. The passage of excessive or inadequate amounts of urine, blood in the urine, backache in some instances, or puffiness of body tissues may be an indication that kidney function is impaired. Regardless of the cause, such symptoms should result in a visit to a physician for checking.

The physician has at his disposal the facilities for making numerous tests to assist him in determining the nature and extent of kidney disease. One of the most valuable means of detecting kidney disorders is by an analysis of the urine to determine its chemical composition as well as its specific gravity or density. Examination of the urine includes testing to discover the degree of alkalinity or acidity and determining whether or not it contains albumin, sugar, pus or blood cells, sediment, or casts. Urinalysis is a routine procedure in most examinations conducted by a physician because the urine provides information about malfunction of other organs of the body besides the kidneys. Albumin, a simple protein substance found in many animal and vegetable tissues, is present in the blood as a part of the blood protein. Normally the urine is practically free of albumin. The presence of albumin does indicate possible malfunction of the nephrons, but additional tests must be made to confirm the cause.

Bacteriological examination of the urine to determine the nature and extent of any pathogenic (disease-producing) organisms is an extremely important aspect of a complete urinalysis. The presence of casts in the urine is another clue which aids in the detection of nephritis. Casts are small, threadlike masses of protein material formed by an accumulation of such material in the tubule of the nephron. Different types of cast can be detected by the laboratory technician.

X-ray pictures provide information relative to size, shape, and position of the kidney, and by use of liquids which are opaque to the X ray the physician obtains information regarding the internal structure of the kidney. In addition, harmless dyes are injected into the muscles or veins, and the time required for their passage is measured to determine the ability of the kidney to excrete materials. Fortunately, instruments such as the cystoscope and catheters may be used as an approach to the pelvic cavity of the kidney without resorting to surgery.

On the basis of information which the physician gathers by means of the above procedures, he is able to direct treatment at the specific cause of the difficulty. The individual must realize that proper diet, adequate rest, and control of infections in the body are important in both preventing and treating kidney diseases.

Cancer

Cancer is being treated effectively in the patient who seeks the advice of his physician while the cancer is in its earliest stages. Therefore, it is important to understand something of the nature of cancer in order to aid in early detection and to appreciate the need for complete cooperation with the physician.

Despite the fact that treatment can be effective in a high percentage of cases, cancer is the second leading cause of death. Because malignant growths are more frequently a disease of older persons, the death rate is likely to continue to be high as the number of older persons in the population increases. Cancer is not limited to the elderly, however. It is third among the causes of death in the fifteen- to twenty-four-year-olds and second only to accidents in the one- to fourteen-year-olds [14].

What is cancer? "Cancer" is the name used for a group of diseases which have the common characteristic of abnormal cell growth. "Malignant neoplasms" and "malignant tumors" are other terms used to designate this abnormal cell growth. Neoplasm or tumor means a swelling, or lump. "Malignant" defines the lump as being harmful. Malignant tumors have the ability to continue to grow and to spread from the original site to other parts of the body. They rarely cease growing of their own accord but must be stopped by external means. Benign tumors are harmless in the sense that they do not spread to other parts of the body but are localized. They may, however, be harmful to the extent that they interfere with normal functions in the local area of the body.

Normal cell growth. Normal cell growth is an orderly process. The individual develops from a single cell or ovum to a mature adult person. As he develops through the periods of infancy, childhood, and adolescence, the growth of different body tissues speeds up and slows down in a regulated manner. Finally the individual reaches his maximum height, but growth and repair of the various body tissues continue in order to maintain the efficiency of the organism. Millions of cells are destroyed and replaced each day. An example of the normal replacement of tissue is the healing of an incision or cut on a finger. The replacement of destroyed cells continues until the wound is healed, and then replacement or growth of cells ceases.

When man is able to solve the secret of what starts and stops the growth of cells in a normal manner, he undoubtedly will have the answer to the riddle of abnormal cell growth, which occurs in cancer.

Cancer does spread. Control of cancer at the present time is based on detection of the malignant tumor before the abnormally growing cells break from their original site and establish "colonies" elsewhere in the body. This ability to spread to other tissues and establish new growth centers is called metastasis. Metastasis occurs by direct extension to adjacent tissues, by spreading through the blood stream, and by transfer of cells through the lymphatic system.

Once a malignant tumor reaches the stage where metastasis occurs, treatment is relatively ineffective because of the difficulty of locating all the new growth centers and destroying them by the treatment techniques available.

Cancer cells are different. Cancer cells differ from normal cells. Diagnosis of cancer is based upon detection of abnormal cells by microscopic examination of suspected tissue. The pathologist, a medical specialist, is able to detect malignant tissue by this means, which is called a histological test.

Cancer in the different tissues of the body is referred to by names such as (1) sarcoma, a malignant tumor of connective tissue (bone, muscle); (2) carcinoma, a malignant tumor of epithelial tissue (skin, membrane linings, and glandular structures); (3) melanoma, a malignant tumor arising in the pigment cells; (4) lymphoma, a group of tumors affecting lymphatic tissues (Hodgkin's disease and lymphosarcoma); and (5) leukemia, a malignant tumorlike disease of the blood-forming tissues causing abnormal growth of the white blood cells.

Cause of cancer. The exact cause of cancer has defied the best efforts of research workers. Many contributing or predisposing factors are known, and man is able to produce cancer in animals in the laboratory. Chronic or prolonged irritation is recognized as one of the exciting factors. This irritation may be produced by chemical, thermal, or mechanical means.

Chemicals capable of producing cancer are known as carcinogenic agents. Cancer of the bladder among aniline-dye workers, cancer of the bone in luminous-dial painters, cancer of the skin in asphalt workers, and cancer of the scrotum among chimney sweeps provide examples of the cancer-inciting ability of some chemicals [1]. The danger to miners and smelter workers from uranium ore and other similar substances is not understood completely, but apparently they can be considered as possible cancer-inciting substances. Examples of malignant growths caused by thermal, or heat, irritation are lip cancer associated with the heat of the pipe stem and skin cancer due to excessive exposure to sunlight. Malignant growths resulting from irritation of certain types of mole by clothing indicate the possible danger of mechanical irritation as an inciting agent.

There is no conclusive evidence to show that cancer is caused by germs or virus, and cancer is not considered to be communicable. Helping with the care of a cancer patient does not expose an individual to the danger of "catching" the cancer.

Common sites of cancer in the body. The frequency with which cancer occurs in specific organs differs between the sexes. Table 11 compares the incidence of cancer by site and sex. Cancer of the digestive tract is the most common site in the male, accounting for over one-third of the cases. Cancer of the breast and the genital organs accounts for one-half of the cancer cases among females.

Cancer of the skin. Skin cancer can be cured in 95 per cent of the cases if proper treatment is undertaken in the early stages. Skin cancer is visible to the naked eye and therefore can be detected early enough to allow for effective treatment. However, each year many individuals die of this type of malignant condition simply because they fail to observe the growth or delay in seeking medical assistance until the cancer has metastasized. The skin is an organ, and any condition which affects the skin can have an effect on other organs of the body. To assume that a growth

Table 11. Cancer Incidence by Sex and Site *

Site	*Males,* %	*Females,* %
Skin	17	11
Mouth	10	2
Respiratory tract	8	2
Breast	..	24
Digestive tract	36	23
Urinary tract	7	3
Genital tract	12	27
All others	10	8
Totals	100	100

* Based on information provided by the American Cancer Society.

on the skin cannot cause severe damage or even death is but to invite disaster if the growth is malignant.

Moles or skin blemishes which increase in size or undergo changes of any kind should be examined by a physician. Self-treatment or treatment by a "quack" is dangerous because of the delay in correct diagnosis if the mole becomes malignant. Fortunately most moles do not become cancerous. The type of mole most apt to develop into a malignant tumor is dark brown or bluish black and is slightly raised. This type of mole, if irritated by the clothing, may show signs of growth after being dormant for years.

Any skin sore or lesion which resists normal healing and persists for a longer period of time than is usual should be referred to a physician. He is best qualified to determine the nature of the growth or lesion and to prescribe the best treatment.

Cancer of the respiratory tract. Cancer of the respiratory tract shows a steady increase during recent years, according to statisticians of the Metropolitan Life Insurance Co. [10]. More men than women are affected by respiratory cancer. A portion of the increase in incidence is attributed to better means of detecting and diagnosing malignant growths in heretofore inaccessible organs. The bronchoscope for examining the respiratory tract, improved X-ray procedures for detecting growths, and laboratory tests of respiratory secretions provide the physician with more adequate means of making an early and accurate diagnosis.

The part that smoking plays in the onset of lung cancer is subject to disagreement among authorities [25]. The incidence of lung cancer is greater among heavy smokers than among nonsmokers, but there is no definite proof at present that smoking is the specific cause. Likewise, the role of air pollution as a cause of lung cancer has not been established.

Some individuals who develop lung cancer are being saved. However, as with other types of cancer, early detection is absolutely essential. A hacking cough which lasts for a period of time, persistent hoarseness, coughing up blood, and obscure chest pains are indications that the individual should see his physician. The cause of the symptoms should be diagnosed and treated by a physician.

Cancer of the digestive tract. Cancer of the digestive tract causes many deaths because it is difficult to detect in its early stages. Men over forty are more susceptible to cancer of the digestive tract. Therefore, they should be especially alert to detect any indications of deviation from the normal.

Some of the more specific symptoms which may be indicative of the presence of cancer of the digestive tract are (1) difficulty in swallowing food; (2) persistent indigestion or a vague uneasiness after eating; (3) persistent change in bowel habits, toward either diarrhea or constipation; and (4) a bloody discharge from the anal opening, black or tarry stools. Bleeding from the anal opening can be caused by hemorrhoids. Self-diagnosis of hemorrhoids (commonly called piles) is especially risky because of delay in detecting the presence of cancer in the rectum or lower part of the digestive tract. The danger of hemorrhoids, a form of varicose veins, should not be minimized. They are a common ailment which can be treated by one's physician to prevent serious complications.

Regular medical examinations are essential in early detection of malignant tumors of the digestive tract. Loss of weight, anemia, and fatigue are general symptoms which should result in a special visit to a physician.

Cancer of the breast. Breast cancer is common in women and rare in men. As a result of the educational campaign to inform women about breast cancer, many lives are being saved. However, cancer of the breast still causes thousands of needless deaths each year.

An early indication of breast cancer is a lump. The lump is painless in most cases, at least in the early stages of growth. Most lumps of the breast are not cancerous, but they should be examined by a physician as soon as they are detected. Other signs which may indicate the presence of a malignant condition are alteration in shape of the breast, elevation or retraction of the nipple of the breast, puckering of the skin, bleeding or discharge from the nipple, or a swollen lymph node or gland in the armpit. Cancer of the breast frequently is associated with the menopause. Women undergoing this change should be alert to detect symptoms noted above. Single women have higher death rates from breast cancer than do married women. The nursing of a child is believed to be a factor in reducing the chances of breast cancer [19].

The influence of heredity on the occurrence of cancer varies with the type of cancer and is not understood fully at the present time. However, the chance of developing breast cancer is greater in a girl whose mother had it than in one whose mother did not [26].

Cancer of the female genital organs. The reproductive organs are the most common site for malignant conditions in women. Over one-half of the total number of cancers of the reproductive organs occur in the cervix. Fortunately, cancer of this area of the uterus is relatively easy for a physician to detect and, if located in its early stage, responds readily to treatment.

The most important sign which serves as a warning is irregular or abnormal bleeding from the vagina. However, in many cases, such bleeding does not occur until the growth is in its advanced stages. Therefore it is important for a woman particularly from about thirty-five years of age on, to have regular examinations by a physician.

Cancer of the male genitourinary tract. Cancer of the genitourinary tract causes about one-fifth of the male deaths from cancer. The prostate gland is more likely to be the site of cancer than is any other organ in the male genitourinary tract. It is estimated that at least 2 to 3 per cent of all males past fifty years of age develop cancer of the prostate.

The most specific symptom indicating possible cancer in the genitourinary tract is the presence of blood in the urine. In addition, any change in normal habits of urination should be sufficient reason for seeking the advice of a physician.

Means of detecting cancer. Control of cancer is dependent upon early detection. Current means of treating cancer are effective only if they are used early. Therefore each individual should take responsibility for arranging regular examinations by his physician for observing common symptoms which might indicate the presence of a malignant tumor, and for reporting such symptoms to his physician.

Common symptoms. Early symptoms may or may not be detected easily. Unfortunately, pain is seldom an early sign of cancer. The following danger signals are stressed in the educational campaign carried on by the American Cancer Society [18]:

1. Any sore that does not heal.
2. A lump or thickening, in the breast or elsewhere.
3. Unusual bleeding or discharge.
4. Any change in a mole or wart.
5. Persistent indigestion or difficulty in swallowing.
6. Persistent hoarseness or cough.
7. Any persistent change in normal bowel habits.

The appearance of any one of these symptoms may mean cancer, or it may mean some other condition. The individual is not capable of diagnosing for himself. He should not put off the visit to his physician until more symptoms appear. Delay may be fatal.

A physician diagnoses cancer. The physician has at his disposal various means for determining whether or not a growth is present and if so whether or not the growth is malignant. Among the procedures which are of assistance to the physician are (1) observing and feeling for growths, (2) a microscopic examination of secretions from the lining of the respiratory and genital tracts, (3) X-ray pictures of inaccessible areas of the body, and (4) microscopic examination of suspected tissue.

Treatment of cancer. Recognized means of curing cancer which are accepted by the medical profession at the present time are surgery, X ray, and radium. The principle involved in each of these treatments is the complete removal or destruction of all cancerous cells.

All cancers do not respond to the same type of treatment. X ray is effective for use with some cancers, while for others it is relatively ineffective. X ray or radium must be used under the supervision of specialists. Radiotherapy causes damage to normal cells as well as to cancerous cells, and care must be taken to concentrate the rays on malignant tissue for a sufficiently long period of time and at the same time to avoid excessive exposure of normal cells. Improvements in equipment and in technique for using X ray and radium make such treatment more effective at present.

Even though surgery, X-ray, and radium treatments are started early, the physician is cautious about claims for a cure. Only if the patient is free from recurrence for a five-year period is the malignant condition considered to be arrested. Following this five-year period regular examinations are essential, because a cancer can reappear at or near the same site or in other parts of the body. Recovery from cancer does not indicate immunity against further malignant conditions.

In addition to the three above-mentioned specific treatments, some palliative measures which are used include radioactive isotopes, hormones, and chemical substances such as nitrogen mustard [1, 4].

Despite the claims made by many individuals outside the medical profession, there is no evidence that unorthodox treatments have cured a cancer. The great danger in seeking the advice of such individuals lies in delaying proper treatment until it is too late.

Diabetes Mellitus

Individuals with diabetes occupy important positions and take part in nearly every phase of life in our country today. Doctors, lawyers, political leaders, businessmen, professional athletes, and laborers are represented among the diabetic cases. It has been only within the last thirty years that effective treatment for diabetic individuals has been realized. It is significant that at the present time the average life expectancy of a diabetic individual has been raised until it is approximately three-fourths of that of the general population. The significance of these figures is appreciated more when one realizes that at the turn of the century diabetic patients had an average life expectancy of approximately three years [6].

Diabetes remains as a major health problem in the United States despite the improvements in treatment. It is ninth among the leading causes of death. In addition to the estimated 1 million diabetic cases under treatment in the United States, it is estimated that there are approximately another million undiagnosed cases of diabetes.

What is diabetes? Diabetes results when the pancreas, an endocrine gland located near the stomach, fails to supply a sufficient amount of the hormone, insulin. As a result of the insufficient supply of insulin, the storage of sugar in the liver is inhibited, the formation of sugar from glycogen stored in the liver is speeded up, and the utilization of sugar by the tissues is depressed.

As a consequence of the changes listed above, (1) the blood sugar level is abnormally high, (2) the kidneys excrete sugar in the urine, (3) the excretion of sugar results in an excessive loss of salt and water, (4) increased utilization of protein and fat sources of heat and energy is required to compensate for the inability of tissues to oxidize sugar, and (5) the system is poisoned by products of incomplete combustion of proteins and fats [16].

Cause of diabetes. No single factor is responsible for the development of diabetes mellitus. In some, specific injury due to infection or the presence of growths causes the islands of Langerhans in the pancreas to produce insufficient amounts of insulin. In many, the onset of diabetes is gradual, with many factors contributing to the development of the disease.

Heredity is recognized as an important factor in the causation of diabetes. Scheinfeld notes that one out of four diabetic patients in this country has diabetic relatives, and the American Diabetes Association reports that about 50 per cent of diabetic children come from families in which there is or has been diabetes. A pair of simple recessive genes are responsible for most cases of diabetes, according to Joslin and his coworkers, who have made extensive studies of the disease [26].

Obesity is a contributing factor in the onset of diabetes. The American Diabetes Association points out that twenty stout persons develop diabetes for every thin person. A study by the Metropolitan Life Insurance Co. showed that 85 per cent of the diabetic patients who were forty years of age or older when they developed diabetes were overweight prior to the onset of the disease [11]. It is not known whether or not overeating causes diabetes in an individual who does not have an inherited susceptibility. There is little doubt, however, that the strain placed on the islands of Langerhans of a susceptible person by overeating is a contributing factor.

Joslin reports that two-thirds of the cases of diabetes develop after the age of forty-five is reached [6]. Diabetes, however, is not limited to older persons. It is estimated that more than 50,000 children under fifteen years of age are victims of this chronic disease. Women are more likely to develop diabetes than are men. After the age of forty years a woman has about one-third more chances of developing diabetes than a man has. It is not known whether the increased rate for women is due to differences in eating habits, glandular changes during menopause, or some unknown factor or factors.

Detecting diabetes. Diabetes can be detected by the physician in its incipient stages prior to the time when symptoms are apparent to the individual. Regular physical examinations, including a urinalysis, provide the opportunity for early detection. In addition, the appearance of the following symptoms may indicate the onset of the disease.

Symptoms of diabetes. An increased output of urine may be one of the first indications that diabetes is present. The increase occurs because the kidneys eliminate excess amounts of sugar which accumulate in the blood. The demand for fluid to aid in the elimination of excess sugar causes an increased feeling of thirst. Owing to the inability to oxidize sugar properly, the tissues lack an adequate energy supply. The result is a constant feeling of hunger. The use of protein and fat supplies as a source of energy results in a weight loss. Closely allied with these symptoms is the tendency to tire easily.

Other symptoms appear in varying degrees of intensity. The person may be annoyed by excessive itching, he may begin to notice a change in vision, and he may discover that wounds do not heal readily.

Screening tests. Because of the estimated 1 million or more undetected cases of diabetes in the United States, attempts are being made to conduct screening tests of large numbers of individuals. The screening tests for tuberculosis by means of portable X-ray units are an example of mass screening which has proved to be valuable. The American Diabetes Association, working in cooperation with other interested groups, is emphasizing the desirability of regular tests for diabetes through a year-round educational program and by having one week set aside as Diabetes Detection Week. During this week a special effort is made to provide facilities and encourage individuals to take advantage of the opportunity to be tested.

Interested organizations and individuals are stressing the advantage of "multiphasic screening," which would provide for tuberculosis testing, blood testing for venereal disease, and testing for diabetes to be carried on at the same time. Mass testing programs for these three diseases would result in the early detection of many cases.

Results of testing over 3,000 students at the University of Southern California provide information relative to the effectiveness of screening tests [12, 15]. On the basis of these findings it is suggested that a blood-sugar test performed 2 hours after the individual ingests 50 grams of dextrose provides a simple but effective screening method for detecting diabetes.

Controlling diabetes. Under the supervision of a competent physician, diabetes is the most readily controlled of the chronic diseases. Diabetic persons are fortunate compared with victims of some of the other chronic diseases, because diabetes can be treated effectively. When the diabetic person is able to maintain relatively sugar-free urine and to prevent other symptoms, his diabetes is said to be "controlled." However, diabetes is not cured in the sense that a communicable disease is cured. Regulation of diet, exercise, and insulin must be maintained, or symptoms of the condition appear once again.

Complications of diabetes. Before insulin became available, diabetic coma ranked as the primary cause of death in diabetic cases. Diabetic coma occurs when the individual does not have enough insulin. As a result, products from the incomplete combustion of proteins and fats cause an acidosis which is fatal if untreated. Overdoses of insulin cause a reaction, or insulin shock as it is called sometimes. The individual suffering from insulin reaction may exhibit symptoms of intoxication. An identification card indicating that a person is a diabetic case saves considerable embarrassment and may avert a real disaster. A physician should be called immediately if diabetic coma or insulin reaction is suspected.

Rheumatism

Rheumatism is a general term for a group of diseases which produce an inflammation of body tissues. Rheumatic diseases are not one of the newer afflictions of mankind. The Java man, who lived some 500,000 years ago, and the Neanderthal man, of some 25,000 years past, were both victims of arthritis [9]. Lewin [4] emphasizes the extent to which this group of diseases is a current problem:

> About seven and a half million Americans are chronic sufferers from one or another of the rheumatoid diseases. This is twice as many as have heart disease, ten times as many as have tuberculosis, ten times as many as have diabetes, and seven times as many as have cancer. It is forty times as many as have infantile paralysis, or polio, as it is more commonly called.

Arthritis. Arthritis is classified commonly as being of two general types. Osteoarthritis, a degenerative joint disease sometimes called hypertrophic arthritis, is primarily a disease of older persons. It seldom occurs before the age of forty years. Rheumatoid arthritis, sometimes called atrophic arthritis because of its wasting-away effect on the joints, is a disease of active life. Most of the victims of rheumatoid arthritis are under the age of fifty years.

Osteoarthritis. This disease of older individuals is most likely to be found in persons who are overweight, have faulty posture, or have poor muscle tone. Joints literally show signs of wearing out because of the burdens placed upon them. Joint injury is another factor which contributes to the onset of osteoarthritis. The weight-bearing joints are affected by the conditions mentioned above. As a result, the knees, ankles, hips, and vertebrae frequently are altered by this degenerative process. The most likely point to show signs of osteoarthritis is the joint at the tip of the fingers; women are more likely to be so affected than are men [9].

[4] Philip Lewin, *Arthritis and the Rheumatic Diseases,* p. 4. New York: McGraw-Hill Book Company, Inc., 1951.

X-ray examination of a joint affected by osteoarthritis shows calcium deposits or bony outgrowths. The cartilage at the joint shows signs of aging. These permanent changes in joint structure produce some pain and stiffness and result in enlarged, knobby joints.

Osteoarthritis, or degenerative arthritis, responds to treatment and is not the crippler that rheumatoid arthritis is. Early recognition and treatment of the condition make the prognosis much more favorable.

Rheumatoid arthritis. The victim of rheumatoid arthritis usually suffers considerably. In the early, or prearthritic, stage, vague and fleeting joint pains and joint stiffness after periods of rest may be noticed. During the active stages of the disease, swelling of the joint occurs. The characteristic swelling usually is associated with weakness of the joint, pain which may be constant or may be noticed only with movement, stiffness, restriction of movement which may appear gradually, muscular atrophy resulting from disuse of muscles, and cracking when the joint is used. Despite the localized symptoms, rheumatoid arthritis is not a localized disease. It is a disease of the entire system and is commonly preceded by a period of general ill health.

Although the actual cause of rheumatoid arthritis is not understood clearly, there are some factors which contribute to its onset. Infection is perhaps the primary villain, although the specific manner in which it accomplishes its mission is as yet not clear. Cold and exposure, endocrine imbalance, excess weight, worry, and digestive disturbances are suggested as factors which predispose to rheumatoid arthritis [2, 9, 22, 23].

Heredity, age, sex, and climate apparently influence the nature and extent of the arthritic affliction. The degree to which environmental factors and hereditary susceptibility contribute to the onset of arthritis is not clearly understood at present. The majority of individuals who have arthritis are in the older segments of the population, although it is possible for even the very young to develop the disease. Women are more likely to develop rheumatoid arthritis than are men. The sex factor also influences the location of arthritis. The more frequent occurrence of arthritis in the hips, feet, or spine of men may be due to injury or occupational damage. Endocrine changes common to pregnancy, childbirth, and menopause frequently are the forerunners of arthritis of the knees, spine, fingers, and hands of women. Although all the reasons are not understood, rheumatoid arthritis flourishes more in the cooler climates than in warm climates.

Gout. Gout has some characteristics which make it stand out among the rheumatic diseases. In a high percentage of cases, gout affects the big toe, although fingers and the knee may be affected. Approximately 95 to 97 per cent of the cases are men [2, 9]. Gout most frequently is found in inactive, heavy eaters and usually occurs after age forty-five. The condition is associated with the presence of excess amounts of uric acid in the body. The excess uric acid which is produced by improper protein metabolism causes the formation of crystal deposits of the acid in a joint. Fortunately for the relatively small number of sufferers, gout usually responds to treatment which is available at present.

Fibrositis. Fibrositis is a general term used to designate inflammation of the soft tissues. Pain, tenderness, and stiffness are common symptoms of this condition. Inflammation of specific soft tissues is indicated by such terms as neuritis, lumbago, sciatica, torticollis (wryneck), and bursitis.

Rheumatic fever. Rheumatic fever is one of the four major divisions of the rheumatic diseases and in clinical classifications is sometimes referred to as acute rheumatism. It is discussed in detail in connection with heart diseases.

If one has rheumatism. Rheumatism provides a lucrative field for the "healer" who promises relief from pain but whose primary interest is in relieving the victim of his money and not his illness. An individual who suspects the onset of arthritis should seek the help of a competent physician immediately and should avoid the advice of well-meaning friends, dispensers of "wonder" drugs, and quacks who make extravagant claims about curing the ailment. Early treatment by a competent physician offers the best chance for alleviating the effects of arthritis. Most of the drugs advertised as being helpful to individuals suffering from the pains of arthritis contain aspirin or some other pain-killing substance which may give relief but will fail to get at the cause of the disease.

The mental state has a profound influence on physical health. One's attitude regarding arthritis is an important factor in determining the extent to which he is incapacitated. Because worry tends to aggravate difficulties associated with rheumatism, one's thinking should be reorganized so that worry is decreased to a minimum. Regular periods of complete rest should be planned for each day. Proper diet and the maintenance of good habits of elimination are a prime responsibility of the individual. In addition, control of weight is helpful in relieving stress on joints.

At present there is no specific treatment which is effective for all individuals with arthritis. Types of treatment which offer some degree of effectiveness under the supervision of a qualified physician include glandular or endocrine therapy, chemotherapy, biological therapy, physiotherapy, and orthopedic surgery [9].

Allergies

An allergic individual who is sneezing, wheezing, or itching is one of the most miserable people in the world. Fortunately, allergies seldom are the cause of death. However, they constitute a definite health problem because of the misery and suffering of the allergic person, his decrease in efficiency, and the cost of relieving allergic reactions.

An estimated 10 million Americans are victims of allergic complaints such as hay fever, asthma, hives, eczema, allergic rhinitis, gastrointestinal allergies, allergic headaches, contact eczema, drug allergy, and eye inflammations [3].

What is an allergy? Allergic reactions are of many different types depending upon the substance which precipitates the reaction and the body tissues involved. The reactions vary considerably, but the basic process which produces the reactions is essentially the same in all cases.

Allergens. The chemical substances responsible for allergic reactions are called allergens. Allergens are antigens that induce the body to develop specific antibodies (see Chapter 13, page 297). The antibodies produced by the reaction of body tissues to antigens from disease-producing organisms serve a definite protective function. The antibodies produced by the reaction of body tissues to allergens do not serve a protective function. Instead, they in turn react with additional amounts of the same allergen to release histamine. The histamine produces typical allergic results with which the victim is familiar.

Although allergens for a long time were thought to be exclusively protein in nature, it has been demonstrated that other chemical substances are capable of causing allergic reactions.

How do allergens enter the body? Allergens make their way into the human organism by different routes. An individual who is constitutionally predisposed to allergic reactions may become sensitized by inhaling or breathing, by ingesting or swallowing, by injection, or by contact with a particular allergen.

Allergens taken in through the respiratory tract include dusts, mold spores, animal danders, and pollen from a variety of plants. Hay fever is an allergic reaction in the nasal membrane resulting from exposure and sensitization to allergens of this type. Hay fever symptoms may make a seasonal appearance when due to pollens, an irregular appearance when due to animal dander (dog, cat, horse) that the person contacts only occasionally, or a regular appearance when due to house dust.

Symptoms of hay fever include obstruction of nasal passages due to swelling of membranes, nasal discharge, and sneezing.

Allergens which enter the body through the respiratory tract, as well as by other means, may produce their effect in the bronchial tubes and cause asthma. The asthmatic person has difficulty in breathing because of the constriction of the bronchial tubes. He may make a wheezing sound as he breathes, and he is likely to discharge sputum by coughing as the attack begins to terminate. The symptoms tend to vary with individuals. They may be mistaken for other conditions, especially in children.

Immune serums obtained from animal sources can produce an allergic reaction when injected into individuals. Because of the danger of extreme allergic reactions, testing of individuals commonly is practiced prior to the use of such serums. The replacement of serum treatment by the sulfonamides and penicillin reduces the danger from this source. However, these drugs in turn can cause an allergic reaction. With some persons the reaction is so severe that the use of these drugs is dangerous and must be avoided.

Allergies resulting from ingestion of foods are common. The results may be no more than a feeling of discomfort, or they may be definite and pronounced. Hives, eczema, asthma, and migraine headaches are symptoms which are sometimes produced by allergic reaction to foods. Wheat, milk, eggs, nuts, fish, peas, beans, potatoes, and cocoa are some of the foods most likely to produce allergic reactions.

Poison ivy causes a distinct and severe allergic reaction in many as a result of contact of the oily residue from the plant with the skin. First exposures serve to sensitize the person, and subsequent exposures produce the characteristic inflammation of contact dermatitis. Failure to develop the allergic reaction following an exposure is not definite proof of immunity. Instead, it can mean that the individual is being sensitized and that through additional exposures he may develop an allergic reaction. Other plants, various chemicals, metals (mercury in particular), and dyes used in clothing are some of the common offenders which produce allergic reactions through contact with the skin.

Something can be done. Detecting an allergy is not always a simple matter for the physician, and self-diagnosis is likely to result in error. Fortunately, the family physician or the allergist has at his disposal the means for determining whether or not an allergy is present, the substances responsible for the allergy, and effective means for relieving or curing the condition.

Determining the cause. Once an allergy has been diagnosed, it is essential to discover all the substances causing it. Testing for sensitivity by means of skin and mucous-membrane tests is effective in most instances, although it may take a long time to complete the extensive number of tests to be made. The tests are based on the fact that the sensitized individual has developed antibodies which react locally with allergens being injected.

Avoiding the allergens. Avoiding the allergens responsible for producing the allergy is an important method of treatment. Unfortunately, this method is not always practical. A vacation away from his home area for a period of time during the pollen season may be practical for one person and impossible for another. Devices for filtering the air coming into the home are effective for relieving the symptoms for some individuals. In general, however, air-filtering devices are not a satisfactory means of avoiding exposure. The Council on Medicine of the American Medical Association makes recommendations helpful in evaluating air-filtering devices, many of which are ineffective.

Food allergies are alleviated by planning a diet which avoids the particular foods responsible for the allergy. Unless the person is allergic to a number of foods, the elimination of such foods from the diet is the most successful treatment available. In most instances, careful planning of substitute foods allows the proper balance of nutrients to be maintained.

If the source of the allergen is the household pet, either cat or dog, the most effective procedure for avoiding exposure is to find a new home for the pet. Recognition of poison ivy and care in avoiding exposure to it provide the most practical control measure for most individuals. In some instances, avoiding the allergen is difficult or even impossible. Fortunately, there are other methods which can be used effectively in cases where exposure is certain.

Building up resistance. The basic principle of building up resistance is an active immunization process. Preparations of the offending substance are injected underneath the skin in increasing quantities. After a period of time a tolerance is developed which permits an ordinary exposure without the allergic reaction. Unfortunately, all allergies do not respond to this type of desensitization. The physician determines whether or not this treatment is effective for specific individuals. In general, this protection lasts only for a limited period and may have to be repeated.

Relieving symptoms. Relieving symptoms is only a stopgap measure, and the continued treatment of an allergy by relieving the symptoms is not always recommended by a physician. There are effective means for relieving allergies which endanger the life of the individual or which cause extreme discomfort.

The use of preparations for constricting blood vessels in the nose to reduce nasal discharge may be effective, but the indiscriminate use of nose drops is not recommended and may be harmful. Many individuals simply add to their difficulty by using commercial preparations without seeking the advice of their physician.

Antihistamines, which provide relief from the symptoms of some allergies, are an example of a drug which can produce dangerous reactions in some persons.

The influence of emotional factors in producing allergic reactions should not be overlooked. In some cases, the most effective treatment for allergic conditions involves the elimination of nervous tensions which are the inciting factor.

What lies ahead? Many of the answers relative to allergies are not known. Some allergies defy the best efforts of specialists to discover the cause or to provide relief. Studies indicate an extremely close relationship between allergies and many disease conditions which affect mankind [3]. One of the factors slowing down the discovery of fundamental facts relating to allergies is the lack of funds for extensive research. The number of victims testifies to the nature and extent of the problem. In comparison with money spent on other types of research and on relieving symptoms, research concerning allergies is lagging far behind.

Summary

Diseases of the heart and circulatory system, cancer, diabetes, kidney diseases, rheumatism, and allergies are among the chronic diseases which kill or disable many individuals in the United States. Early detection is essential in effective control of the chronic or degenerative diseases. Both the individual and the physician have responsibilities for the early detection and for delaying the onset of these diseases. Although chronic diseases are more prevalent among older persons, college-age individuals also are affected. Health practices which maintain and improve the health status aid in delaying and reducing the disabling effects of some of the chronic diseases. The preventive aspect of chronic-disease control is being recognized, and the geriatric specialist is working with his patients to delay the onset of these diseases.

Suggested Activities

1. Investigate the contributions made to the understanding and control of chronic or degenerative diseases by the work of such men as William Harvey, Richard Bright, and Frederick Banting.

2. Contact the local, state, or national office of one of the voluntary health organizations to discover the contributions which the organization is making in terms of education, service, and research. The American Cancer Society, the American Rheumatism Association, the American Diabetes Association, and the American Heart Association are examples of organizations to contact.

3. Write for information to an individual or organization advertising "wonder" remedies for treatment of cancer, diabetes, or rheumatism. On the basis of scientific information available in the Suggested Readings, critically evaluate the claims made.

4. Investigate programs being carried on in your community to decrease the effects of any of the chronic diseases. What organizations are involved in the community program, and what specific activities are being undertaken?

5. Use models, charts, pictures, and slides to improve your understanding of the body organs and systems and the effect which specific chronic diseases have on them.

6. Investigate the part that laboratory experimentation with animals has played in improved methods of treatment for the chronic diseases. Examples of such experimentation are mice for cancer and dogs for heart surgery and for diabetes.

7. Have the college physician or some other physician discuss cancer control and show the film *Breast Self Examination* (sound, 20 minutes), American Cancer Society, 1950.

8. Preview, show, and discuss audio-visual aids pertinent to the chronic diseases, such as the following: (*a*) *Traitor Within* (sound, 11 minutes), American Cancer Society; (*b*) *Guard Your Heart* (sound, 27 minutes), American Heart Association; (*c*) *The Story of Wendy Hill* (sound, 20 minutes), Public Health Service.

Suggested Readings

1. American Cancer Society, *A Cancer Source Book for Nurses.* New York, 1950.

2. American Rheumatism Association, *Rheumatic Diseases.* Philadelphia: W. B. Saunders Company, 1952.

3. Feinberg, Samuel M., *Allergy: Facts and Fancies.* New York: Harper & Brothers, 1951.

4. Heller, John R., "Recent Progress in Cancer Research," *Public Health Reports,* 68:309–316, March, 1953.

5. Hench, Philip S., and Howard M. Odel, "The Kidney: Its Diseases and Disturbances," in Morris Fishbein (Ed.), *Modern Home Medical Adviser*, pp. 418–463. New York: Doubleday and Company, 1949.

6. Joslin, Elliott P., "Diabetes," in Morris Fishbein (Ed.), *Modern Home Medical Adviser*, pp. 563–606. New York: Doubleday & Company, Inc., 1949.

7. Kahn, Harold A., "Changing Causes of Death in Childhood," *Public Health Reports*, 66:1246, September 28, 1951.

8. Kiser, Clyde V., "The Demographic Background of our Aging Population," *The Social and Biological Challenge of Our Aging Population. Eastern States Health Conference Proceedings*, Mar. 31–Apr. 1, 1949, pp. 44–66. New York: Columbia University Press, 1950.

9. Lewin, Philip, *Arthritis and the Rheumatic Diseases*. New York: McGraw-Hill Book Company, Inc., 1951.

10. Metropolitan Life Insurance Co., "Continued Rise in Respiratory Cancer," *Statistical Bulletin*, 31:7–9, March, 1950.

11. Metropolitan Life Insurance Co., *Influence of Overweight on Health and Disease*. New York, 1951.

12. Millmore, B. K., "Diabetes Control Activities in California," *California's Health*, 9:57–60, Oct. 31, 1951.

13. National Health Assembly, *America's Health*. New York: Harper & Brothers, 1949.

14. National Office of Vital Statistics, "Estimated Number of Deaths and Death Rates for Specified Causes, United States, 1950," *Current Mortality Analysis*, 8:1–17, May, 1952.

15. Reinberg, Martin H., Paul O. Greeley, and Mary S. Littlefield, "Early Diagnosis of Diabetes Mellitus," *Journal of the American Medical Association*, 148:1177–1181, Apr. 5, 1952.

16. Wilder, Russell M., *A Primer for Diabetic Patients*. Philadelphia: W. B. Saunders Company, 1950.

17. Wright, Irving S., *Diseases of the Arteries*. New York: American Heart Association, 1950.

Popular Readings

18. American Cancer Society, 101 *Answers to Your Questions about Cancer*. New York, 1951.

19. American Cancer Society, *Who, What, Why, Where, When of Cancer*. New York, 1951.

20. Blakeslee, Alton L., "Arthritis—and the Miracle Drugs," *Public Affairs Pamphlet* 166. New York: Public Affairs Committee, 1952.

21. Crosby, Alexander L., "Your Blood Pressure and Your Arteries," *Public Affairs Pamphlet* 168. New York: Public Affairs Committee, 1951.

22. Hagman, Patricia E. (Ed.), *Good Health for You and Your Family*. New York: A. S. Barnes and Company, 1951.

23. Metropolitan Life Insurance Co., *Arthritis*. New York, 1950.

24. Metropolitan Life Insurance Co., *Your Heart*. New York, 1951.

25. Riis, Roger William, *The Truth about Smoking*. New York: Grossett & Dunlap, Inc., 1951.

26. Scheinfeld, Amram, *The New You and Heredity*. Philadelphia: J. B. Lippincott Company, 1950.

15. Understanding Depressants and Stimulants

The American public is contentedly consuming more kinds and quantities of stimulants and depressants than at any time before in its history. Right or wrong, this is undeniably an expression of a way of life during the last half of the twentieth century. Americans are heavy consumers of stimulants and depressants such as coffee, tea, cola beverages, tobacco, alcoholic beverages, and some narcotics.

A substantial number, including college students, lack either the ability or the interest to distinguish between the serviceable and the harmful commercial forms of depressants and stimulants. Some are influenced by new testimonials, advertising, and opinions of so-called "authorities" on these products. When compiled, these data become a formidable array of truth, half truth, and untruth. They either reinforce attitudes and practices already formed or increase the perplexities of those who find it difficult to discriminate.

As indicated in Chapter 2, college students consider stimulants and depressants a major concern, one of the important health factors. Also, from the point of view of interests of college students, this area ranks high. Lantagne found that this area, which he termed "habit-forming substances," was rated the first interest of college students.[1] It was even ahead of mental health and family health. The subsequent discussion is presented to assist the student in making an intelligent appraisal of the available data pertaining to the problem. The following questions are designed to aid the student in such an appraisal: (1) What are stimulants and depressants? (2) What are the properties of alcohol, tobacco, and narcotics? (3) How do these products affect the body? (4) What are the problems created by undisciplined use of these products? (5)

[1] Joseph E. Lantagne, "An Analysis of Health Interests of 1,000 Junior College Students in California," *Junior College Journal*, 21:429–433, April, 1951.

What decisions should the individual make concerning the use of stimulants and depressants?

STIMULANTS AND DEPRESSANTS DEFINED

For purposes of this discussion, depressants may be defined as substances that produce relaxation, profuse perspiration, reduced ability to move and think, and reduced action of the vital organs of the body. Acetylsalicylic acid, bromide, barbiturate, chloroform, cocaine, ethyl alcohol, ether, and opium and its derivatives are typical depressants.

Stimulants may be defined as substances that produce the opposite effect from depressants. They also serve to irritate body tissue. Nicotine,[2] caffeine, Benzedrine, tannic acid, and theobromine are typical stimulants.

However, such classification means little unless one can identify these products or substances in their commercial form. Table 12 should help to make such identification possible.

Table 12. Substances Which Depress or Stimulate

Product	*Depressant*	*Stimulant*
Brewed liquors (beer)	x	
Distilled liquors (brandy, gin, rum, whisky)	x	
Wines (dry, fortified, heavy, light, sparkling, sweet)	x	
Elixirs (cordials, *crèmes*, liqueurs)	x	
Nicotine	First stimulant, then depressant	
Acetylsalicylic acid	x	
Barbiturates	x	
Bromides	x	
Chloroform	x	
Demeral	x	
Ether	x	
Heroin	x	
Marihuana	x	
Morphine	x	
Opium and derivatives	x	
Benzedrine	...	x
Cola beverages	...	x
Cocaine	...	x
Coffee	...	x
Maté	...	x
Tea	...	x

[2] Nicotine first acts as a stimulant, then becomes a profound depressant.

In order to report the amount and kind of stimulants and depressants the American public is consuming, it will be necessary to depart, temporarily, from specifics such as those listed on Table 12 and to study four principal groups, namely:

1. Beverage alcohol (depressant).
2. Tobacco (both stimulant and depressant).
3. Narcotics (depressant).
4. Benzedrine and "stay-awake" substances (stimulants).

Beverage Alcohol

Historically, the drinking of beverage alcohol is a very old custom the origin of which is lost in antiquity. Because of the simplicity of producing a drink which caused intoxication, its first appearance probably occurred simultaneously in many parts of the world. When primitive peoples first caused grain mash, fruit mash, mare's milk, or palm-tree sap to ferment, an ingredient was discovered which became evident to the consumer and to the observer alike. It gave to the consumer temporary pleasure and to his community unhappiness. The drinker believed he had the answer to his feelings of fatigue and anxiety. His inhibitions were released. He became aggressive and delighted in fighting. As a result of this type of behavior, it became necessary to develop controls for both the manufacturing and the consumption of alcoholic beverages.[3]

Types of drinker. Haggard and Jellinek define the moderate drinker as one who does not seek intoxication and does not expose himself to it. "He uses alcoholic beverages as a condiment and for the milder sedative effects. Alcohol constitutes neither a necessity nor a considerable item in his budget."[4]

The intemperate drinker extends the limits of moderation and purposely exposes himself to the intoxicating effects inherent in alcohol. Intemperate drinkers are called inebriates. The inebriate may follow any one of four patterns of drinking, namely, normal excessive, symptomatic, stupid, and alcoholic addiction [10].

The normal (occasional) excessive drinker is motivated essentially by the feeling of well-being produced. He drinks because he enjoys it. Symptomatic drinkers are those who drink because of mental deviations. Stupid drinkers are those who drink because of low mental ability and because they cannot rise any higher in their periods of leisure. An alco-

[3] Lloyd E. Webster, lecture notes, Workshop on Alcohol Studies, Yale University.

[4] Howard W. Haggard and E. M. Jellinek, *Alcohol Explored*, p. 12. New York: Doubleday & Company, Inc., 1945.

holic addict is one who has no control over his desire for alcohol [10]. This means he is a person who cannot stop drinking. He is so frequently intoxicated that he does not lead a normal life. McCarthy classifies drinkers as occasional, frequent, regular, alcohol-dependent, and alcoholic (see Table 13).

There was a time when it was believed that the desire to drink alcoholic beverages was transmitted biologically. Today it is accepted that the desire to drink is acquired [10, 14]. Recent research studies have tried to establish a common denominator for cases of chronic alcoholism, that is, to determine whether there are similar basic physical and mental characteristics occurring frequently enough in alcoholics to identify an "alcoholic personality pattern." Buhler and LeFever [5] believe that, from a statistical standpoint, the alcoholic's inability to endure strain and tension is the most significant and consistent trait:

> The alcoholic personality appears to have the following characteristics: significantly low tension tolerance, therefore need to escape tension; low inner directivity in the sense of lack of imagination in setting up goals and insufficient motivation by such goals; instead, strong motivation by instinctual needs. While these traits are common to the alcoholic and social psychopath, discriminating characteristics are the alcoholic's critical self-awareness, guilt feelings and anxieties, and more adequate rationality and emotionality.

Consumption of alcohol. At present there are no accurate records on the total consumption of brews, distilled liquors, wines, or elixirs used in this country. The figures which are available make the record accurate only as indicated by taxes paid. The amount of home-brew and wines made for home consumption is difficult to estimate.

Out of the total population of the United States, the users of beverage alcohol who are fifteen years of age and over number approximately 65 million. Over 3 million of these are excessive drinkers. Of this group, 800,000 are chronic alcoholics. Haggard and Jellinek estimate that these 65 million persons consume 3 to 4 gallons of absolute alcohol per year [10]. The total expenditure for beverage alcohol in 1934 was $2,080,000,000. In 1949, it had risen to $8,550,000,000, according to the United States Department of Commerce. In 1953, the figure was estimated to be over $9,000,000,000.

Advertising is an important part in the program of selling alcoholic beverages. In 1945, 40 million dollars was spent to advertise beer, wine,

[5] Charlotte Buhler and D. Welty LeFever, "A Rorschach Study on the Psychological Characteristics of Alcoholics," *Quarterly Journal of Studies on Alcohol,* 8:198–260, September, 1947.

Table 13. Facts about Drinkers *

Type of drinker	*Occasion and frequency*	*Reason for drinking*	*Effects of alcohol*
I. Occasional:			
Medicinal	For minor physical ailments such as a cold or toothache	To reduce physical discomfort	Drug action like that of aspirin
Social....	Holiday or family celebration	Custom, tradition	Mild animation or gaiety
II. Frequent:			
Medicinal	Prescribed for some heart or artery ailments	To reduce physical discomfort or anxiety	Sedative action
Dietary..	With certain foods or dining occasions	Flavor	Minor increase in satisfaction with meals
Social....	Depends on number of social affairs—maybe 1 to 3 times weekly	Custom, relaxation	Mild animation or gaiety, conversational ease
III. Regular:			
Dietary..	Frequent or daily use with meals	Custom. Considered important in diet	Minor, except to increase enjoyment of food
Social....	Several times weekly or less	Considered important in social relations	Feeling of physical and psychological well-being. Mild animation or gaiety
IV. Alcohol-dependent	Daily whenever possible but not to avoid meeting responsibilities of life	Limited personal assets. To find satisfaction in drinking. To remove tension	Dulls feelings of inferiority, frustration, personal failures. Blocks possibility of emotional growth. Intoxication may occur
V. Alcoholic:			
Regular..	Frequent, sometimes daily, intoxication	Dissatisfaction with self or environment	Major changes in behavior
Periodic..	Drinking sprees at intervals		Indication of a severe emotional illness

* Raymond G. McCarthy, *Facts about Alcohol*, pp. 32–33. Chicago: Science Research Associates, Inc., 1951.

and distilled liquors over the radio and in newspapers and magazines. In 1951, this amount, including advertising over television, had risen to nearly 100 million dollars. Such figures are significant to show trends.

The Properties of Beverage Alcohol

Brewed liquors. As previously stated, if the student is to make wise decisions in matters of beverage alcohol, he should know some of the facts about its properties. Perhaps the most commonly used alcoholic beverages are the brewed liquors. This group comprises liquors such as beer, ale, porter, and stout, made from cereal grains.

Distilled liquors. Brandy, gin, rum, and whisky comprise the distilled liquors. Until 500 years ago, these drinks were unknown. To satisfy the increasing demand for a drink stronger than beer and wine, brewers developed the process of distillation, and hard liquors had their inception.

Brandy is distilled from fermented grapes or other fruits. It was probably the first of the hard liquors to be distilled. Its alcohol concentration is usually 100 proof, or 50 per cent alcohol. Gin is a colorless distillation from fermented rye. Like brandy, it is usually 100 proof. Because molasses is the base for rum making, no malt is necessary. Rum is also 100 proof. Grains such as corn, rye, or barley are used to produce whisky. Modern as well as ancient wine making results primarily from the natural fermentation of sweet fruit juices. Liqueurs, cordials, *crèmes,* and the like are the elixirs. They are sweetened alcoholic beverages.

Effects of Alcohol on the Body

Research reveals, in part, what happens when beverage alcohol is taken into the body. In spite of the fact that extensive time and effort have been allotted to the study of alcohol and its physiological effects on tissue, there are still many gaps to be filled. It is thought that alcohol passes directly from the stomach or intestines into the blood stream. It requires no digestion. A few minutes after ingestion, it can be found circulating in the blood, and it continues to circulate throughout the body until it is oxidized or eliminated by the lungs or kidneys. Once in the stomach, alcohol causes an increased flow of digestive fluids. This is probably due to the fact that it sets up a chemical action as it passes through the walls of the stomach.

Because beverage alcohol is oxidized and energy is liberated, it is sometimes classified as a food. It is, however, a misnomer to classify alcohol with such important foods as proteins, fats, carbohydrates, vitamins, and mineral salts. Its chief value is to yield approximately 7 calories per gram. It cannot create new tissue, nor can it repair broken tissue. It has no protective or regulating functions as have vitamins and minerals. Hence, alcohol should never be recommended as a food.[6]

It is not uncommon for heavy drinkers to suffer from malnutrition and constipation, probably because the drinker tends to be careless about his diet and ingests little or no roughage. Diarrhea may also result because of excessive intake of fluids or oils used in flavoring such drinks as gin.

Man does not build up an immunity to alcohol. It takes exactly the same amount of alcohol to kill a nondrinker as to kill a chronic alcoholic.

Alcohol causes small blood vessels in the skin to expand, thus permitting larger quantities of blood to flow close to the surface, creating a feeling of warmth. Much body heat may be lost. This can be dangerous to health, especially in cold weather.

It is thought that alcohol has no direct action, injurious or otherwise, on the kidneys. It does tend to increase the flow of urine, which is probably due to the action of the pituitary gland [10].

When large amounts of alcohol are ingested in a short period of time, the liver becomes enlarged and inflamed. After the alcohol is oxidized, the liver returns to its normal functioning with no apparent injury. The serious pathological conditions of the liver which are frequently found in some alcoholics are thought to be produced by malnutrition rather than by direct action of alcohol [10, 14].

Perhaps the most obvious physiological effect of alcohol is its effect on the brain. Because of the rich supply of blood flowing to that organ, alcohol reaches it rapidly and affects it markedly. For example, reaction time is lengthened; there is an obvious loss of inhibitions; the optic center is dulled, and vision is distorted; and the centers which control muscular coordination become affected. When the concentration of alcohol in the blood reaches 0.4 or 0.5, it acts as an anesthetic and causes unconsciousness. Should the concentration increase, the cardiac and respiratory centers can become affected and death may follow.

Beverage alcohol has no value in curing snake bites or head colds. It should never be used by one who is suffering from shock. Shock is primarily a state of extreme depression, and alcohol acts as a depressant; the combined effect of alcohol with a state of shock is likely to produce very serious results.

After large amounts of alcohol have been drunk, there is a definite disturbance in body chemistry. This tends to bring on what is known

[6] Lloyd E. Webster, lecture notes, Summer School on Alcohol Studies, Yale University.

as a hang-over. The chief symptoms of this state are headache, thirst, and fatigue. The headache is caused by disturbance in the liver and by impurities found in alcoholic beverages. The thirst comes from dehydration which is produced by a shifting of the water within the body cells to the extracellular areas. Fatigue probably results from loss of sleep, tensions, undernourishment, and careless living in general.

The following diseases can be brought on by excessive use of beverage alcohol:

Polyneuropathy—burning sensation in the soles of feet, pain in legs, difficulty in walking.

Wet beriberi—swelling of legs, swelling of the heart, so-called "beer heart."

Dry beriberi—excessive mental states of anxiety.

"Alcoholic" pellagra—spotty reddening of the skin. The tongue, lips, gums, and palate may take on a scarlet hue, and ulcers may develop.

Cirrhosis of the liver—increase in fibrous connective tissue.

Pneumonia—chronic alcoholics are more susceptible [10].

The following physical conditions are often associated with the use of beverage alcohol:

Tuberculosis—any association between tuberculosis and inebriety results not from direct action of alcohol but from neglect of hygienic conditions often characteristic of the families of inebriates.

Venereal disease—those who are intoxicated become irresponsible and are more frequently exposed to venereal infection.

Infant mortality—mortality of children is much higher in alcoholic families than in temperate families, in fact, nearly twice as high, probably owing to environment [10].

Feeblemindedness, epilepsy, and mental disorders—such states are more frequent in the offspring of abnormal drinkers than in the offspring of those practicing moderation or abstinence. Alcohol does not make for poor heredity, but many alcoholics come from the group which has poor heredity. The offspring inherit the defects of the parents; and the defects may predispose to alcoholism [10].

Personality and Alcohol

There is no evidence to show that an emotionally mature person, that is, one who gets on well with his fellows, who has a sense of security, who accepts responsibility, who handles his problems well, and who is interested in his position as a citizen of the community, is likely to become addicted to the use of beverage alcohol. He may drink, but the appeal is limited and alcohol is not used as an escape, nor does it become an important item in his budget [25]. There is evidence, much evidence, to show that the emotionally immature person, that is, one who does not face issues squarely, who seeks ways of escaping responsibilities, who feels insecure and lacks faith in himself, often seeks pseudo security in drinking: [7]

> He may discover that he can push his insecure feelings way off into some never-never-land if he drinks enough. Alcohol, the sedative, blurs anxieties. In fact, it can make him feel he is admired, heroic, feared—anything he'd like to be. But like any other means of escape, drinking is unsatisfactory because it prevents him from doing anything constructive about his problems. And what's more, it creates new and serious problems.

Such immature action actually puts to sleep the very forces which could be of greatest help.

In the world of science, ethyl alcohol is classified as a crude form of anesthetic [14, 18]. The physiological reactions of one undergoing anesthesia are not difficult to recognize. Because ethyl alcohol acts primarily on the brain and the central nervous system, the behavior of the individual ingesting such alcohol undergoes change. In drinking which produces a mild intoxication, there appears a wide variety of behavior changes. In prolonged drinking which produces profound intoxication, the variations are slight. Early Asiatic philosophers described it by saying:

> When the evil one gave man alcohol he added the blood of a fox, a wolf, and a pig. Thus when man takes beverage alcohol into his body and becomes mildly intoxicated, his voice is smooth like velvet, his words are soft and oily, and his eyes are sharp like the fox's. When he is well under the influence of alcohol, he becomes cruel like a wolf and when he is in the state of severe drunkenness, he becomes filthy as a pig.[8]

Modern observers are more factual and scientific in reporting behavior changes. For example, behavior common to mild intoxication may be classified as follows [10, 14]:

1. Mild intoxication.
   a. The emotional expressions are heightened and expanded.

[7] Raymond G. McCarthy, *Facts About Alcohol,* p. 37. Chicago: Research Associates, Inc., 1951.

[8] Haggard and Jellinek, *op. cit.*, p. 114.

b. The individual has a feeling of complete well-being and a notion that the time has arrived for the solution of all his problems.
c. He shows great interest in his immediate environment.
d. Motor expressions become overvigorous and he tends to be aggressive.

2. Moderately severe intoxication.
a. There is no doubt that the individual is intoxicated.
b. There is an inhibitory effect upon his senses.
c. He cannot concentrate, and his thinking is superficial.
d. He repeats over and over again a single thought (overemphasis on one idea).
e. He is incapable of using sound judgment.
f. There is a gap between his feeling of competence and his ability to perform.
g. His behavior may take a violent turn.
h. There is an obvious failure of muscle coordination.

3. Severe drunkenness.
a. The individual has lost control over thought, perception, muscular action, speech, and vision. From this stage, it is easy to pass into unconsciousness and even death.

Perhaps the most significant contribution experimental psychology has made to the studies of alcoholism is to reaffirm the conclusion that ethyl alcohol is a depressant and not a stimulant. As a depressant, it inhibits all body processes.

Much has been written on and many case studies have been made of mental diseases brought about by excessive drinking. Most authorities in the fields of psychology, sociology, and medicine agree that prolonged drinking may produce one or more of the following mental disorders [10, 14]:

1. Simple alcoholic deterioration. The important symptom is a degeneration of the ethical sense. That is, the individual shows a progressive tendency toward brutal behavior to those with whom he has the closest association.

2. Chronic alcoholic deterioration with psychosis. Chief among the symptoms are the increasing fits of rage and delusions.

3. Pathological intoxication. Pathological intoxication reactions are not commonly observed. The individual's control over his emotions has diminished to the vanishing point. Suicides are frequent among individuals in this classification.

4. Delirium tremens. This is a mental disorder occurring in about 4 per cent of compulsive drinkers. It appears to be the end result of ten to fifteen years of excessive indulgence in alcoholic beverages. The chief symptom is an in-

creasing activity of the entire body; the head, tongue, face, fingers, and legs tremble. Various types of hallucinations occur. The condition may last for as many as five days and usually is not fatal.

5. Korsakoff's psychosis. This mental disorder is characterized by failure in memory. The individual spends most of his time trying to fill in the gaps.

6. Alcoholic paranoid states. This condition, brought on by excessive drinking, is not uncommon. The chief symptom is feelings of persecution, arising from the most harmless acts of others. This state is exceedingly dangerous. Many murders have been committed by individuals suffering delusions of persecution.

7. Acute alcoholic hallucinosis. Individuals in this classification are probably showing early symptoms of schizophrenia. The drinking of beverage alcohol is largely symptomatic.

If a person drinks for a bracer, or to escape worries and troubles, or when he feels blue, or the first thing in the morning, or if he feels uncomfortable unless he has had a drink, or if he often drinks alone, it is time to call a halt and seek ways and means of controlling the practice.

Rehabilitation of Alcoholics

The first and most important move in controlling compulsive drinking is to recognize it as a problem which one cannot solve alone. The drinker must recognize the need for help, which can come from a variety of sources, namely, physicians (psychiatrists), clergymen, clinics, and through group therapy such as that offered by Alcoholics Anonymous. Alcoholics Anonymous is a comparatively new movement and a highly successful one. Its unique contribution is made when the individual adheres closely to the all-important twelve steps. These steps are:[9]

1. Admit that we were powerless over alcohol and that our lives had become unmanageable.
2. Come to believe that a Power Greater than Ourselves could restore us to sanity.
3. Make a decision to turn our will and our lives over to the care of God as we understand Him.
4. Make a searching and fearless moral inventory of ourselves.
5. Admit to God, to ourselves and to another human being the exact nature of our wrongs.
6. We are entirely ready to have God remove all these defects of character.
7. Humbly ask Him to remove our shortcomings.

[9] *Alcoholics Anonymous,* Alcoholics Anonymous Publishing, Inc., 1952.

8. Make a list of all the people we had harmed and become willing to make amends to them all.

9. Make direct amends to such people wherever possible, except when to do so would injure them or others.

10. Continue to take personal inventory and when we are wrong, promptly admit it.

11. Seek through prayer and meditation to improve our conscious contact with God as we understood Him, praying only for knowledge of His will for us and the Power to carry that out.

12. Having had a spiritual experience as the result of these steps, we try to carry this message to alcoholics, and to practice these principles in all our affairs.

A guide developed by Alcoholics Anonymous has proved highly successful in rehabilitating both men and women who want to be helped [1].

Alcohol and Traffic Accidents

Is it safe to drive after indulging in beverage alcohol? This question was asked of a group of 500 college freshmen. The answers were revealing: [10]

1. Fifteen per cent said yes, unless you are drunk. There is no reason why you cannot drive if you are careful.
2. Two per cent said one or two cocktails are OK but no more.
3. Thirty-three per cent said it is safe to drive after one has consumed two or three bottles of beer.
4. Forty per cent said let your experience be the judge. If you start to drive and find you are not sure of yourself, stop.
5. Ten per cent said if you have been drinking, don't drive.

The study was informal. Out of this group of 500, few were prepared to give a statement based on established fact. The majority expressed an opinion that they thought it was safe to drive if the indulgence in alcohol was mild. Unfortunately, the most dangerous driver on the highway is the person who takes his automobile out, believing that the small amount of alcohol he has drunk makes him a more skillful driver. The laboratory, the clinics, and the record books have proved him to be wrong. Bjerver and Goldberg, Swedish scientists, after meticulous research both on the highway and in the laboratory, concluded that the drinking of three bottles of beer having 4 per cent alcohol by volume caused a deteriora-

[10] Lloyd E. Webster, unpublished material.

tion in the driving of experienced drivers of between 25 and 30 per cent. They also reported on a test to determine the ability of the eye to distinguish a flickering light and a test to determine the blink reflex. The subjects consumed between 100 and 130 cubic centimeters of distilled spirits containing 40 per cent alcohol by volume. The result showed a deterioration of 34.2 per cent on the flicker test and 35.0 per cent on the blink-reaction test. These scientists concluded that the part played by alcohol in causing traffic accidents is greater than that which appears on official statistical records. They further concluded that the threshold of impairment of driving ability is an alcohol concentrate of 0.035 to 0.04 per cent in the blood [8].

The National Safety Council of this country believes all persons having a concentration of alcohol in the blood above 0.15 per cent to be unsafe drivers. Goodwin Joss has an interesting chart on the percentage of alcohol in the brain and the expected physiological effects thereof (see Table 14). It would appear that the zone between 0.05 to 0.15 per

Table 14. Percentage of Alcohol in Brain and Accompanying Physiological Effects *

Alcohol in brain, %	*Class*	*Physiological effects*
0.005–0.02	Trace	No noticeable effect
0.02–0.10	1 plus	Somewhat stimulated; no other noticeable effect
0.10–0.25	2 plus	Decreased inhibitions; emotional instability; some incoordination; loss of sense of care; talkative or taciturn behavior; aggressive or retiring behavior; slowing of response to stimuli and decreased reaction time
0.25–0.40	3 plus	Unstable equilibrium; disturbed senses; slurred speech and staggering gait
0.40–0.60	4 plus	Deeply intoxicated; pronounced difficulty in locomotion; alcoholic coma; death

* Goodwin Joss, "Contribution of Alcohol to Accident Fatalities in Hennepin County during a One-year Period," *Quarterly Journal of Studies on Alcohol*, March, 1947, p. 589.

cent concentration of alcohol in the blood might be considered a questionable one for safe driving. Below 0.05 per cent might be questioned only as a point on the threshold of impairment of driving ability. However, once the 0.05 per cent has been reached, the driver has probably exceeded the lowest "speed limits" for alcohol [10].

Alcohol and Crime

Ralph S. Binay,[11] psychiatrist at the Sing Sing Prison in New York State, reports a study of over 3,000 men inmates and the part alcohol played in their crime and incarceration. His report is as follows:

1. Sex crimes—alcohol as the entire cause, 22 per cent; alcohol as partial cause, 9 per cent.
2. Murder—alcohol as the entire cause, 16 per cent; alcohol as partial cause, 8 per cent.
3. Grand larceny—alcohol as the entire cause, 11 per cent; alcohol as partial cause, 5 per cent.
4. Robbery—alcohol as the entire cause, 17 per cent; alcohol as partial cause, 4 per cent.
5. Burglary—alcohol as the entire cause, 18 per cent; alcohol as partial cause, 12 per cent.

Economic Losses Caused by Beverage Alcohol

The two chief causes of arrest by police officers in the United States are traffic violations and being intoxicated in public. Over 70 per cent of the cost in maintaining the 4,000 jails in this country is for taking care of men and women who have been drinking. This amounts to 26 million dollars annually [18].

It is difficult to give an accurate estimation of the total economic losses due to alcohol. There are many factors which are not accessible for study. For example, an accurate accounting of a traffic accident must take into consideration:

1. Loss of time from job.
2. Repair of automobile or its replacement.
3. Repair to city property.
4. Cost of hospitalization and medical care.
5. Cost of litigation—insurance adjustments.
6. If there is a death, many of the items just listed, plus funeral expenses.

Because there is no central reporting, these important facts are seldom recorded. Further, there is a need for studies to determine losses which result from fires set by careless drinkers and also deaths and accidents which occur in industrial plants where alcohol is involved. Few, if any, reliable studies have been made which cover all these details. Needless

[11] Ralph S. Binay, "Alcoholism and Crime," *Quarterly Journal of Studies on Alcohol,* 3:686–716, 1942.

to say, when these studies have been made, they will show that the total sum lost because of alcohol will be huge. Spalding and Montague [18] have given a conservative estimate of $2,400,000,000 annually; probably it is much more.

Beverage Alcohol and Business

Part of an assignment to freshman men registered in a university health education course was to interview men and women who had attained leadership in motion pictures, transportation, the steel industry, department stores, the oil industry, government, law, medicine, dentistry, education, engineering, and religion. One of the twenty-five questions asked in the interview was, Of what significance is the drinking of beverage alcohol to success in your business? Between the years 1937 and 1943, 2,000 interviews were conducted. Ninety-nine per cent of these people in high positions stated that the use of beverage alcohol played no role in achieving success in their respective fields.[12]

Most businessmen make it apparent that, when one is entrusted with the responsibility of the welfare of his fellows or is in charge of precision instruments or of dangerous machinery, he does not drink—at least not on the job. Railroads do not permit drinking among their personnel while on duty. Commercial air lines make it grounds for dismissal if a pilot indulges in any form of drinking twenty-five hours before a flight.

In his lectures and discussions at the Yale School of Alcohol Studies, E. M. Jellinek emphasizes the point that industry loses heavily each year because of the drinking practices of the workers. He believes that, of the 1 million workers who are more than moderate drinkers, each is likely to lose twenty or more days annually from his job. This is a staggering loss of man-hours. It is estimated that industry would stand to gain over 1 billion dollars a year if workers who drink would avoid indulging while on the job and would control their drinking practices so that the familiar hang-over does not take its heavy toll of absenteeism.

Beverage Alcohol and the College Student

Bacon and Straus, completing a five-year study of the drinking practices of 17,000 American college youth in twenty-seven colleges, believe that 4 out of 5 college men who drink began their drinking before entering college and 65 per cent of the college women who drink began before entering college. They concluded that the probability that col-

[12] Lloyd E. Webster, unpublished study.

lege students will drink at all is closely related to the practice of their parents. Ninety per cent of the college men who drink and 83 per cent of the college women who drink came from homes where both parents drink [3].

Further, the study shows an interesting correlation between family income and drinking. For example, where the annual income is $10,000 or over, 86 per cent of the men and 79 per cent of the women drink. Where the income is under $2,500, 66 per cent of the men and 30 per cent of the women drink.

There appears to be a difference in the type of beverage most frequently used by the students answering the questionnaire. Seventy-two per cent of the men preferred beer. Forty-two per cent expressed a preference for distilled liquors, but only 21 per cent could afford to purchase them. Forty-one per cent of the college women who were studied drank beer, but only 17 per cent preferred it. The preferred drink for the woman students was wine.

In comparing veteran and nonveteran students, it was found that veterans had had more frequent and intensive drinking experiences. When age and other factors were accounted for, the veterans showed no major differences in drinking practices.

Perhaps the most striking finding of the study was the fact that customs and attitudes of college students with regard to drinking are already well determined before matriculation.

In 1950, Berezin and Roth [13] made a study of drinking among college women. A report of their summary and conclusions follows:

1. College women who do not drink had a higher average number of dates than those who do drink; and no definite association was found between drinking or not drinking and degree of attachment.

2. Religious affiliation appears to be definitely associated with drinking practices. Jewish girls were found to begin their drinking at an earlier age than did non-Jewish girls. Certain Protestant denominations were shown to have a lower drinking average than other Protestant groups. This may be related to the varying teachings about drinking in the respective churches.

3. Membership in a sorority is an effective index of drinking practices. Sorority girls drink more frequently in the course of their social engagements than do non-sorority girls. These findings require further study before any causal explanation can be suggested.

[13] F. Berezin, and Norman Roth, "Some Factors Affecting the Drinking Practices of 383 College Women in a Coeducational Institution," *Quarterly Journal of Studies on Alcohol*, 11:212–221, June, 1950.

4. Place of residence was found to be associated with the individual's choice of a setting for social engagements. Out-of-town girls drink in taverns and bars more frequently than do those whose homes are in the college town.

The college men and women who do not drink are challenged often by their colleagues to do so. They are asked to drink as a symbol of fellowship. Sometimes the appeal is to learn how to appreciate appropriate wines with food. Then again they are urged to drink at initiations. Some feel that drinking is necessary to acquire status; others drink as a symbol of rebellion against school and home authority. In spite of this wide range of motivations, there are many men and women on the campus who do not drink. Apparently they have established their fellowship and status without the benefit of alcohol.

The fact that beverage alcohol is a depressant, that it can interfere with basic nutrition, that it can produce an impressive array of physical and mental disorders, that it can cause a variety of accidents, that it contributes to much crime and unhappiness, and that it is a constant threat to efficiency and progress in industry should be sufficient reason for the college man or woman to consider its consumption wisely or to abstain. After a thorough appraisal of his own strong and weak points, his ambitions, and his objectives for living, and after an analysis of beverage alcohol and its many and varied effects, the student is in a strong position to decide what part it should play in his college living and in his life after college days are ended.

Tobacco

The smoking of tobacco is a very old practice. Archaeologists have found a variety of implements in the ruins of early cultures—English, Chinese, and Roman—which indicate that people even before the first century were using some form of mixture and implements for transmitting smoke through the nose and mouth, for the purpose of pleasure.

The present-day use of tobacco probably had its inception among the Indians of America. Early explorers of the Americas who observed the practice and returned to Europe with Indian pipes and tobacco were Captain Phillip Amardas, Captain Arthur Barlow, Sir Francis Drake, Sir John Hawkins, and Sir Walter Raleigh [18].

After 1600 the use of tobacco in Europe and elsewhere became widespread. Opponents of the new practice sprang up everywhere. Smoking was denounced by the clergy, by medical men, and finally by the rulers of England, Turkey, and Russia. King James of England issued the edict

Contre Blaste which forbade smoking. Amurath IV of Turkey prohibited the use of tobacco and sentenced all smokers to death. Michael III of Russia ordered that all men and women found guilty of smoking were to have their noses cut off. In spite of these vigorous and cruel efforts to stamp out smoking, it continued to flourish, and today, in the United States, it is estimated that 75 per cent of the men and 40 per cent of the women use tobacco in some form.

Over 3 million pounds of tobacco plants is produced annually in this country. In 1916, the American public smoked 25 billion cigarettes. In 1951, the figure had risen to 450 billion cigarettes annually. (A small decrease occurred in 1953, the first decrease in 18 years.) Increases in cigar smoking and the chewing of tobacco and the use of snuff follow a similar trend. This rapid growth in the use of tobacco and its products has been accelerated by extensive advertising. It is not unusual for a tobacco company to spend 1 million dollars annually to advertise over television and radio, in motion pictures, and in newspapers and magazines. However, much of the advertising should not be taken seriously. For example, the Federal Trade Commission [14] reports:

Scientific evidence in the record establishes that there is no significant difference in the acid in the tobacco used in the manufacture of popular brands of cigarettes or in the smoke therefrom. Furthermore, contrary to claims made in advertising, there is no difference in the effect of the acidity on the persons smoking any of the popular brands of cigarettes.

Testimony of medical witnesses, as well as reports of tests and experiments conducted by chemists, establish the fact that there is no significant difference in either the tars and resins or the nicotine in the smoke from all the leading brands of cigarettes. The testimony of medical experts also establishes the fact that the smoke from all the leading brands is irritating to the mucous membrane of the respiratory tract and that the differences in the chemical constituents of different brands of cigarettes, as shown by reports of tests, are so slight that the smoke from one brand of cigarettes is no less irritating than is the smoke from other brands.

No manufacturer attempts to remove all the nicotine from the tobacco. To do so would destroy the tobacco for commercial purposes.

The smoke from all the leading brands of cigarettes contains throat irritants "in essentially the same quantities and degree." There is no known practical process by which the nicotine, tars and resins in the tobacco leaf "may be removed or substantially reduced" without at the same time denaturing the

[14] Federal Trade Commission, *Orders* 4827, 4795 *and* 4922. Washington, 1950–1951.

tobacco and rendering it unsatisfactory for use in the manufacture of cigarettes.

In the "cease and desist" orders, the Federal Trade Commission[15] had further directed the major tobacco companies to stop claiming:

1. That smoking cigarettes encourages the flow of digestive fluids or that it aids digestion in any respect.
2. That smoking cigarettes relieves fatigue.
3. That smoking does not affect or impair the "wind" or physical condition of athletes.
4. That such cigarettes or the smoke therefrom will never harm or irritate the throat, nor leave an aftertaste.
5. That the smoke from such cigarettes is soothing, restful or comforting to the nerves, or that it protects one against nerve strain.
6. That their cigarettes are less acid than other popular brands of cigarettes.
7. That their cigarettes offer one throat protection.
8. That their cigarettes are less irritating to the throat than competing brands.
9. That their tobacco is better than and higher priced than the tobaccos used in competing brands of cigarettes.
10. That one has protection against coughing in smoking their brand.
11. That their brand of cigarettes has twice as many exclusive smokers as have all other cigarettes combined.
12. That the superiority of their particular brand is recognized by eminent medical authorities.
13. That the throats and mouths are as fresh and comfortable and the breath as pure and sweet after a day of smoking their cigarettes as in the morning.

Interest is often expressed in the effectiveness of filter-tip cigarettes. Recently, the American Medical Association conducted a series of tests to determine how much, if any, nicotine was removed from the main stream of cigarette smoke by this means. The conclusion was that "filters are responsible for removing very little of the total nicotine in the smoked portion of the cigarette. The bulk of the nicotine, about 75 per cent in the case of the 'regular' cigarette, is lost in the side stream or is destroyed by the burning coal."[16] Advertisers often claim that there is a low percentage of nicotine in the main-stream smoke if filters are used. The American Medical Association reports state that this is misleading, "that widely divergent values can be obtained from the same analytical data by choosing different bases for the calculations."[17]

[15] *Ibid.*

[16] Walter Wolman, "A Study of Cigarettes, Cigarette Smoke, and Filters," *Journal of the American Medical Association,* 152:917–920, July 4, 1953.

[17] *Ibid.*

Why People Smoke

In spite of the fact that tobacco can become a sizable item in the budget, that it may be a contributing factor in the cause of serious physical ailments, and that it can become a fire hazard, millions of people smoke, with thousands of new converts springing up each year. Finnegan [18] summarizes the reasons for this popularity as follows:

1. Nicotine craving.
2. Optical perception of the smoke.
3. Agreeable smell and taste.
4. Manipulation and sucking of cigar or cigarette somewhat resembling the influence of the nipple on the infant.
5. Pleasurable irritation of the laryngeal and tracheal sensory branches of the pneumogastric nerve.
6. Relief of tension.
7. Stimulation.
8. Sociability.
9. Gives people something to do.
10. Permits one to do "nothing" gracefully.
11. Satisfies a desire or craving.
12. Sense of "grown-upness."
13. Feeling of self-confidence.
14. Pyromania.
15. Pleasure.

Once the practice of using tobacco has been established, it is difficult to stop. This was attested to during World War II by the long lines in front of stores selling a limited supply of cigarettes. Arutzen [2] observed the strength of the practice or habit among the Germans during 1946–1947. At that time tobacco was rationed; men were allowed forty cigarettes a month, and women were allowed twenty. In order to obtain something to smoke, the majority of men and women preferred to go without food in order to have money to buy cigarettes.

Why People Do Not Smoke

Not all people smoke. Throughout the country perhaps 60 per cent of the adult women and 25 per cent of the adult men do not smoke. Their reasons are: [19]

[18] J. K. Finnegan, "The Role of Nicotine in the Cigarette Habit," *Science*, 102:94, July 27, 1945.

[19] Laurence E. Morehouse, University of Southern California, unpublished material.

1. Education (knowledge of harmful effects).
2. Religion (contrary to church doctrines).
3. Expensive.
4. Fire hazard.
5. Lack of desire.

The Effects of Smoking on Health

It is difficult to prove that smoking brings about any permanent change in one's well-being. In the case of beverage alcohol, the social and physical reaction can be readily observed. In the case of tobacco, one may have to resort to the laboratory to determine what, if any, action substances within the tobacco plant have on the body.

The chief toxic element resulting from combustion or burning of tobacco is nicotine. It is an oily substance and is poisonous. There is enough nicotine in one cigar to cause quick death to an adult should he receive the full concentrated dose into his circulatory system. Tobacco smoke contains not only nicotine but carbon monoxide, pyridine bases (collidine, a strong irritant), hydrocyanic acid, and ammonia. When absorbed into the body through the smoke, nicotine first stimulates the cerebrum and autonomic nervous system and then acts as a depressant. Beginning smokers and those who have smoked too heavily at any one time may suffer dizziness, nausea, diarrhea, and, in some cases, excitement and insomnia.

Pyridine bases are local irritants. Hydrocyanic acid interferes with the normal oxidation process in body tissue. Ammonia is a local irritant. Carbon monoxide, having a high affinity for hemoglobin of the blood, can interfere seriously with blood oxygenation. The amount of nicotine and its companion substances in tobacco smoke varies. For example, no two cigarettes in the same brand contain the same amount of nicotine. This is due to variations in the soil and methods of processing the leaf. The so-called "denicotinized" cigarette made from tobacco leaves is largely a myth. At present, there is no satisfactory method of substantially reducing nicotine and at the same time maintaining a high quality of tobacco for the manufacturing of cigarettes.

The amount of by-products which enter the body in smoking depends upon several factors, namely, the size of the cigarette, the pack of tobacco within a given cigarette, dryness of the tobacco, and the rate at which the cigarette is smoked. The shorter and thicker the cigarette, the more nicotine passes out with the inhaled smoke. The looser the tobacco within the cigarette, the more available becomes the nicotine. The drier the tobacco, the greater the amount of nicotine. The faster the cigarette is smoked, the greater the amount of nicotine.

Tobacco smoke taken into the mouth deposits its substances on the mucous membrane lining of the nose, mouth, and throat for absorption into the blood stream. When smoke is inhaled, the coverage is large and absorption of nicotine may be as much as ten times greater than when the individual does not inhale. A cigarette smoked down to the butt end gives a higher percentage of nicotine than one discarded earlier.

There is no scientific evidence to support the belief that cigarette paper contains substances which are harmful to the body.

Many scientists have tried to determine whether there is any relationship between efficiency of animal tissue and the use of tobacco. Most agree that some change takes place when tissue is exposed to the by-products of burning tobacco. However, this change varies with the sensitivity of the individual to tobacco smoke. It is also possible that an immunity to the effects of tobacco may gradually be acquired if the practice of smoking persists. Following are some of the reactions to smoking which have been accepted by those investigating in the field [11]:

1. Membranes of the throat show varying degrees of inflammation. Scientists agree on the irritability but have not as yet identified the specific which causes this reaction.
2. Heart rate and blood pressure increase markedly in some individuals and but slightly in others.
3. Vasoconstriction of the peripheral blood vessels shows marked individual difference. A decrease in skin temperature, particularly of the toes and fingers, has been recorded.
4. Heavy smoking interferes with good nutrition. Cutting down or eliminating tobacco results in a return of normal appetite and proper nutrition.
5. Smoking may increase gastric acidity. Individuals with stomach ulcers should not smoke.
6. Except in childhood, there is little statistical evidence to show that smoking interferes with one's height and weight. It appears that heavy smoking has an adverse effect on longevity.
7. In many people, the metabolic rate is increased by smoking.
8. Smoking tends to bring a rise in respiratory rates.
9. Smoking tends to bring about a drop in external body temperature and an increase in internal body temperature.
10. The taste threshold tends to rise rapidly after smoking. This is probably transient.

Tobacco smoking and physical performance. For many years tobacco smoking has been considered to have a definite effect on athletic performance. It has been reported recently that the exact knowledge of the effect of tobacco on athletic performances is inadequate. Much more research is needed on this problem. However, two series of experiments with subjects performing on a bicycle ergometer showed that abstinence from smoking for one week caused improvement in tobacco-sensitive subjects and had no effect on nonsensitive ones. Since a relatively large proportion of an athletic team may consist of tobacco-sensitive men, the nonsmoking rule is a wise precaution.[20] The effect of tobacco smoking on physical performance may depend on individual differences to the extent that no uniform effects can be shown. Future studies will no doubt be made on this problem.

Tobacco and Lung Cancer

Another point which is being investigated is the role of tobacco in the rapidly increasing incidence of lung cancer. At present there is evidence to show that smoking tobacco contributes to the cause of lung cancer. Wynder,[21] writing in the *New England Journal of Medicine,* states:

> There is, . . . strong evidence that the great increase in the incidence of lung cancer can be explained largely by the use of tobacco—in particular, of cigarettes. The following points may be brought forth:
>
> It is rare for a nonsmoking male to develop epidermoid or undifferentiated cancer of the lungs. Among 760 male lung cancer cases, 1.4 per cent were nonsmokers compared to 14.6 per cent among 780 controls. Doll and Hill found 2 nonsmokers among 649 male lung cancer cases. In countries where the consumption of tobacco is low, the incidence of lung cancer is also low (Iceland).
>
> The lung cancer patients smoked significantly more than the average population. Of 760 male patients with lung cancer 51.3 per cent smoked more than one pack of cigarettes a day for at least twenty years, compared to 19.1 per cent of 780 controls. Doll and Hill's data have shown that the likelihood of a person's developing cancer of the lungs increases with the amount of tobacco smoked.
>
> The present-day sex ratio corresponds well to the long-term smoking habits of the two sexes. About 95 per cent of lung cancer patients had smoked for at least twenty years, 85 per cent for more than thirty years. A very few females in the cancer age have smoked for this length of time.

[20] Peter V. Karpovich and C. J. Hale, "Tobacco Smoking and Physical Performance," *Journal of Applied Physiology,* 3:573–636, April, 1951.

[21] Ernest L. Wynder, M.D., "Some Practical Aspects of Cancer Prevention," *New England Journal of Medicine,* vol. 246, Mar. 27, 1952.

Lester Breslow [22] observes that there is a growing belief among medical personnel in a positive correlation betwen lung cancer and cigarette smoking. Edgar Mayer, a medical authority, believes there is a possibility that smoking plays an important part in causing cancer of the lungs. In a recent address before the Los Angeles County Medical Association, he pointed out that in New York City there has been a 400 per cent increase in lung cancer since 1920.[23] Other authorities believe that there is a possibility that heavy smoking may be one of many factors causing lung cancer. Still others feel that too few cases have been studied to draw any sweeping conclusions at this time.

After a careful perusal of all the points just discussed, plus any additional information which can be found in the references at the end of the chapter or in current research material, the college student is in an excellent position to decide what he should do about using tobacco, whether he should start smoking, or cut down on his daily consumption, or eliminate the practice entirely.

Depressant Drugs

In discussing the use of beverage alcohol and tobacco, it is important to appraise all the scientific facts faithfully, so that the millions of consumers of these products, as well as those who abstain, can be accurately informed of their effects. This is even more important in the case of habit-forming drugs, whose use is governed by law. Public opinion vigorously opposes the use of these drugs except as prescribed by the medical profession. At present the law in most states is so strict that even physicians are not granted a free hand in writing prescriptions for them.

Depressant drugs act on the central nervous system and in turn affect all the physiological processes of the body. They have no curative value. They are used primarily for purposes of escape, such as relief from pain, unpleasant memories, insomnia, etc.

The "painkillers," or analgesics, include such drugs as alkalizers, aspirin, and Anacin. The hypnotic drugs, or sedatives, are used essentially to induce sleep (barbituric acid) [12, 18]. Any drug which produces stupor or sleep and at the same time relieves pain is a narcotic. Cocaine and opium and its derivatives are typical of the narcotic class.

[22] Lester Breslow, M.D., "Does Cigarette Smoking Cause Lung Cancer?" *California's Health,* July 15, 1951.

[23] Edgar Mayer, M.D. An address before the Fourth Annual Chest Disease Symposium, Los Angeles County Medical Association, Jan. 22, 1953.

The analgesics, or painkillers, are probably the least harmful. However, prolonged use may result in unfavorable physical symptoms as well as in delaying the proper treatment until it may be too late.

Barbituric acid. The barbiturates should be used only upon the prescription and counsel of a reputable physician. In the home, the source should be carefully controlled by a responsible member of the family who is not using them. The fact that, in 1940, 70 tons of the salts of barbituric acid was manufactured in the United States and that by 1950 the figure had risen to 300 tons is evidence that a portion of the American public should take a serious look at their mental and social well-being. Why has there been such a great increase, and why is the tonnage figure still climbing? It is apparent that people are using an easy, quick, and readily available method of reducing the conscious activity of the brain. The situation is a reflection of widespread tension, fear, and social unrest which preclude relaxation and sleep. Until individuals who depend upon sleeping pills can make satisfying adjustments without the aid of a "crutch" and can gain control over themselves and their environment and its attendant problems, the consumption of salts of barbituric acid will continue to rise.

Barbituric acid compounds are taken in either capsule or pill form. Upon prescription, they may be purchased under a variety of names, such as Sodium Amytal, Allonal, barbital, phenobarbital, Seconal, Nembutal, Tuinal, and Veronal. When a reputable physician prescribes one of these compounds, he does so for a specific purpose and usually permits only two to twelve capsules or pills per prescription. Once the prescription has been completed, it cannot be refilled. This is in accordance with recent legislation, which is observed in all states in the Union. However, this law is broken many times by addicts who appeal to unscrupulous physicians or who make their purchases on the black market.

The danger in using barbiturates lies in both long-continued use and in overdosing. If a person lacks self-control and wants an easy escape into sleep, he resorts to a sleeping pill. If he is an addict, he uses a pill each time he feels nervous or uncomfortable. Such undisciplined action can produce serious physical and mental conditions. An overdose can result in death. The deaths attributed to accidental or purposeful overdosing have increased during the past few years. It is unwise to have a bottle containing sleeping pills adjacent to one's bed. It is better to have sleeping pills controlled by someone in the family who is not using them and administered according to prescription by this same individual.

Marihuana. Marihuana is a renegade hypnotic drug. It has been outlawed by both medicine and law. Its action on the body is unpredictable. Swallowing a small amount of the smoke may leave one person unaffected but may produce serious personality changes in another. Marihuana is one of the oldest of the drugs used for narcotic purposes. Ancient history records the use of hemp plants (hashish) in Arabia and in Persia. Over 4,000 years ago, Persian outlaw bands were given hashish when their raids called for rashness and cruelty. These criminals were known as hashish users, or *hashshashin* [12]. The English word "assassin," meaning "killer," stems from this term.

By the year 1545, the hemp plant was being grown in Brazil primarily for the purposes of making rope. Soon the Brazilians began smoking the dried tops of the hemp plant. This practice spread north, and before 1600 it was widespread among the Indians of Mexico. It was here that the plant became known as marihuana [12]. By 1920, marihuana smoking had spread farther to the north, and for the first time the American public became aware that it was being used in this country. The practice became so widespread that by 1937 the Marihuana Act was passed by the United States Congress. This act forbids the importing, manufacturing, producing, compounding, selling, prescribing, administering, or giving away of marihuana in any form, including the seeds.

As previously stated, the effect of marihuana on the individual is unpredictable. Some can smoke it without apparent reaction; to others, it may become a drug leading to heroin addiction. It is not difficult to recognize someone who has recently been smoking marihuana. Usually the eyes are bloodshot, the speech is rapid and high-pitched, the breath has an odor of marihuana (it is sometimes said that marihuana smells like musty hay), and the throat will be so dry it may be difficult to expectorate.

Swallowing the smoke may produce a reaction which highly distorts the senses. Time, space, and movement are confused. For example, in attempting to ride a motorcycle, one is quite likely to turn a corner while still in the middle of the block. One may step out of a second- or third-story window thinking that the street is only a few inches below him. One may kill a member of his family or his friend on an uncontrolled impulse. The marihuana smoker is usually a maladjusted individual and needs psychiatric help.

Marihuana has no legal, medical, or social standing. To grow the plant, to have a bush in one's yard, to have a single seed of a marihuana plant in an automobile or on one's person is a felony. It can be bought wherever the peddler chooses to sell it, which is often in a pool hall, malt shop, drive-in, or shoe-shining parlor.

Perhaps the most sinister problem in relation to marihuana smoking is that it serves as a stepping stone to the use of heroin.

Heroin. Heroin, a habit-forming drug, is a morphine derivative (diacetylmorphine). It is a white, bitter crystalline powder. At one time it was used by physicians as a sedative. Today, it is illegal to use it or to manufacture it.

Those using heroin either sniff it or inject it into the blood stream. The effects are similar to those of morphine. The individual finds himself greatly elated. He loses his sense of pain. He forgets unpleasantness and for a few hours appears to be at peace with the world. As soon as the body fluids have neutralized the heroin, which takes between three to six hours, the addict is in need of another shot. An addict of a year's standing or more requires between $25 to $75 a day to satisfy his desires. Heroin is sold illegally in 1-grain capsules, usually at $5 a grain.

Addiction to heroin often follows closely upon the repeated use of marihuana and is a rapid and vicious process. Within a few weeks, one can become a full-fledged addict—a "main liner." Placing the needle into a large vein of the arm gives a fast, jolting reaction. Usually the first four or five shots cause illness. It is at this point that the individual is most susceptible to efforts to turn him away from the drug. After two to four weeks of injections, the body builds up a tolerance, and the desire or ability to stop is lost. When an addict is deprived of the drug, he suffers the agonies of withdrawal pains. They are very real and are caused by dehydration of the body. The only temporary release is another shot.

The heroin addict is a pitiful specimen. His face has a gray pallor. He is restless, nervous, and suffers auditory and visual hallucinations. He is constipated and malnourished. His appetite for food is unstable. He is a sick person—mentally, morally, and physically.

There are two Federal government hospitals in the United States where drug addicts are treated. They are located at Fort Worth, Tex., and Lexington, Ky. The personnel of these hospitals believe a high percentage of the patients can be cured [26]. The rest of the unfortunates are incurable. One of the great dangers accompanying the so-called cure is that it takes only one shot to put the "cured individual" back on the addict list.

The number of heroin addicts under twenty-one years of age who have been admitted to the Federal government hospitals for treatment rose over 2,000 per cent between 1947 and 1950. In June, 1951, there were

139 boys and 19 girls undergoing treatment in these institutions. Thirty-eight of the patients were white, and 120 were Negroes. Eighty-seven were from New York, 24 from Chicago, 15 from Washington, D.C., and 32 from other parts of the United States [26].

Other habit-forming drugs. Barbituric acid, marihuana, and heroin were given prominence in this chapter because they form the bulk of habit-forming drugs being used by young people today.

Opium and its derivatives are a menace to the health of the American people but are not used to the same extent as are barbituric acid and marihuana. Opium comes from the *Papaver somniferum* poppy. It has many useful functions in medicine. Its illegal use, however, has brought nothing but suffering and great harm to mankind. The chief alkaloid from opium is morphine, from which codeine and heroin are derived. Codeine's chief use is in medicine, and it is not considered important as a habit-forming drug. It is a white crystalline alkaloid and is used as a substitute for morphine.

Cocaine is a crystalline alkaloid, methyl benzol ecgonine. It is made from coca leaves. Pizarro, in 1537, was the first to note its effects as he observed the Indians of South America chewing coca leaves. By 1855, cocaine had been extracted from the coca leaf by German scientists. Its chief use in the United States is for local anesthetics. Because it is habit-forming, science has developed two powerful non-habit-forming drugs which are taking its place—novocaine and procaine.

Stimulants in Modern Society

Research gives no dictum on stimulants such as Benzedrine, cola beverages, coffee, and tea. Findings relative to the effects these products have on the human body are considered as trends in research data and not as final evidence.

Caffeine. The stimulant which is common to cola, coffee, tea, and maté is caffeine. In most cases of normal indulgence, caffeine tends to retard fatigue and aids in rapid recovery from "that tired feeling." As yet, science has not produced evidence to show that moderate ingestion of drinks containing caffeine is harmful to the normal adult.

The United States Navy, Office of Naval Research, collaborating with Tufts College, Institute for Applied Experimental Psychology, has gathered together interesting research data about the effects of caffeine on physiological functions. This study [7] shows that in the matter of:

1. Circulation—the pulse is increased 5 to 10 per cent thirty minutes after drinking coffee. Blood pressure is increased about 5 per cent.

2. Respiration—there is little or no effect on the rate of respiration.

3. Sleep—1 to 4 grains of caffeine has no appreciable effect on the sleep of most normal people. Five to six grains produces a marked disturbance in the sleep of most individuals.

4. Temperature—caffeine has little effect on body temperature.

5. Diuresis—before tolerance of caffeine has been developed, there is a marked increase in the amount of urine.

6. General well-being—4 or more grains of caffeine can produce dizziness, a feeling of numbness, headache, indigestion, diarrhea or constipation, and irritability in many people.

7. Motor effect—caffeine usually increases motor response.

8. Sensory effects—it is believed that sensory responses are favorably affected.

9. Higher mental processes—small amounts of caffeine, that is, under 4 grains, have a more favorable effect on mental processes than do large amounts.

It appears from the foregoing data that small amounts of caffeine cause but slight reactions in normal individuals. However, large amounts of caffeine may produce unfavorable reactions such as indigestion, heartburn, dizziness, headache, irritability, insomnia, numbness of extremities, and peripheral coldness [11]. It has been found that drinks containing caffeine taken on an empty stomach or late in the evening have more general effects than if taken in the forenoon or with food in the stomach [11].

Benzedrine. There is a belief among some college students that the taking of Benzedrine pills results in greater physical and mental efficiency. The facts as reported by research studies [11] are:

1. Benzedrine has more effect on lightweight people than those of heavier build.

2. Women are more likely than men to be stimulated by Benzedrine.

3. Benzedrine produces a rapid rise in blood pressure.

4. There is a 9 per cent increase in respiratory rates.

5. Motor processes are stimulated, with an accompanying feeling of reduced fatigue.

6. Visual acuity is enhanced; however, hearing will not be affected.

7. Higher mental processes are not affected.

8. After ingesting Benzedrine, some individuals will have an increased feeling of "pep" and well-being, while others may be depressed and become dizzy.

9. The normal person is likely to be wakeful, with no desire to sleep, after taking Benzedrine pills.

It is unwise for the college student to resort to drugs in any form to obtain high grades. Scholastic achievement is likely to be better when a balance is established between periods of work, rest, relaxation, recreation, and sleep. Add to that wholesome food, and one possesses a success formula superior to any known concoction of pharmaceutical skill.

Summary

Stimulant and depressant drugs are used universally. Beverage alcohol is consumed because of custom and tradition, for purposes of relaxation and reducing physical discomforts, for its pleasant taste, and from a desire to escape from problems.

Tobacco is used to give pleasure through smell and taste, to relieve tension, for sociability, stimulation, etc.

Science finds that an excessive use of stimulants and depressants in any form is harmful to the body.

Suggested Activities

1. Compile arguments in favor of and opposed to (*a*) moderation in the use of beverage alcohol; (*b*) total abstinence.
2. Compile data showing the trend in the use of beverage alcohol, tobacco, and sleeping pills by the American public. List reasons for such trends.
3. Discuss the physical, social, mental, and economic results when alcohol and tobacco are used intemperately.
4. Compile arguments gathered from your associates indicating why they drink or smoke or why they abstain.
5. Report on an interview with the police department covering such questions as: (*a*) Has there been an increase or decrease during the past year in traffic accidents caused by drunken driving? (*b*) What means are used to determine the extent to which a driver is under the influence of alcohol? (*c*) What is the law governing driving when intoxicated? (*d*) What does the police department recommend for the cutting down of accidents due to drunken driving?
6. Report on an interview with a psychiatrist or a superintendent of a mental hospital on: (*a*) relationships between the use of beverage alcohol and mental illness; (*b*) types of psychosis which can result from the use of alcohol; (*c*) the prognosis of a psychosis caused by abnormal drinking.
7. Study the laws in your state governing the manufacture and sale of intoxicating beverages. How is the tax revenue from such sales used?
8. Discuss reasons why people use tobacco or do not use it.
9. Cite recent research studies showing the effects of tobacco on performance, length of life, and health.
10. Interview a prominent obstetrician on the question, should women stop smoking during pregnancy and lactation?
11. Why do some people show signs of nausea, dizziness, and headache after smoking for the first time? Discuss.

12. Interview a prominent dentist, and ask him whether or not there is any relationship between mouth health and the use of tobacco.

13. Suggest ways by which a person can break himself of the practice of smoking. Refer to Chapter 5 for suggestions on breaking a habit.

14. State reasons why the smoking of marihuana is a dangerous practice.

15. What are the laws in your state governing the possession of and use of narcotics?

16. Interview a narcotics agent on the use of heroin, its distribution, its methods of use, its effects on the body, how one becomes an addict, and the possibilities of a cure.

17. Report on the two Federal hospitals which treat narcotic addicts and discuss the methods used to effect cures.

18. View and discuss the following films: (*a*) *Problem Drinkers* (sound, 18 minutes), available from Text-Film Department, McGraw-Hill; (*b*) *I Am an Alcoholic* (sound, 16 minutes), available from Text-Film Department, McGraw-Hill; (*c*) *Alcoholism* (sound, 22 minutes), Encyclopaedia Britannica, 1952; (*d*) *No Smoking* (sound, 10 minutes), Sid David Production, 1952; (*e*) *Drug Addiction* (sound, 22 minutes), Encyclopaedia Britannica, 1952.

Suggested Readings

1. Alcoholics Anonymous, *An Interpretation of the Twelve Steps of the Alcoholics Anonymous Program.* Minneapolis: Coll-Webb Co., 1952.

2. Arutzen, F. I., "Some Psychological Aspects of Nicotinism," *American Journal of Psychology,* July, 1948, Vol. 61.

3. Bacon, Selden, and Robert Straus, *Drinking in College.* New Haven: Yale University Press, 1953.

4. Bacon, Selden, and Robert Straus, "Alcoholism and Social Stability," *Quarterly Journal of Studies on Alcohol,* 12:231–259, 1951.

5. Benay, Ralph S., "Alcoholism and Crime," *Quarterly Journal of Studies on Alcohol,* 3:686–716, 1942.

6. Berezin, F., and Norman Roth, "Some Factors Affecting the Drinking Practices of 383 College Women in a Coeducational Institution," *Quarterly Journal of Studies on Alcohol,* 11:219–220, June, 1950.

7. Buhler, C., and D. W. LeFever, "A Rorschach Study on the Psychological Characteristics of Alcoholics," *Quarterly Journal of Studies on Alcohol,* September, 1947.

8. Bjerver, K., and Leonard Goldberg, "Effects of Alcohol Ingestion on Driving Ability," *Quarterly Journal of Studies on Alcohol,* 1:1–20, March, 1950.

9. Grigg, Walter H., "Prevention and Control of Addiction to Narcotics," *American Journal of Public Health,* October, 1952.

10. Haggard, Howard W., and E. M. Jellinek, *Alcohol Explored,* New York: Doubleday & Company, Inc., 1945.

11. *Handbook of Human Engineering Data for Design Engineers.* Tufts Institute for Applied Experimental Psychology, 1949.

12. Hesse, Erich, *Narcotics and Drug Addiction.* New York: Philosophical Library, Inc., 1946.

13. Lemere, Frederick, and W. L. Voegtlin, "An Evaluation of the Aversion Treatment of Alcoholism," *Quarterly Journal of Studies on Alcohol,* 2:199–204, June, 1952.

14. Quarterly Journal of Studies on Alcohol, *Alcohol, Science and Society.* New Haven, 1945.

15. Reeves, W. E., and L. E. Morehouse, "The Acute Effect of Smoking upon the Physical Performance of Habitual Smokers," *Research Quarterly,* 21: 245–248, October, 1950.

16. Rice, Thurman, and R. N. Harger, *Effects of Alcoholic Drinks, Tobacco, Sedatives, Narcotics.* Chicago: Wheeler Publishing Company, 1949.

17. Riley, John W., C. F. Marden, and Marcia Lipshitz, "The Motivational Pattern of Drinking," *Quarterly Journal of Studies on Alcohol,* 3:353–362, December, 1948.

18. Spaulding, Willard, and John R. Montague, *Alcohol and Human Affairs.* Yonkers, N.Y.: World Book Company, 1949.

19. Secretariat, Department of Social Affairs, United Nations, *Bulletin on Narcotics,* Vol. 1, October, 1949.

20. Williams, Jesse F., *Alcohol—The Study of a Current Problem.* Sacramento: California State Department of Education, 1953.

21. Williams, Roger J., *Nutrition and Alcoholism.* Norman, Okla.: University of Oklahoma Press, 1951.

22. Wolman, Walter, "A Study of Cigarettes, Cigarette Smoke and Filters," *Journal of the American Medical Association,* 150:917–920, July 4, 1953.

Popular Readings

23. Anderson, Dwight, *The Other Side of the Bottle.* New York: A. A. Wyn, Inc., 1950.

24. Hecht, Carol A., Ruth J. Grine, and Sally E. Rothrock, "The Drinking and Dating Habits of 336 College Women in a Coeducational Institution," *Quarterly Journal of Studies on Alcohol,* 2:252–258, September, 1948.

25. McCarthy, R. G., *Facts about Alcohol.* Chicago: Science Research Associates, Inc., 1951.

26. Vogel, Victor H., "Our Youth and Narcotics," *Today's Health,* October, 1951.

PART SIX

Effective Living in the Community

16. Living Safely in a Community

Most people have a deep affection and sincere loyalty for their "home town" regardless of its size or fame. It is a great thrill to be away from home, especially at the other end of the country, and meet someone from the home town; immediately a strong bond is established. A similar loyalty exists for one's home state. No matter where a person moves later in life, the home state where he grew up remains the best state in all of the United States.

Next to individual loyalties such as those for parents, sweethearts, wives, and husbands are those pertaining to groups. This is true also of larger groups making up a community, a state, and a nation. For example, during World War II several thousand men volunteered to work on battle-damaged ships in the Navy Yard at Pearl Harbor, Honolulu. Though they lived together in large housing areas in comfortable quarters and were furnished an extraordinary recreation program in terms of a variety of activities and fine equipment, they were nevertheless not happy. After a few months one recreation leader thought of organizing them into groups according to some natural common bond. Hence state clubs were formed, representing almost every state in the Union, from Maine to Texas and from Florida to Washington. It was not long before the men were happier on the job, enjoyed more thoroughly their leisure time, were engaged in civic enterprises in a new land, and were showing eagerness to make their housing area a better place in which to live.

National loyalties are even stronger. Citizens of the United States are positive that no land compares with theirs, symbolized by the Statue of Liberty. Canadians argue that their part of North America is superior to any other land. Across the sea the British Isles are home to the English; and it is difficult, if not impossible, to dispute 20 million or more Frenchmen when they extol the wonders of their native land. These individual and group loyalties are the result of the personal experiences of the individual interacting in his own environment. They represent the individual's interest in his community, both small and large.

What Is a Community?

Most people today live in a community, if the word "community" is used in its broadest sense to mean a group of people living in a given area under the same unit of government. As such the community may be a neighborhood, a rural district, a small town, a city, the state, and even the country. More specifically, a community is a group of people living together in a particular area who have organized to meet common interests and problems.

Regardless of the size of the area, the word "community" implies the idea of shared purposes among its people. In a democracy, a person living in a community has certain civic responsibilities as well as responsibilities to himself personally. This idea is in keeping with the present-day health philosophy that health is both an individual and a group responsibility.

Health and Safe Living in a Community

The definition of health with its safe-living implications stated in Chapter 1 emphasizes the point that the individual has the opportunity and the responsibility to help shape his environment. Reference was made to the fact that the student's health potential is multiplied when he joins a group endeavor in the interest of a safer and more healthful community. Effective living in society implies that the individual makes a contribution to society. This means that he functions best when he is working for a cause greater than himself. Improving community health and safety are some of these great causes. They too are public functions. No longer is it thought that professional groups, such as physicians, dentists, educators, engineers, and others, alone can give health and safety to the public. Just as the individual earns his health status by the way he uses his innate capacities and participates in life activities, so does the public, through its individual and cooperative effort, assist in determining the health and safety of the community.

Where does the college-age group stand in the matter of safe living in the community? From the record book comes a fact that is disturbing. The age group fifteen to twenty-four leads all others in number of automobile accidents, fatal and otherwise. One could deduce from this fact that many college men and women have set aside the philosophy of safe living while motoring and have substituted the philosophy of greater freedom—freedom to do what seems to give the most pleasure. Looking back, one finds that the primary objective of the founding fathers of this country was the right to greater freedom. However, this was freedom to think, to believe, and to move according to one's inner sense of values. Two hundred years have brought no basic change in this early concept, only a different emphasis on making life more secure and more rewarding. There was a time when this freedom and security of life depended largely on native resistance to disease, skilled use of weapons, fleetness of limb, and keenness of eye. This was the versatility of the individual in a physical setting. Today, security of life, including the freedom to act, to worship, to think for oneself, depends less on somatic strength and skills and more on tolerance, motivation, constructive skills, and education. This is the versatility of the individual in a social setting. Once man lived independently apart from his fellows and close to dangers inherent in the world of water, sky, forest, and earth. Today he has harnessed these natural destructive forces for his increased security and richness of living. Out of these forces he has created new implements, new vehicles, and new weapons, many of which are now becoming threats to his security.

At one time education for security was a matter of mastering a few fundamental practices in a simple environment. Today, education for living safely accepts these practices merely as points of departure and goes further. It picks up significant strands in the areas of commerce, industry, farming, traffic, homemaking, sports, conservation, and law. It weaves these into a positive pattern of safety, of security which becomes a strong protective and creative force for all, a force which not only makes individual and community life more secure but helps to give it scope, depth, and meaning. Man has always lived with danger. However, to make danger his ally and to exchange needless risks and poor adventure for adventure with proper controls is the modern concept of safe living [11].

To ensure an understanding and appreciation of living safely, an insight into present-day safety education, and a knowledge of how to do something about the problems of safety, both on the campus and in the community, the student in health education should be able to discuss intelligently such questions as: (1) What are the significant problems in safety education and how are they determined? (2) Do one's attitudes and practices influence his safety behavior? If so, how? (3) What are some of the effective ways of teaching safety education to adults? (4) If society is to develop ways and means of preventing accidents and death, how can accident facts and statistical information help? (5) What are some of the causes of accidents and accidental death? (6) What can the college student do to prevent accidents? (7) What information should the college student have about first aid to the sick and injured? (8) How important is it for the student to carry accident insurance?

Safety Problems

Problems of safety in the year 1754 and problems of safety today have about as much in common as have the respective modes of living and mores of people then and now. When a man became drunk two centuries ago, the chief danger to society was a personal one, that is, injury or death to the individual. Today the drunken pedestrian, the drunken driver, the drunken smoker, pilot, engineer, factory worker, inspector, physician, lawyer, politician, or diplomat not only runs the risk of limiting or destroying his own rights, security, and freedom but also endangers the well-being of his fellows.

Intoxication from beverage alcohol in the world of work or play is perhaps the first major problem in safety education. The college student should not have to learn this the "hard way." (For a more detailed discussion, see Chapter 15, Understanding Depressants and Stimulants.)

The daily carnage along city streets and open highways presents a second major problem. It stems from the speed and ease with which America travels to and from business and pleasure. It is expressed in the annual death of 35,000 to 38,000 people killed and over 1 million injured in automobile accidents. Preventing these accidents and saving lives is as much a problem for the student as for the specialists in safety.

Accidents occurring in the home, on the farm, or at school contribute a third major problem. Twenty-nine thousand to 35,000 people die and over 4 million are injured each year from home accidents. There are relatively few accidental deaths on the college campus. However, each school does have an impressive record of painful injuries, a high percentage of which are preventable. Accidents occurring on the farm account for over 13,000 fatalities and over 1 million injured annually [9]. The prevention of these accidents and deaths is primarily a matter of eliminating environmental dangers and of educating careless or ignorant individuals.

A fourth problem in safety deals with fire. More than 10,000 people die each year in fires the great majority of which are preventable [9]. Twenty per cent of these casualties are children. The greatest cause of death by fire is carelessness. The best ally for prevention is safety education and an alert adult population.

A fifth major problem in safe living is concerned with accidents in industry. Many students will enter industry upon graduation, and they should know that there has been a substantial decline in the frequency of industrial accidents since 1930 [9]. This has occurred in spite of the fact that thousands of inexperienced men and women were employed during the war years. Much of the credit for this decline can be given to sound safety practices encouraged by labor and management alike. However, there are still between 17,000 and 18,000 occupational deaths and over 2 million occupational injuries each year [9]. Again, prevention is not merely eliminating danger but creating an emotional climate and environment which produce a happier and more efficient workman, that is, one who takes pride in a job safely done, who is educated in the skills of his trade, who knows and observes common safety practices, and who willingly participates in the planning of safety rules.

Safety Attitudes and Practices

There is no single cause for accidents, nor is there a single cure. Mechanical and personal failures, physical conditions of the environment, and emotional instability are of prime significance. In this discussion, accidents due to personal factors will receive the greatest emphasis. From accident reports, research studies, and observation comes a fact which sheds light on at least one primary cause of accidents—emotional instability.

Instability, emotional or otherwise, is often a factor in poor judgment and subsequent accidents and is a common characteristic of the immature adult. Usually such a person is one who resents change and whose knowledge of facts does not always result in sound behavior. His likes and dislikes are based on emotion. He can be counted upon to make unrealistic and unwise adjustments to his environment. He may possess the strength, power, and position of an adult, but all too often these forces are employed to satisfy unstable emotional urges. Behind the wheel of an automobile he can quickly become a class A force for destruction.

It was Demosthenes who remarked that it is impossible to have wholesome attitudes toward one's fellow men while one is engaged in planning "petty and mean employment" [18]. This ancient adage illustrates an attitudinal principle which can be applied to the problem of modern accidents. When one is angry, tense, worried, or hilarious, he is in no mood to act with care or courtesy.

Safe living, whether in the home, on the farm, on the playing field, in the factory, or any other part of the community, requires mature control of emotions, thoughts, and actions. If accidents due to unstable control are to be prevented, studies such as those conducted by Weinerman [13], Arbous [3], Dunbar [5], and the Center for Safety Education at New York University should be reviewed carefully. These studies and others point the way to a better understanding of why the unstable, the immature, and the social and emotional malcontents, as well as those with physical anomalies, are the accident repeaters and accident-prone individuals.

Safety Education

There is little need to speculate on the importance of education as a factor in controlling and preventing accidents. It has been shown repeatedly that where there is cooperative action in safety education, whether it be in school, community, home, or industry, an improved record of accident prevention has been achieved [11].

Education has at least three unique teaching opportunities which have a significant bearing on the prevention of accidents: (1) cooperation in all its aspects; (2) the assuming of civic responsibilities; (3) developing a creative attitude [19]. These three need not be confined to the course in health education but can be employed with great profit throughout the total curriculum. For example, authorities in safety education agree that a safety rule or a safe environment cooperatively planned has great potential strength. This is the democratic way of putting purposeful action to practical ends.

Some time ago a large university campus was bisected by a busy city street. Numerous accidents occurred. Some were fatal. During a discussion of the situation in a health education class it was determined to make a critical study of the problem. After two weeks of day and evening observations by students and faculty, facts were assembled and presented to the proper authorities. The result was a permanent closing of the street and the prevention of further accidents and possible death. The study required the cooperative efforts of students, professors, president, board of trustees of the university, and city-government officials. It was a cooperative venture, and the university and community at large shared in the profit. Cooperation need not be confined to the campus. The student who believes in safety, both for himself and others, cooperates with authorities and his associates in his community, during activities at the beach and swimming pool, on hunting or fishing trips, at the theater, on the highway, in fact, everywhere he goes. He is willing to assume the role of a responsible citizen whether he is under authority or acting under his own control.

The study of political science and allied subjects presents a unique opportunity for broadening the student's concept of government and for

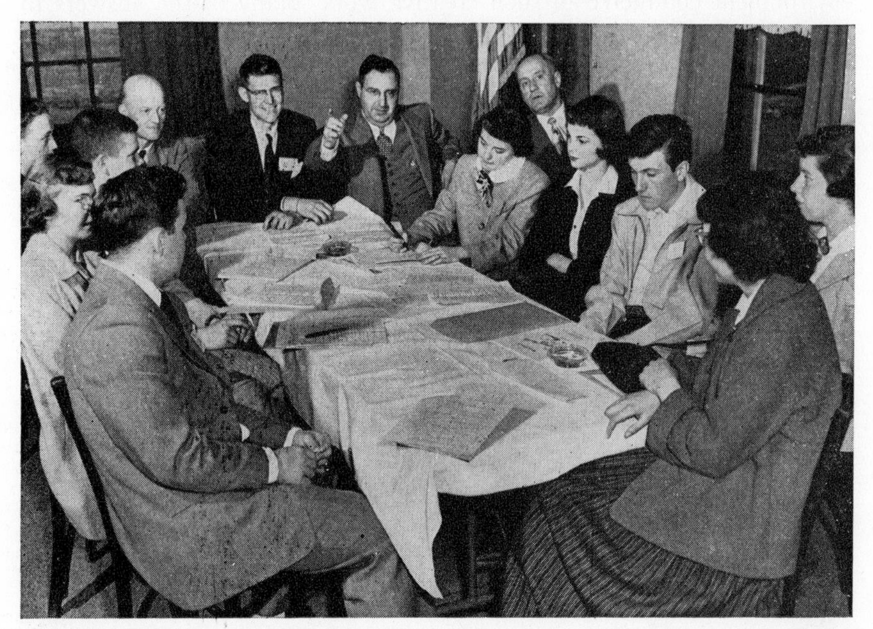

Fig. 16.1. Community planning with student representation is important to living safely. (*Racine County Safety Council, Racine, Wis.*)

creating a feeling of pride in and responsibility for a safe environment in his community. It is a worthy extension of these courses when students and others become actively interested in keeping the immediate environment safe. They also may express their interest by calling attention to safety hazards in the community and by working for rules, city ordinances, and state and national laws which both eliminate hazards and widen areas for safe living.

The essence of creativeness is freedom—freedom to think, to feel, and to move according to one's sense of values and the compulsion of both extrinsic and intrinsic disciplines. Too often the word "creative" has been reserved for the fields of literature and the fine arts. It is commendable when one originates a work that adds to the culture and pleasure of his fellow men. Likewise it is commendable when one originates a plan or constructs a vehicle or machine which breaks through the barriers of routine and imitation and gives to the community a safer and freer way to make a living and to spend leisure time. For example, it was a young college student who conceived the idea of equipping all four wheels of an automobile with brakes. Another developed the small light reflectors one finds on most highway curves. The college student moves in an environment conducive to such creative work, Many of the answers to the five major problems in safety, and the factors which contribute to them, lie somewhere within the scope of creative effort.

Accident Facts

The National Safety Council, with headquarters in Chicago, is a reliable source of information on accident facts. Its prediction of the number of people who will be killed and injured over certain holidays or week ends is familiar to all. These predictions are based on statistical evidence covering many years of research. Each year the council gathers data on accidents and accidental deaths from national, state, and local agencies. These data are classified and published in an annual report called *Accident Facts.* It is significant to note that a recent edition opens with an editorial on the number of lives saved, not of those destroyed.

Instead of showing the number of people killed in accidents through the year, Figure 16.2 shows the number who were not killed, that is, the

Table 15. Death and Injury Rates, 1953 *

All accidents:	
Deaths	One every 5 minutes
Injuries	One every 3 seconds
Motor vehicle:	
Deaths	One every 14 minutes
Injuries	One every 23 seconds
Occupational:	
Deaths	One every 35 minutes
Injuries	One every 16 seconds
Workers off job:	
Deaths	One every 15 minutes
Injuries	One every 12 seconds
Home:	
Deaths	One every 18 minutes
Injuries	One every 7 seconds
Public non-motor-vehicle:	
Deaths	One every 32 minutes
Injuries	One every 15 seconds

* Data from National Safety Council.

number who were saved from accidental death by an organized attack on this social problem.

From 1900 until 1913, the year of the formal organization of the safety movement, an average of nearly 75,000 persons per year were killed in accidents—a rate of eighty-five deaths per 100,000 population. If this rate had prevailed in the following year, 1914, the accidental death toll would have reached 84,000. But the rate was reduced to seventy-nine, and the death toll

THEY DIDN'T DIE

The chart below is a different kind of a chart. Instead of showing the number of people killed in accidents through the years, it shows the number who were not killed — the number who were saved from accidental death by the organized attack on this social problem.

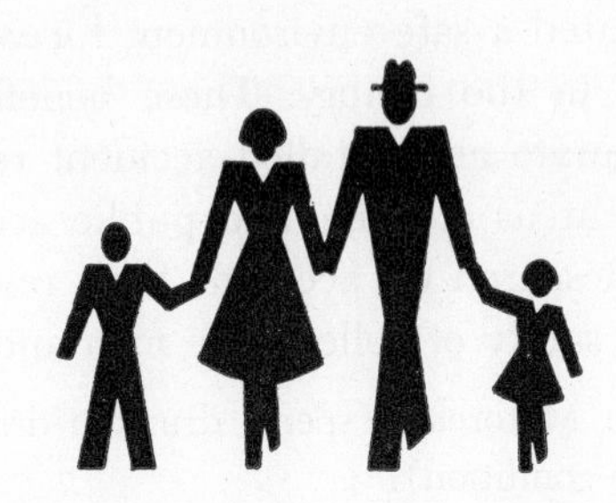

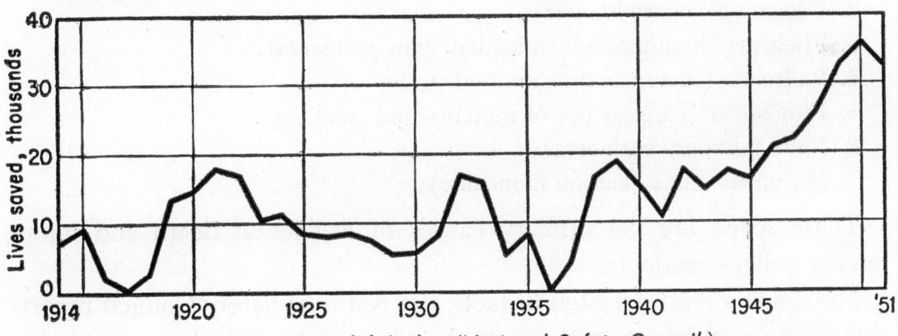

Fig. 16.2. They didn't die. (*National Safety Council.*)

was only 77,000, a saving of about 7,000 lives. Similar comparisons based on the rates for succeeding years are plotted on the chart, and accumulate to a total of about 500,000 lives by 1951.[1]

In view of the fact that nearly 100,000 accidental deaths and over 9 million injuries occur each year, such a positive statement is both unique and challenging. Even this large death and injury figure is not discouraging when one realizes that both active and potential causes of accidents have greatly increased in scope, while the mortality rate remains constant. These facts help to give encouragement to those interested in living safely.

Accident facts, accurately compiled, can be useful not only in determining the cause of accidents but in giving important leads toward

[1] National Safety Council, *Accident Facts,* p. 2. Chicago, 1952.

accident prevention. For example, recent records show that industrial accidents have been greatly reduced since 1935. This reduction was in part the result of many years of keeping accurate accident records and then doing something about them. Each accident was investigated and recorded. Through the years an immense amount of statistical information was compiled. With these data at their command, employer and employee, government agent and safety educator, working together, brought about much-needed safety legislation, installed safe machinery, created a safe environment for working, and adopted rules for safe living in the factory. These beneficial changes had their beginnings in accurate and detailed accident reporting. Similar studies are needed in the areas of home and public accidents.

Research on accident facts reveals the following as major threats to the safety of college-age men and women [9]:

1. Motorcars (speed, drunken driving, drivers falling asleep, vehicle in unsafe condition).
2. Drowning (nonswimmers).
3. Firearms (hunting and "unloaded" gun accidents).
4. Railroads (motorcar collision with trains).
5. Fire burns (careless use of matches and smoking).
6. Falls (slippery surfaces).
7. Poisonous gases (carbon monoxide).

These seven are the primary causes of accidental death and injury among college students.

For the student interested in facts, the National Safety Council reports that while a 10-minute safety speech is being given, 2 persons probably will be killed and 180 injured. The costs will amount to $165,000.

Causes and Prevention of Accidents

In explaining the cause of a poor grade to his father, a college freshman began his explanation, "Well, Dad, it was this way. I . . . etc., etc." After patiently listening to the lengthy defense, the father interrupted by remarking, "Now, son, what was the real cause?" All too often the basic cause of accidents is obscured by lengthy rationalization. For every accident there is a fundamental cause, and until that cause is discovered and corrected, accidents and their multiple "reasons" will continue to fill the record books. (See Table 16.)

Determining the cause of accidents by place and related data is simplified when a program of adequate reporting is in force. Developing preventive measures is slower and more difficult.

Table 16. Causes and Prevention of Accidents *

Causes	*Prevention*
Occupational Accidents	
Mechanical (manual skills):	
Occur most frequently when employee is handling objects, working with machinery, working with vehicles, or using hand tools or falls on slippery surfaces or from heights	Less likely to occur when employee is adequately trained and proficient in skills of his trade and is protected from dangers, including falls
Personal:	
Likely to occur when employee is fatigued or ill, is upset emotionally, disobeys safety rules, has physical disabilities, is maladjusted socially, is ignorant of job to be done, or lacks recreational skills	Less likely to occur if employee has adequate psychological counseling and medical services, receives precise preemployment screening by personnel office, practices sound discipline both on and off job, helps plan rules of safety, understands requirements of job, and has opportunity to engage in wholesome recreational programs
Traffic Accidents	
Mechanical (manual skills):	
Occur most frequently when motor vehicles collide with pedestrians, with each other, or with trains, street cars, animals, or fixed objects, overturn, or run off highway	Less likely to occur if operator of motor vehicle possesses up-to-date license to drive, knows and obeys traffic regulations of state and community, respects rights of others, and is skillful in operating vehicle
Personal:	
Likely to occur when pedestrian or operator of vehicle, or both, are under influence of alcohol, fatigued, sleepy, careless, discourteous, upset emotionally, or ignorant of traffic regulations or have serious physical disabilities	Less likely to occur if pedestrian and vehicle operator keep off highway when under influence of alcohol and when physically, mentally, or emotionally incapable of good judgment
Aquatic Accidents	
Mechanical (manual skills):	
Likely to occur when one falls out of boat or canoe and is unable to swim, collides with objects in water, dives or steps into unknown depths, lacks adequate training in water-rescue techniques, or lacks skill in handling boat or canoe	Less likely to occur if one is skilled in handling boats and canoes, knows skills of swimming and diving, knows where these skills can be practiced safely, and is trained in techniques of water rescue
Personal:	
Likely to occur when one is overfatigued or under influence of alcoholic beverages, becomes frightened while swimming, ignores safety rules, or has uncompensated physical disabilities	Less likely to occur if one stays out of water when overfatigued or when one has been drinking alcoholic beverages, obeys rules established for safety, recognizes physical strengths or handicaps, and stays within safe limits while swimming, diving, or boating

Table 16. Causes and Prevention of Accidents (*Continued*)

Causes	*Prevention*
	Home Accidents
	(Firearms)
Mechanical (manual skills):	
Most likely to occur when one lacks skill in handling a gun (cleaning, pointing, etc.) or knowledge of correct ways to handle a gun while hunting	Less likely to occur if one possesses skill in handling firearms (cleaning, shooting, etc.) and never points a gun at another person when on a hunting trip or elsewhere
Personal:	
Likely to occur when one leaves an unused gun loaded, is upset emotionally, is careless in handling a gun, is ignorant of or disregards laws of his state governing hunting, or uses firearms while under influence of beverage alcohol	Less likely to occur if one makes sure unused firearms are left unloaded, never looks down barrel of a gun, never lets snow get into muzzle of gun, never gets into an automobile with loaded gun, never moves about in boat with loaded gun, understands regulations governing hunting in his state, and avoids using firearms when under influence of beverage alcohol
	(Burns)
Mechanical (manual skills):	
Likely to occur when one smokes in bed or while lying down, is careless or ignorant of safe manner of handling fireworks, or lacks skill and understanding of safe ways to handle inflammables	Less likely to occur if one does not smoke in bed or while lying down, if only skilled operators are permitted to handle fireworks, and if there is skilled and safe use of inflammables
Personal:	
Likely to occur when an individual working with fire or inflammable chemicals is overfatigued, has been drinking beverage alcohol, is upset emotionally, or is careless about an open fire	Less likely to occur if smokers who are intoxicated are kept under supervision, if proper safeguards are used around open fires, and if there is constant protection of children against misuse of fire or inflammable materials
	(Falls)
Mechanical (manual skills):	
Most likely to occur when good housekeeping techniques are lacking, floors are slippery, passageways and stairs are poorly lighted, or an unstable support is used in reaching for high places	Less likely to occur if good housekeeping techniques are practiced, floors and stairs are not slippery, all passageways are kept free from articles, steps are in good repair, steady hand rails are available on stairways, ladders and other articles used for climbing to high places are made secure and are appropriate for bearing desired weight, and white line is painted on top and bottom steps

Table 16. Causes and Prevention of Accidents (*Continued*)

Causes	*Prevention*
(Falls, *cont.*)	
Personal:	
Likely to occur when one is careless or lacks proper safety attitudes, is intoxicated, or is not alert to environmental hazards	Less likely to occur if one has proper safety attitudes, if intoxicated persons are kept under control, and if members of household receive sound instruction on home safety
(Poisonous Gases)	
Mechanical (manual skills):	
Likely to occur when gas appliances are defective, when gas heaters are burning with windows of room closed, when coal-burning furnace is defective, when carbon monoxide is not permitted safe escape, or when one searches for gas leaks with lighted match or candle	Less likely to occur if all heating and cooking appliances are correctly installed and inspected regularly, if room heated by gas has fresh supply of oxygen, and if flashlight is used when searching for gas leaks
Personal:	
Likely to occur when there is carelessness or ignorance about safe heating and cooking facilities in house, about importance of fresh air in room heated by gas, or about importance of protecting against fatal monoxide gas or when one is careless in determining source of gas leakage or is overfatigued or intoxicated and unable to use gas appliances properly	Less likely to occur if members of household receive adequate instruction on safe use of all gas appliances and individuals realize dangers of carbon monoxide (as in working on running motor with garage door closed)
School-Campus Accidents	
Mechanical (manual skills):	
May occur in physical education program when pupils engaged in body-contact sports and games use improper and unsafe equipment or play on slippery surfaces or in unprotected and unsafe areas May occur in shops, laboratories, and classrooms when pupils are not properly instructed in use of hand tools, fast-moving machinery, explosives, and other dangerous chemicals	Less likely to occur if there is proper instruction in skills, if adequate and safe equipment is used, if playing areas are made safe, if there is intelligent supervision of all physical activities, if proper instruction and supervision in use of dangerous equipment is provided in all shops, laboratories, and classrooms, and if dangerous machinery and chemicals are properly safeguarded.
Personal:	
May occur in physical education program when pupil lacks game and sport skills, is overtense, has uncompensated bodily disabilities, is overfatigued or careless, or uses inadequate or unsafe equipment	Less likely to occur if there is adequate medical examination and counseling of all students, if recreation program is provided for entire student body, and if pupils are properly instructed in the skills and safe-

Table 16. Causes and Prevention of Accidents (*Continued*)

Causes	*Prevention*
School-Campus Accidents (*cont.*)	
May occur in shops, laboratories, and classrooms when pupil lacks skill and understanding about proper use of assigned materials and equipment, fails to exercise proper safeguards while working with dangerous materials, or is fatigued or sleepy	guards necessary for safe use of dangerous equipment in shops, laboratories, and classrooms.

* Data from National Safety Council, *Accident Facts* (annual publication); and H. J. Stack, F. B. Siebrecht, and J. D. Elkow, *Education for Safe Living*. New York: Prentice-Hall, Inc., 1951.

Authorities in safety education agree that the majority of accidents involve persons who are emotionally unstable, socially maladjusted, selfish, or careless or who have some physical anomaly. When to one or more of these conditions is added excessive speed, inattention, poor judgment, discourtesy, intoxication, or fatigue, there is likely to be an accident.

One must not lose sight of the fact that the prevention of accidents under supervision is easier and probably more effective than it is without supervision. In other words, it is easier to prevent an accident in a controlled environment such as a school, a factory, or a patrolled highway than in the home, where the individual is king and is acting under his own orders.

The problem of accident prevention, then, must take all these facts into consideration. Prevention that saves lives as well as provides for safe living becomes a matter of raising a generation of healthy people [3] and of providing them with adequate laws on safety, sound safetv engineering, and purposeful safety education [17].

Safety in Recreation and Sports

The concept of safety can be so well integrated with the recreation and sports program that players are seldom conscious of safety per se. For example, in baseball, dropping the bat as one starts for first base is as easy to learn as hurling it to the right or to the left. Protecting oneself while tackling or being tackled in football is as easy as are undisciplined movements. Leaving a game before one is overfatigued can be taught as a safe and correct form of participation. Learning to fall without injury is a desirable skill and is applicable to all sports. By a thorough understanding of what to do and what to avoid, by using only acceptable equipment, by seeking the advice of skilled leaders, by staying within the limits of one's ability, by maintaining a sound physical body, and by avoiding hazardous playing conditions, one can make safety so much a part of participation that it is thought of only when its absence is apparent.

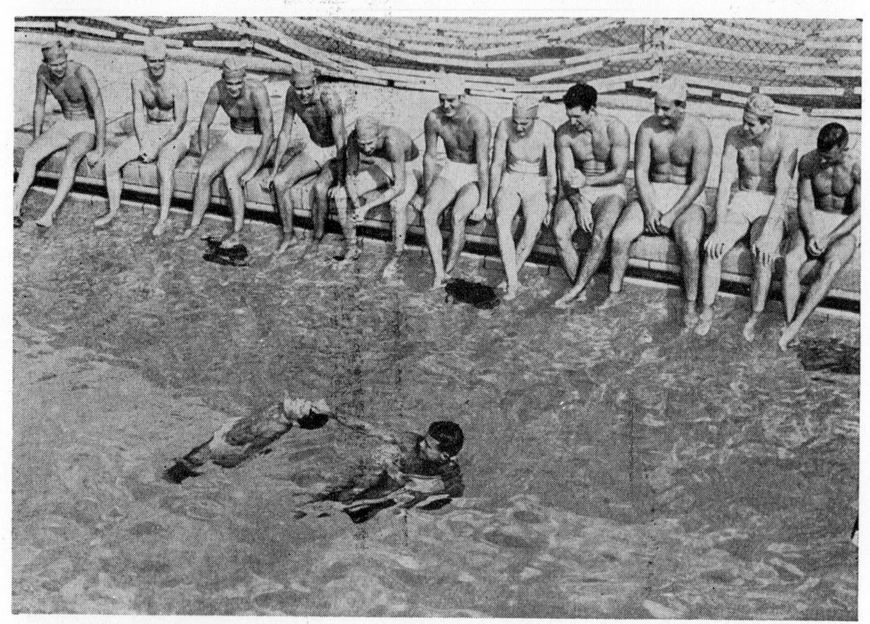

Fig. 16.3. Lives can be saved when people are adequately prepared for emergencies. (*Photo by Lee Hansen.*)

Stack, Siebrecht, and Elkow summarize safety procedures for participation of sports as follows: [2]

1. Proper player equipment.
2. Safe space facilities.
3. Adequate conditioning and training of all participants.
4. Adequate knowledge of proper procedure for all activities.
5. Sufficient skill for performing the activity.
6. Equal competition and adequate reserve strength.
7. Adequate officiating.
8. First aid in case of injury and follow-up for all injuries.
9. Athletic injury insurance.
10. Formulating an individual code of safe conduct for sports participation (by the students under the guidance of the instructor).

[2] H. J. Stack, E. B. Siebrecht, and J. D. Elkow, *Education for Safe Living,* p. 116. New York: Prentice-Hall, Inc., 1951.

Fire Prevention

Over 10,000 people die each year by fire, and of this number 300 are in the college-age group [9]. A regrettable factor is that most of these deaths result from careless use of fire, and carelessness is a preventable cause. Fatality and accidents by fire could become unimportant items in causes of death if users of matches and tobacco and others would faithfully practice the following:

1. Avoid smoking in bed, or when sleepy, or while lying down.
2. Put out every live cigarette or cigar butt before discarding it.
3. Always break a match in half before throwing it away.
4. Keep intoxicated smokers under constant surveillance.
5. Keep matches in covered containers, inaccessible to children and rodents.
6. Avoid carrying loose matches in clothing.
7. Safeguard young children against fire at all times.

Pouring kerosene or gasoline on an open fire; standing too close to an open fireplace or gas heater, or looking for the source of a gas leakage or determining the amount of gasoline in the tank with a lighted match may result in serious, even fatal, burns.

The number of accidents and deaths among college students because of fire is statistically insignificant. Most fatal fires and serious burns involve young children. The fact that children are the chief victims is a challenge to adults to accept the responsibility of providing a safe environment for children and to educate them in the wise use of fire.

First Aid

Rendering first aid to the sick and injured is one way of recognizing the importance of the human personality. When a child or an adult has an accident and receives an injury, those first on the scene, whether stranger or friend, stop to render aid. Sometimes the assistance is good, and sometimes it is unwise. For many years organizations such as the American Red Cross have been instructing people in the proper methods of first aid. A complete and comprehensive understanding of first aid to the sick and injured can be obtained by studying the *American Red Cross First Aid Textbook* or by enrolling in the first-aid classes taught by the American Red Cross.

During World War II, the adult civilian population of this country stormed the American Red Cross for instruction in first aid. This proved most beneficial. Where a chapter formerly gave a few hundred first-aid

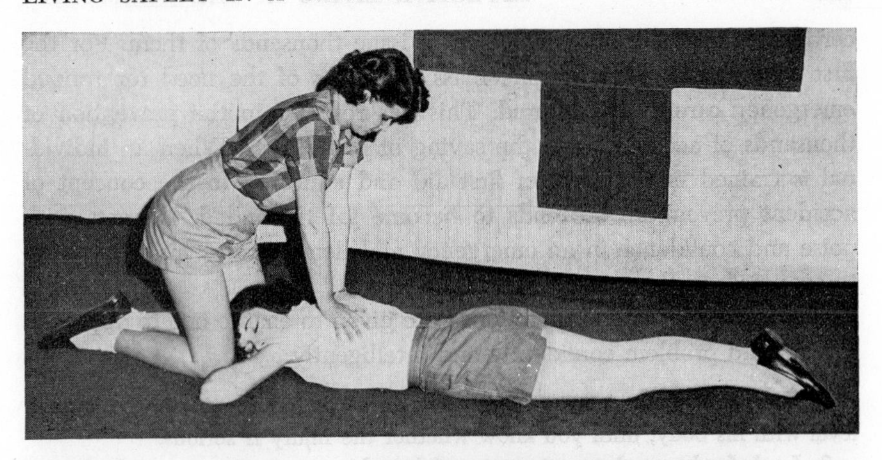

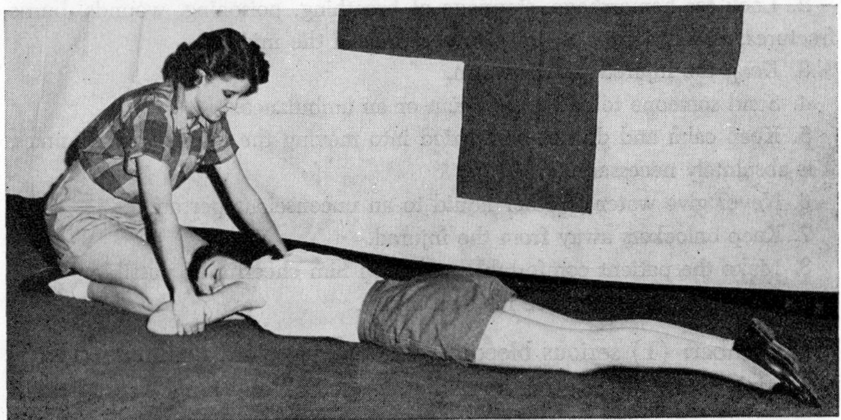

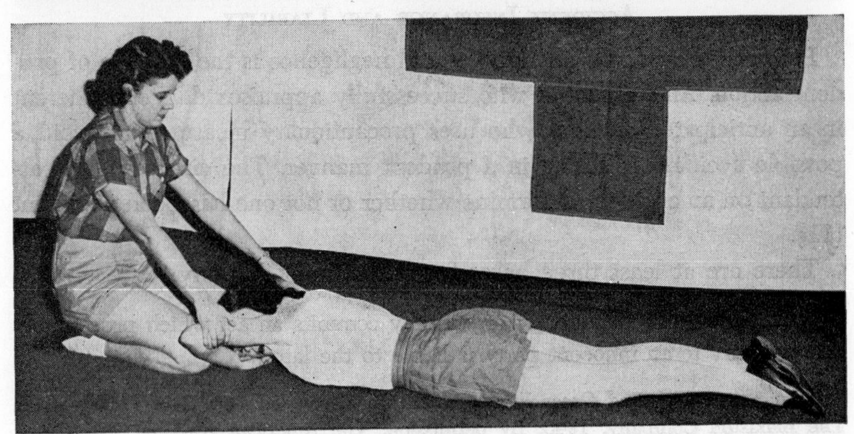

Figs. 16.4, 16.5, and 16.6. Correct technique for executing the back-pressure–arm-lift method of artificial respiration, recently adopted by the American National Red Cross. (*American Red Cross.*)

certificates annually, it soon began to issue thousands of them. For the first time this country became mass conscious of the need for trained emergency care of the injured. This has resulted in the prevention of thousands of accidents and the saving of many lives. When an individual is trained in the skills of first aid and educated to the concept of accident prevention, he tends to become safety-minded. He acts with poise and confidence in an emergency and demonstrates his willingness to cooperate in the area of living safely.

The following general directions [3] are given to enable one to approach the first-aid problem confidently and intelligently:

1. Keep the injured person lying down in a comfortable position, his head level with his body, until you know whether the injury is serious.
2. Look for hemorrhage, stoppage of breathing, poisoning, wounds, burns, fractures, and dislocations. Be sure you find all the injuries.
3. Keep the injured person warm.
4. Send someone to call a physician or an ambulance.
5. Keep calm and do not be hurried into moving the injured person unless it is absolutely necessary.
6. Never give water or other liquid to an unconscious person.
7. Keep onlookers away from the injured.
8. Make the patient comfortable and keep him cheerful, if possible.
9. Don't let the patient see his own injury.

Remember: (1) serious bleeding, (2) stoppage of breathing, and (3) poisoning must be treated immediately before anything else is done.

Accident Insurance and Liability

Liability is based on negligence, and negligence is the absence of prudent action. An individual who successfully appraises dangers inherent in an anticipated act and who uses precautionary measures to avoid a possible accident is acting in a prudent manner. The circumstances attendant on an accident determine whether or not one has been negligent [11].

There are at least three bases for determining liability: [4]

1. A person who negligently or willfully commits an act which proximately causes injury to an innocent party is liable to the latter.

[3] From *American Red Cross First Aid Textbook,* rev. ed., pp. 2–6. Philadelphia: The Blakiston Company, 1945. By permission, The American National Red Cross, Washington.

[4] Suggested by the general counsel of the Automobile Club of Southern California, 1953.

2. In the event a person injured by the negligence of another is likewise guilty of negligence contributing to his injury, such injured person cannot recover.

3. In the event there is no negligence on the part of any person for the injury of a particular person, the latter has no right of recovery.

Whereas the aim of safety education is to prevent or reduce accidents, it is the part of wisdom to be protected against possible liability action resulting from accidents. This can be done by carrying liability insurance.

From the point of view of the college student who drives an automobile, carrying automobile liability insurance is a necessity. Such a policy provides insurance, subject to policy agreement, conditions, and exclusions, against claims arising from accidents resulting from ownership, maintenance, or use of the insured automobile.

If one multiplies the actual cost of protection by his life expectancy, the total will in all probability not be as large as the amount of an average judgment against him. The fee for an attorney to represent one in a damage suit is likely to exceed the amount of the premium which he would pay for several years. In short, a judgment rendered against a defendant, plus attorney's fees, could prove an economic disaster to both himself and his family. Few college-student drivers of automobiles can afford to take this risk. It may be of interest to the college group to know that automobile insurance rates are much higher for those under twenty-five than for older persons. This is due in part to the high accident rate incurred by the fifteen- to twenty-four-year age group. The record shows that this group has the highest number of (1) collisions between motor vehicles, (2) collision with railroad trains, (3) collisions with fixed objects, and (4) noncollision accidents such as overturning and running off the highway.

Realizing the importance of carrying liability and accident insurance, many states are making it compulsory for all drivers of automobiles to have this protection.

Civilian Defense

During the summer of 1953 the USSR was reported to possess not only the atomic bomb but the hydrogen bomb as well. This fact was given wide publicity. It served to stimulate an increased interest in national and local civilian defense. As early as 1945, the Federal government began setting up a pattern of civil defense and encouraged states and local groups to establish appropriate legislation for the organization of defense and disaster relief. This has been done, and in most communities there are at least ten major volunteer services which students can join:

1. *Warden service.* To prepare citizens for emergencies and offer leadership in case of attack.
2. *Fire service.* To teach householders how to fight fires in the emergency.
3. *Police service.* To assist local police in controlling traffic, etc., and maintaining law and order.

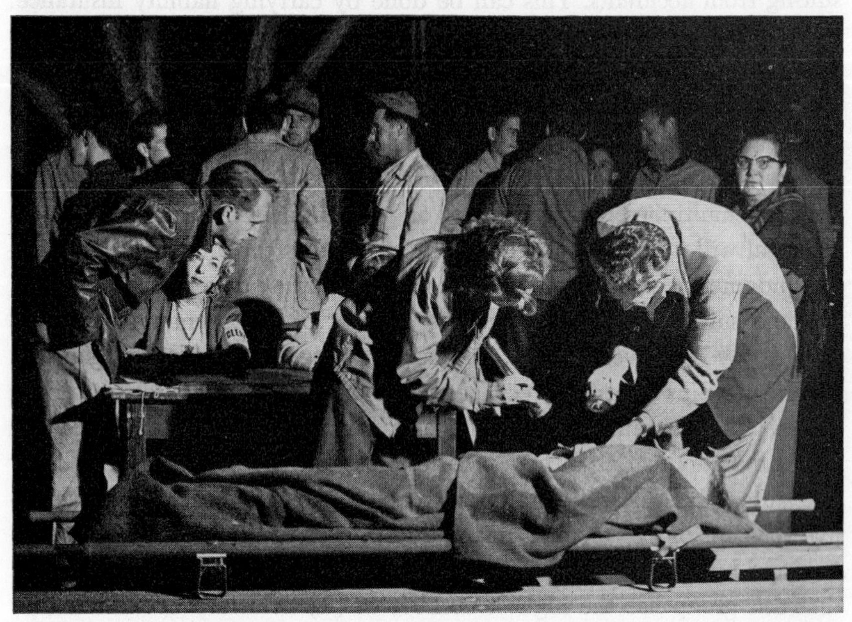

Fig. 16.7. A civil defense "dry run." First-aid-station registration and medical examination for determination of next step in treatment. (*Los Angeles City Health Department.*)

4. *Health service.* To assist in first aid, transport the wounded, repair equipment, and prevent radiological contamination.
5. *Welfare service.* To provide housing, food, clothing, and money and to assist in locating missing persons.
6. *Engineering service.* To restore damaged installations and clear away debris after an attack.
7. *Rescue service.* To rescue trapped persons.
8. *Transportation service.* To move the injured and also food and medical supplies.
9. *Staff service.* To keep records, send out printed materials and letters, do typing, and operate switchboards.
10. *Communication service.* To communicate through radio, television, telegraph, and telephone.

Civilian defense is a vital link in total defense. It is the cooperative effort of the community to withstand emergency and disaster. It is a necessary function of safe living in the community and the nation.

Summary

Learning to live safely is one of our major college and community problems.

Safety educators and safety engineers will continue to have a difficult time preventing accidents, saving lives, and extending the scope of safe living until the public is fully aroused. It is essential to influence people to (1) assume the role of responsible citizens; (2) cooperate with authorities and others in upholding the law; and (3) work to make the home, school, community, factory, and highway safe places for all.

Suggested Activities

1. Work out a sociodrama depicting "making danger an ally and exchanging needless risks and poor adventure for adventure with proper controls."
2. Discuss the causes and prevention of any one of the five major problems in reference to accidental death as they affect the college student.
3. Make a study of accidents in your college or in your community. Point out cases resulting from emotional instability.
4. Pick one of the three suggested methods of safety education, and illustrate, using your campus as the setting.
5. Pick any one of the five major accident areas, and illustrate cause, frequency, and place by means of graphs and charts.
6. Interview a campus official on accident hazards which are present on the campus and how such hazards can be removed.
7. Develop a plan for controlling traffic accidents on or adjacent to the campus.
8. Prepare a set of guide lines for accident prevention in recreational activities.
9. Compare the effectiveness of the Schafer method of artificial respiration with the back-pressure–arm-lift method.
10. Discuss reasons why college students should carry liability and accident insurance.
11. Interview an automobile-club insurance agent on types of insurance a motor-vehicle driver should carry.
12. Preview, show, and discuss the following motion pictures on safety and civil defense: (*a*) *And Then There Were Four* (sound, 20 minutes), General Petroleum; (*b*) *Disaster Control* (sound, 20 minutes), McGraw-Hill; (*c*) *Danger Is Your Companion* (sound, 17 minutes), American Red Cross, 1948; (*d*) *Learning How to Swim* (sound, 28 minutes), American Red Cross, 1953; (*e*)

Heads Up (sound, 22 minutes), American Red Cross; (*f*) *Oars and Paddles* (sound, 22 minutes), American Red Cross.

Suggested Readings

1. American Automobile Association, *Sportsmanlike Driving.* Washington, 1952.

2. *American Red Cross First Aid Textbook*, rev. ed. Philadelphia: The Blakiston Company, 1945.

3. Arbous, A. G., and J. E. Kerrich, "Accident Statistics and the Concept of Accident-proneness," *Biometrics*, 7:340–433, December, 1941.

4. Brightman, I. J., I. McCaffrey, and L. P. Cook, "Mortality Statistics as a Direction Finder in Home Accident Prevention," *American Journal of Public Health*, 42:840–848, July, 1952.

5. Dunbar, F., *Emotions and Bodily Changes.* New York: Columbia University Press, 1946.

6. Kent, F. S., "Engineering Aspects of Home Accident Prevention," *American Journal of Public Health*, 39:1531–1534, December, 1949.

7. Lloyd, F., G. G. Deaver, and F. R. Eastwood, *Safety in Athletics.* Philadelphia: W. B. Saunders Company, 1936.

8. Muller, B., and E. C. Robertson, *Fundamentals of Health and Safety.* New York: D. Van Nostrand Company, Inc., 1948.

9. National Safety Council, *Accident Facts.* (Annual publication.)

10. "Proceedings of the President's Conference on Industrial Safety," *Bulletin* 112. Washington: Government Printing Office, 1949.

11. Stack, H. J., E. B. Siebrecht, and J. D. Elkow, *Education for Safe Living.* New York: Prentice-Hall, Inc., 1951.

12. National Security Resources Board, *United States Civil Defense.* Washington: Government Printing Office, 1950.

13. Weinerman, E. F., "Accident Proneness: A Critique," *American Journal of Public Health*, 39:1527–1531, December, 1949.

Popular Readings

14. Harris, Jennie E., "The Modern Lifesaving Method," *Today's Health*, 31:24–25, 50–55, August, 1953.

15. Damon, Norman, "How Much Further Can We Reduce Traffic Accidents?" *Traffic Quarterly*, October, 1950.

16. General Motors Corp., *ABC's of Hand Tools.* Detroit, 1945.

17. Hunt, Morton M., "The Wellesley Experiment," *Harper's Magazine*, July, 1953, pp. 75–81.

18. Overstreet, Harry, *The Mature Mind.* New York: W. W. Norton & Company, 1949.

19. Travelers Insurance Co., *The Fifth Commandment.* Hartford, 1952.

17. Participating in the Community Health Program

There is widespread interest today in community health. This interest stimulated by World War II has resulted in a number of organized groups. Such groups promote one part or another of the total community health program. Most communities have a program already in existence. For these communities the pertinent questions are these: How effective is the program? Is it serving the needs of the people? Are the total resources of the community utilized? If not, why not? Is there adequate coordination of functions? How can the present program be improved? A number of communities, particularly in rural areas, are getting along without much of an organized program. The questions for these communities then are: How can a community health program be developed? With what groups can cooperation be achieved in order to obtain services and activities to promote and protect the health of all the people? In our changing society new communities are springing up almost overnight. Such communities must "start from scratch" in developing a health program. Whatever the situation in a given community, it is necessary to examine critically what constitutes a community health program in order to understand the individual's civic responsibilities.

The President's Commission on Higher Education,[1] referred to in Chapter 1, agrees with the civic responsibility premise in the statement of its objective for health education. The Commission was aware of the values inherent in community organization for health. The members of the

[1] *Higher Education for American Democracy: A Report of the President's Commission on Higher Education,* Vol. IV, p. 54. Washington, 1947.

Commission not only challenge the college student to maintain and improve his own health but also to cooperate actively and intelligently in solving community health problems. Developing interest in and assuming responsibility for community health by participating in cooperative enterprises are important factors in solving health as a major social problem.

A more complete understanding of the individual's role in community endeavors for better health is made possible by answering the following questions: (1) What makes a good community? (2) What is community organization for health? (3) What are the principles of a community health program? (4) What are the components of a community health program, and how do they function? (5) What are the functions of the state and the national health agencies? (6) How do the state and national health agencies relate to the local communities? (7) What are some specific ways and means by which the student can participate in community activities for improving community health?

What Makes a Good Community?

Sanders [2] believes that there are four factors that go to make up a good community. First, there is a relatively stable economic base with respect to occupational opportunity, diversity of industry, and amount of taxable property to provide essential governmental services, including health services. Second, there is strong community loyalty. As already discussed in Chapter 16, community loyalty is demonstrated by an interest in civic affairs. It is high where there is understanding by members of the community of the projects undertaken and where there is democratic organization. Third, there is a constructive approach to problem solving. Since communities are composed of people, all communities have problems. A good community finds a democratic way of attacking its problems, that is, by means of community organization. Fourth, there are leaders who see the community as a whole. Such leaders are able to do sound planning and engage in community activities for the welfare of the total group, as well as representing their own professions, institutions, or businesses. Thus they produce more agreement than disagreement. According to Sanders: [3]

> A whole community is also a well community in which sore spots are increasingly being healed and in which a unity of purpose pervades the mem-

[2] Irwin T. Sanders, *Making Good Communities Better*, p. 7. Lexington: University of Kentucky Press, 1950.

[3] *Ibid.*, p. 13.

bers. . . . There is a happy medium between a wailing Jeremiah and an unrealistic Pollyanna, between the doleful "this place has gone to the dogs" and the boosterlike "best little town in Michigan."

Community Organization for Health

Community organization is essential in every neighborhood and community regardless of size or kind. In a community the individual alone is powerless to make significant changes for effective group living. However, as a member of a planning group or organization, his influence, with group support, can result in tangible improvements for better living. It must be remembered, too, that health is only one value or one problem confronting society. Through community organization, health is given due recognition along with other existing social values.

Community organization provides a medium by which leaders can view the total community and enables them to work with unity of purpose. Health is not to be considered by itself in isolation; rather it is an integral factor in the total life of the community.

The meaning of community organization. Community organization is a process which attempts to unite the individual members and groups of an area into one group with a common purpose. It stems from the people themselves. It is a process that enables individuals and groups to meet their common needs. The term "process" denotes action and implies that those people who participate in the action are changed. Community organization then is an educational process which favorably influences behavior.

Community organization for health is a process of welding together individual members of the community and the health agencies of an area into one group for the purpose of determining health needs and finding ways and means of meeting those needs to improve the total health of the community [11]. The uniting of individuals and groups for the building of a much-needed hospital in a local community is an example of action through community organization.

The Community Health Program

There are a number of parts that go to make up a total community health program. All these parts together, coordinated and integrated, compose a complete, functional program. This program is designed to promote healthful, effective living for all the people living in the community. A discussion of the components of the program is basic to an understanding of the individual's role in assuming civic responsibility.

The basic purpose of the community health program. The purpose of a community health program grows out of the beliefs or point of view of the people. The major purpose of the community health program or the basic mandate is similar in most states and is often expressed in the legal statutes of states and local communities. The 1869 statute establishing the Massachusetts State Board of Health formulated this mandate as "to take cognizance of the interests of health and life among the citizens." [4] Anderson, in his presidential address to the American Public Health Association at its eightieth annual meeting in Cleveland, Ohio, October, 1952, eloquently presented this objective of public health as the concept that charted the evolution of public health. He pointed out that, at the present time, it also defines its scope of activities. Furthermore, it directs the formation of a community health program, one that "preserves the health and the life of the people" and "keeps people well, not simply keeps them alive." [5] Implied in this objective is the social concept that "society has a responsibility to provide those necessities and protections which individuals cannot provide for themselves." [6]

Anderson [7] developed this point of view still further in the following significant statement:

> Public health is an organized community program designed to prolong efficient human life. It has no artificial limitations that would restrict its activities to certain types of problems. It must deal with and endeavor to combat those forces that tend to impair or to shorten efficient human life and must meet each problem according to its particular needs. The essence of democracy is the concept of rule by the people, who have a right to protect themselves against all forces that lead to illness or to death.

These statements adequately express the modern concepts of the community health program and point out the direction for its development.

Principles of a community health program. The principles of community health are derived from the basic purpose directing the community health program. These principles serve as guide lines in the process of developing the program. Such principles are the following [1, 5, 9, 10, 11]:

1. Access to the means for the attainment and preservation of health is a basic human right.

[4] Gaylord W. Anderson, "Public Health—A Mandate from the People," *American Journal of Public Health and the Nation's Health*, 42:1368, November, 1952.

[5] *Ibid.*, p. 1368.

[6] *Ibid.*

[7] *Ibid.*, p. 1373.

2. The most valuable resource in any community is the people who live there. It is necessary, therefore, to understand the people in the community —the kinds of people, their health status, their health behavior, the types of groups, and their characteristics.

3. Responsibility for health is a joint one, with the individual citizen and local, state, and Federal governments each having major contributions to make to its fuller realization.

4. Plans begin with people and center in their needs and interests. A study of people and identification of their needs and interests precede a program of action. Successful projects and programs are based on the problems of a specific community, not those of a distant community or land.

5. Community action is needed to strengthen the total life of the community. Community organization for health leads to community action by mustering all the resources of the community, human and otherwise.

6. Some form of organization is needed to solve problems and to expedite the use of the scientific method. A health committee or council—some planning body that facilitates fact finding, problem solving, and coordination of functions—is needed to assist in developing a community health program.

7. Problems are best solved by using the scientific method. The procedure for solving community problems follows this method: identify the problem, define it, formulate a hypothesis, gather the facts, classify them, test the findings, draw conclusions, and make interpretations from the data.

8. People learn best when they participate in solving problems. This is the principle of learning by doing. It also includes the principle of involvement. A plan which one has had a hand in making is not quickly cast aside.

9. The American people desire and deserve comprehensive health service of the highest quality, and in our dynamic, expanding economy the means can be found to provide it.

10. The same high quality of health services should be available to all people equally.

11. A health program must take into account the progress and experiences of the past and the realities of the present and must be flexible enough to cope with future changes.

Community health needs. Community health needs include the desires of the people, plus the lacks and inadequacies or the problems pertaining to effective living. Communities, more and more, are determining their own needs as a basis for planning constructive health programs. In addition, they are studying the health needs of the nation as a means of understanding their own problems. The evidence from studies on the health needs in the United States shows a common pattern of health needs. For example, the need for health personnel and improved programs of mental health and dental health are consistent problems throughout the country. Each community contributes to this common pattern. At the same time, the needs of the community in many ways are unique and call for individual study. For these reasons, then, it is important to determine the health needs of the community and to examine examples of local and national health needs.

The specific needs of the community may be determined through a professional survey or through a community self-survey. By the first method, one or more experts in public health evaluation are employed to make the study. The second approach is one in which the citizens themselves, with the leadership of health authorities, make the study. Either method is useful in determining community needs. In assessing the needs of the nation, the United States Public Health Service staff, with cooperating agencies, or a specially appointed commission, with a number of staff members and field investigators, collect the data and report on their findings.

An example of the first method of determining health needs by a public health authority is Hiscock's study of public health in Hawaii. Hiscock is chairman of the School of Public Health, Yale University, and well known for his community health surveys. Illustrative selected findings from his 1950 survey are as follows: [8]

1. Complex housing problems for both official and voluntary health agencies. . . .
2. Cumbersome civic service and budgetary requirements and operation. . . .
3. Personnel shortages. . . .
4. Gaps in services for dental health, mental health, nutrition, physical medicine, and social services, and in community health education resources. . . .
5. Complex water supply and sewage disposal problems. . . .
6. Lack of awareness and understanding by some officials and by many other taxpayers of the organization, purposes and low cost of a modern practical community health program. . . .

The second method enlists the citizens as members of the health team, which tends to make them supporters and boosters for public health. An example of the findings of this second type is illustrated in the preliminary report of the West Los Angeles Self Survey for Health Needs.

The needs of this community were studied jointly by citizens and

[8] Ira V. Hiscock, "Public Health in Hawaii," *Hawaii Medical Journal*, 10:7, November–December, 1950. (Reprints available.)

health authorities, and the following selected findings [9] are the result of this self-survey:

There exists an apparent need for:
1. An emergency hospital.
2. More hospital beds.
3. Improved environmental sanitation.
4. Additional housing units and lower rental dwellings.
5. A health education program to acquaint citizens with health department activities, and to promote community organization.
6. A dental health program, including dental health education and dental clinics.
7. A mental health program.
8. Free or part-pay clinics.

From the authoritative study by the President's Commission on the Health Needs of the Nation, several selected findings are listed to illustrate the major health needs of the wider community—the health needs of the United States. For complete information refer to volumes of the Commission's report (see reference 1). Some specific needs are as follows:

Need for:
1. Health personnel—physicians, dentists, nurses and others.
2. Health facilities—general hospital facilities, health centers, beds for mental disease, chronic disease, tuberculosis, rehabilitation, and research facilities.
3. Improving health and medical services for all people.
4. Research.
5. Immunization against communicable diseases.
6. Rehabilitating the handicapped.
7. Concerted attack on chronic disease.
8. Prevention of mental illness.
9. Dental health programs, including dental health education, dental care, scientific fluoridation of community water supplies.
10. Improved environmental health—water, air, food, shelter.
11. Prevention of accidents.
12. Improved maternal and child health.
13. Improved industrial health to extend medical care plans for workers and their families, and to create more healthful working environments.[10]

[9] Unpublished preliminary findings of West Los Angeles Self Survey for Health Needs, Health Committee, West Los Angeles Coordinating Council, 1953.

[10] A Report to the President by the President's Commission on the Health Needs of the Nation, *Building America's Health.* Vol. II, *America's Health Status, Needs and Resources.* Washington: Government Printing Office, 1952.

Health personnel. The most important component of a community health program is the health personnel who make it function. Many programs look promising on paper but are ineffective because of poor personnel. A functional program, one in which the health needs are being met successfully, has sufficient, competent personnel.

The health officer, physicians, dentists, nurses, research workers, health educators, classroom teachers, hospital administrators, executive secretaries of voluntary agencies, social workers, and other health workers are the people possessing the skills that provide health services, educational experiences, and research findings. Lay citizens join the health personnel in developing a community health education program. Space does not permit a discussion of each of the types of health worker. A brief description of the contributions of five—the health officer, physicians, dentists, nurses, and health educators—serves as an illustration of the members of the health team.

Health officer. The health officer is a doctor of medicine (M.D.) with special preparation in public health. Usually he is in addition a master of public health (M.P.H.) or a doctor of public health (Dr.P.H.), though not all health officers hold such degrees. However, the trend throughout the country is for highly trained personnel well qualified in both the field of medicine and the applied field of public health. The health officer has a unique leadership function in the community health program. He is responsible for the development and maintenance of the health of the general population and for the prevention and control of communicable disease. He cooperates with all agencies and with the public in improving effective living in the community.

Private practitioners—physicians and dentists. Physicians and dentists are considered to be the authorities on health within a community. These men and women are graduates of accredited medical and dental schools. They are licensed to practice within the state in which they reside. They belong to local, state, and national professional societies. They are members of staffs of approved hospitals and clinics in the community. Every few years they enhance their skill and extend their knowledge through postgraduate studies. The cost for the service they render is usually scaled to the mutual advantage of both patient and practitioner. The doctor is the pivotal person in the health team. He is concerned with the total health program, as well as with medical care. The dentist, too, is concerned not only with meeting the dental health problem but in improving all aspects of healthful living.

In addition to providing medical and dental services, doctors and dentists contribute their time and effort by serving on planning committees and community councils. They take active leadership in the formulation and development of programs of action. Through counseling and guidance of patients they educate for better health. Through research they aid in the solution of problems. Their professional associations, the American Medical Association and American Dental Association, provide health education material and individual and group guidance.

Nurses. The supply of nurses, who constitute the largest group of health workers, is most limited. The need for additional nurses is even greater today than the need for doctors and dentists. The skilled nurse relieves the doctor, permitting him to perform duties for which only his training and experience qualify him. She carries out the doctor's orders, enabling the patient to regain his former health status. The bedside nurse is noted for providing physical care and mental comfort for her patients.

One type of nurse considered essential in the community health team is the public health nurse. This nurse provides nursing service and health education in the health department or school where she is employed, as well as in the home. By visiting the home she discovers individual and family health needs, gives demonstrations on maternal and child care to members of the family, and teaches classes for community groups [19]. The nurse serves as a counselor in individualizing health education. She serves as an interpreter of health needs and as a resource person on sources of information and medical care.

Health educator. The health educator in the community, as a staff member of a health department or voluntary agency, plays an important role in the community health program. He is an interpreter to the people and the members of the agencies of the services and activities of the community health program. He assumes leadership, both direct and indirect, in community organization. Primarily, he assists people to help themselves in solving their own problems. He plans, stimulates, promotes, organizes, teaches, coordinates, guides, and evaluates activities and programs [13]. Often he is considered the right-hand man of the health officer or of the executive secretary of a voluntary health agency.

In well-organized state or local health departments there are frequently other professional members on the health team: the sanitarian, nutritionist, medical social worker, laboratory technician, public health dentist, preventive mental hygiene personnel, statistician, industrial hygiene engineer—all who promote and protect the health of the community. Information about their functions can be obtained from the Suggested Readings or through a visit to a health department.

Health services and activities. The actual community health program is planned carefully on the basis of the health needs that have been determined. This program, functioning through the health personnel and lay citizens who work together to meet the needs, consists of health services and educational and other activities as follows: [11]

Promotion of health. Services and activities contributing to the attainment of health:

1. An adequate, safe food supply and distribution.
2. Proper housing.
3. A healthful working environment.
4. Safety outside the home and workplace, as well as inside.
5. Education for health.
6. Recreation.
7. Security, including access to health services.

Prevention of disease. Preventive services:

1. Immunization against communicable disease.
2. Individual and family health guidance, such as maternity care and infant care.
3. Aggressive, early detection of disease, with follow-up to ensure diagnosis and treatment.

Diagnosis and treatment. Personal health services for cure or alleviation of disease:

1. Diagnosis of disease before and after symptoms have appeared.
2. Treatment in the home, office or clinic, and general hospital.
3. Treatment in specialized institutions, *e.g.*, mental hospitals, tuberculosis sanatoria, nursing and custodial homes, teaching and research centers.

Rehabilitation. Services for the restoration of handicapped to total usefulness within their capabilities:

1. In the course of ordinary treatment.
2. In special rehabilitation centers.

The responsibility for developing such a comprehensive program rests with the local health department, the medical, dental, and allied professions, the hospitals, the schools, the voluntary agencies, and, of course, the public in general [2].

Community health resources. The health resources of a community include all the people living in the community. More specifically, the health resources refer to the health agencies and facilities that are engaged in health endeavors, as follows:

[11] *Ibid.*, p. 12.

The official agency: the health department. The local health department or center is a unit of the local government. It is commonly referred to as the official health agency in the community. In keeping with the basic mandate of public health, its purpose is to promote and protect the health of the total community.

The functions of a modern health department include activities relating to (1) vital statistics, (2) sanitation, (3) communicable disease control,

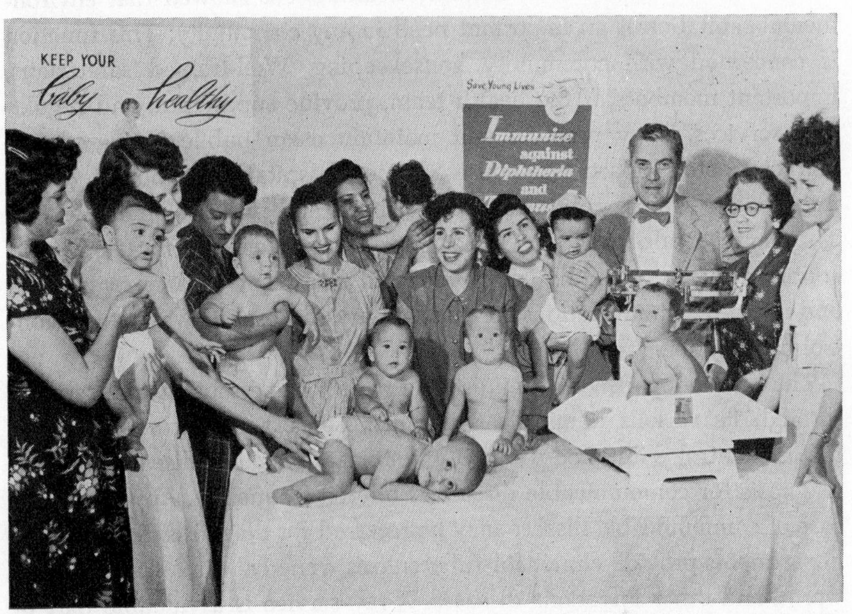

Fig. 17.1. Mothers with their babies participate in a child health conference under the direction of the health officer and director of maternal and child health, an important activity of a local health department. (*Los Angeles City Health Department.*)

(4) laboratory services, (5) maternal and child health, (6) health education, (7) control of chronic disease, (8) accident prevention, (9) hygiene of housing, (10) industrial hygiene, (11) school health services, (12) mental health, (13) medical rehabilitation, and (14) medical care administration. The first six are minimum functions of any local health department, while all constitute present-day optimal services [2]. Examples of these services are discussed below.

Through vital statistics, the health officer keeps his hand on the pulse of the community. The bureau of vital statistics records and analyzes statistics on births, deaths, services, and facilities; many of the health needs of a community health program are found through keeping such data. Any deviation from the normal pattern in the community, such as an increase in deaths in a particular location or an increase in number of cases of one disease, is a significant sign. At once the public health officials are alerted to prevent a serious disease epidemic. The charting of health problems on a daily basis through vital statistics enables the health department personnel and others to plan for an optimum community health program.

The listing of common community health needs showed that environmental sanitation is an important need in any community. This function is concerned with community housekeeping. Well-trained sanitarians, important members of the health team, provide supervision and regulatory services. They promote and maintain clean public eating places, markets, hotels, apartment houses, homes, hospitals, rest homes, swimming pools, camps, public rest rooms, bars, and places of employment. They ensure safe milk and water supplies, prevent rat invasions, and control diseases spread by mosquitoes and flies. They enforce regulations and make recommendations for the sanitary disposal of wastes and control of pollution.

The health department administers a variety of personal health services through its various administrative units. For example, communicable-disease control is initiated through immunization against disease. Medical diagnosis for communicable disease is offered frequently. Any suspected case of communicable disease may be referred for diagnosis. Some health departments provide clinics for tuberculosis, venereal disease, scalp ringworm, and other infectious diseases. X-ray service is a valuable part of the case-finding program in tuberculosis control. Premarital blood tests illustrate a laboratory service provided by the health department.

Personal services also are provided in maternal and child health clinics and child health conferences. Public health nurses conduct adult classes for fathers and expectant mothers. Prenatal examinations and guidance are given for the protection of the mother and unborn child. At least one home visit is made by the public health nurse to all mothers registered in the prenatal conference. Additional visits are made if necessary. Among the helpful services the public health nurse renders are the home demonstrations of infant bathing and preparation of a formula [9].

A public health dentist provides preventive dental service for expectant mothers and young children. Also, a medical social worker offers her services of guidance and counseling to those who need help with social problems arising out of medical-care needs.

Many health departments are providing partial or total support of centers for the detection of such chronic diseases as heart disease, cancer, and diabetes. The health department is interested, too, in programs for mental health and for the rehabilitation of persons afflicted with disease or victims of accidents. Such programs enable these people to live useful, productive lives again.

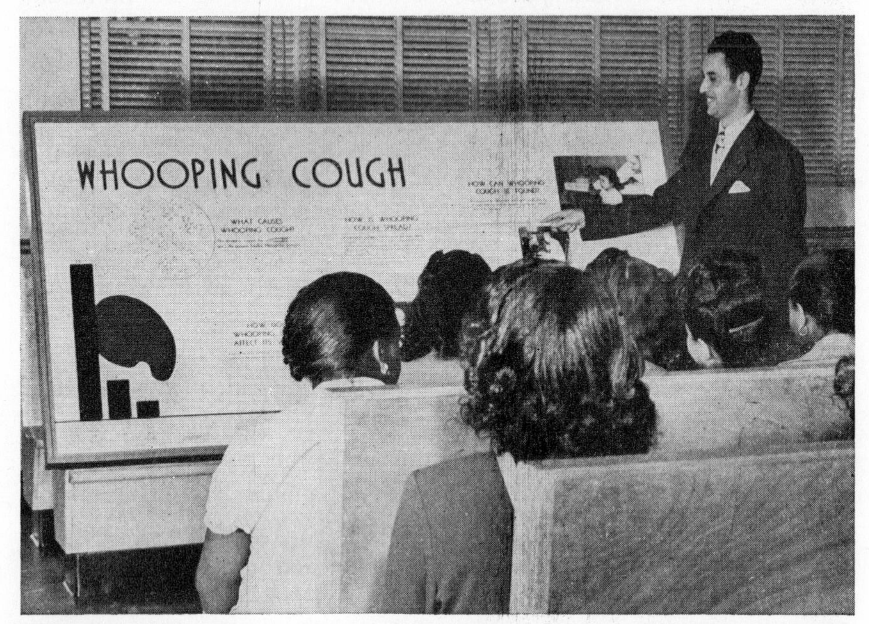

Fig. 17.2. A public health educator instructs a community group. (*Los Angeles City Health Department.*)

Educating the public for effective living is an important function of the local health department. Citizens need to be informed about the services rendered by their health department. They need to understand how they may prevent diseases and defects and how they may live more effectively. The work of the public health educator has been discussed previously.

According to the modern concept of public health, the health department has a community responsibility in the successful operation of its health facilities. It becomes a center for health personnel and citizens interested in the community health program. The practicing physician officially registers his license with the city or county health department. At the time of registration, he receives information about laws, ordinances, regulations, and policies. This procedure serves as a medium for future cooperation between the physician and the department. The two-way cooperative relationship between the private physician and the health department helps to build the health department into a functional health center. An auditorium, classroom, or both assist in bringing the citizen of the community into the health center. In large communities, several well-equipped health centers with administrative offices, clinic facilities, and auditorium space are essential in promoting and protecting community health.

The health department has a major responsibility in assisting in the coordination of the total community health program. The public health personnel must take an active part in coordinating the functions of all agencies and citizen activities to prevent overlapping and duplication of effort. One illustration of coordination is the health department's function in the civil-defense activities. It coordinates these activities, and volunteer personnel maintain a corps ready to serve in any natural disaster or enemy attack. A second example is cooperative planning with school authorities in developing a school health program.

Only a full-time health department with full-time, adequately prepared personnel can provide a community with the above services and assume the responsibilities for health promotion and protection. Health departments must receive community support. A community of 50,000 people or several neighborhoods or communities banded together can receive at least minimum services for $1.50 per year per person. Additional protection can be obtained for a slightly higher per capita cost. It is estimated that some 40 million Americans live in communities or areas without full-time local public health services [6]. This is a challenge to citizens for community action for health.

Voluntary health agencies. Approximately one-fourth of all the money expended in the United States for promotion of health and protection from disease is administered by the voluntary health agencies [4]. A voluntary health agency is an organization operated by private persons without tax-supported funds for the purpose of improving health. Such agencies usually are concerned with alleviating one particular disease or defect. The voluntary health agencies stem from the American tradition of freedom and individual initiative and the desire of people to relieve suffering [7]. They represent the spirit of the American people, who believe in fostering better health through private means over and above their official health agencies. The number and scope of activities of these agencies are peculiar to the United States.

Voluntary health agencies fall into the following three major classifications: (1) agencies devoted to the alleviation of a particular disease, for example, the American Cancer Society, the National Tuberculosis Association, and the National Foundation for Infantile Paralysis; (2) agencies devoted to prevention and rehabilitation of bodily defects, such as the American Heart Association and the National Society for the Prevention of Blindness; (3) agencies concerned with health and welfare of special groups, for example, the American Red Cross, the National Safety Council, and the National Association for Mental Health.

Several of the voluntary agencies that have local branches or affiliated societies or that participate actively in local community health programs are the following:

American Cancer Society, Inc.
American Hearing Society.
American Heart Association.
American National Red Cross.
American Social Hygiene Association, Inc.
National Association for Mental Health.
National Foundation for Infantile Paralysis, Inc.
National Safety Council.
National Society for Crippled Children and Adults, Inc.
National Society for the Prevention of Blindness, Inc.
National Tuberculosis Association.

The functions of these and other voluntary health agencies include: [12]

1. Pioneering—discovering needs and new ways of meeting existing needs.
2. Demonstration—assuming a public health function or subsidizing a project and demonstrating its worth to the citizens, the city council, or county supervisors until the official agency can take over the function.
3. Education—educating for health is considered one of the functions, if not the most important function, of the voluntary health agencies.
4. Supplementation of official agencies—providing funds and/or activities which the official agencies could not provide because of politics, budgetary limitations or legal action.
5. Guarding of citizen interest in health—supporting good official agency health programs and criticizing poor programs, in either case serving the public interest for community health.
6. Promotion of health legislation—supporting legislation for measures im-

[12] S. M. Gunn and P. S. Platt, *Voluntary Health Agencies: An Interpretative Study*, pp. 42–48. New York: The Ronald Press Company, 1945.

proving health conditions, working for the defeat of legislation detrimental to public health.

7. Group planning and coordination—participating in planning a total community health program, assisting in coordination of efforts to avoid duplication and overlapping.

8. Development of well-rounded community health programs—subordinating a vested interest for the welfare of the total community health program.

In most cases the voluntary health agencies are meeting an important need. They make an extensive contribution to education, research, and service relating to the community health program. Since they are responsible only to their own boards of directors, their programs are flexible and they can adapt readily to changing needs. There is evidence to show that they are broadening their scope of activities. For example, the Tuberculosis Association in Los Angeles and also in other communities is called the County Tuberculosis and Health Association, which denotes the addition of other functions than the fight against tuberculosis. The personnel of the voluntary agencies are doing increasingly more work to promote and protect the health of the total community group rather than attempting to alleviate the one particular disease or defect for which their organization was founded. This is an important new trend. A further essential factor is the cooperative relationship between the official agency and the voluntary agency, in which both are working together for the health of all the people.

The community hospital. The community hospital plays an important role in the community health program. Especially is this true as the quantity and quality of medical care increase. People, today, naturally expect to go to the hospital if they are seriously ill. This is the case regardless of economic status. The increase in prepayment health insurance has made it easier for many to pay hospital bills, which in itself has been a factor in increased patronage of hospitals.

The major objectives of hospital care for the patient are to render diagnosis and treatment and restore him again to a productive life. The hospital contributes both to individual and to community health through restoration and rehabilitation of the sick or handicapped person. Many persons are served through the outpatient clinics of the modern hospital.

The hospital contributes to community health also by serving as a facility for the physician as well as for the patient. The modern hospital is a vital part of the physician's medical practice. Actually it is a facility that broadens his skill and medical practice. Not only does the hospital offer the physician equipment that otherwise he might not possess, but it gives him an affiliation with the hospital medical staff and physicians in a number of specialities. This professional association is essential if the physician is to keep up to date and in touch with modern developments in medical practice. Furthermore, the hospital provides a medium by which the physician continues his medical education. For example, he may engage in advanced study for a speciality by fulfilling a hospital residency.

In the past, hospitals were looked upon as "receptacles for the sick." Today the point of view has changed remarkably. The hospital is considered to have a responsibility to the total community health program in fostering and promoting public health and preventive medicine. For illustration, it is considered sound practice for a hospital to have a diagnostic clinic in which physicians employ health examinations as a means of keeping people well. Professor J. M. Mackintosh of the London School of Hygiene expresses this modern concept when he says: [13] "The good hospital is not a structure bounded by four walls or even extended by pseudopodial clinics. It is essentially a sphere of influence reaching far beyond its own curtilage to the homes of the families it serves."

However, over and above that, the physician and the hospital staff are interested in the reasons for the patient's illness. They are concerned with ways and means of restoring him to health so that he can better meet his daily needs after leaving the hospital.

An important modern concept in hospital planning is regional planning and distribution of hospital care. Each area cannot meet all the requirements for hospital care. However, needs can be met by the regional method. The idea is to develop in each region facilities as nearly adequate as is possible. The regional center contains the largest hospitals, most complete facilities, and most specialized medical personnel. General hospitals, community hospitals, and health centers send their specialized cases to the regional center. Each region has its share of general hospitals, tuberculosis hospitals, chronic-disease hospitals, and mental hospitals.

It is essential for good community health that cooperative planning and action take place with the health department, the hospital, the medical societies, the voluntary agencies, the schools, and citizens serving as active participants. One of the responsibilities the student or any other citizen has as a community member today is to work with community agencies to obtain adequate hospital facilities. The specific hospital needs are discussed in Chapter 2 (page 22).

[13] "The Hospital and the Community," *American Journal of Public Health and the Nation's Health*, 41:1412, November, 1951. (Editorial.)

The schools. Some people have never thought of the school as a health agency in the community; yet without a doubt it is one of the important agencies responsible for the health of the people. The opportunity to educate for health is greatest in the schools. The schools constitute the largest organized group. Pupils composing the group spend years in school. These pupils are at a stage in life when behavior is more easily changed than at any other period. Educators recognize health as a major educational objective. To achieve this objective, a health education program is planned and maintained to meet the health needs of school-age children and youth. Such needs were classified by a subcommittee of the Federal health agencies as follows: [14]

All children need:

1. A safe, sanitary, healthful school environment.
2. Protection from infections and conditions which interfere with proper growth and development.
3. An opportunity to realize their potentialities of growth and development.
4. To learn how to live healthfully.
5. Teachers who are equipped by training, temperament and health not only to give specific instruction, but also to help children to mature emotionally.

The school health program planned, organized, and conducted to meet these needs includes administrative divisions of (1) healthful school living—the environmental factors; (2) health service to appraise and improve health status; (3) physical education and recreation for healthful activities; (4) health instruction—planned, direct instruction consisting of meaningful activities to develop scientific knowledge, wholesome attitudes, and practices for healthful living.

Health education furnished in the schools establishes the foundation for health behavior that provides improved living for the individual and strengthens the total community. A successful school health program utilizes the health resources of the community to broaden its scope and increase its activities and personnel. Not only does the school contribute to the health of the community, but the community health program strengthens the school endeavors for health.

The community health council. The reason for a community health council is apparent if one understands human nature. It is only natural that each community agency, like an individual, has its own special

[14] Subcommittee, Governmental Health Agencies, "Health Needs of School Age Children," *School Life,* 28:8, November, 1945.

interest. This is true even though its over-all stated objective is to promote and protect the health of the community. The health council, however, fosters unselfish action by all its members. It serves as a structure to promote democratic action in planning, fact finding, problem solving, and coordination of functions. It makes possible a total program for the health of all the people. The council is a form of community organization

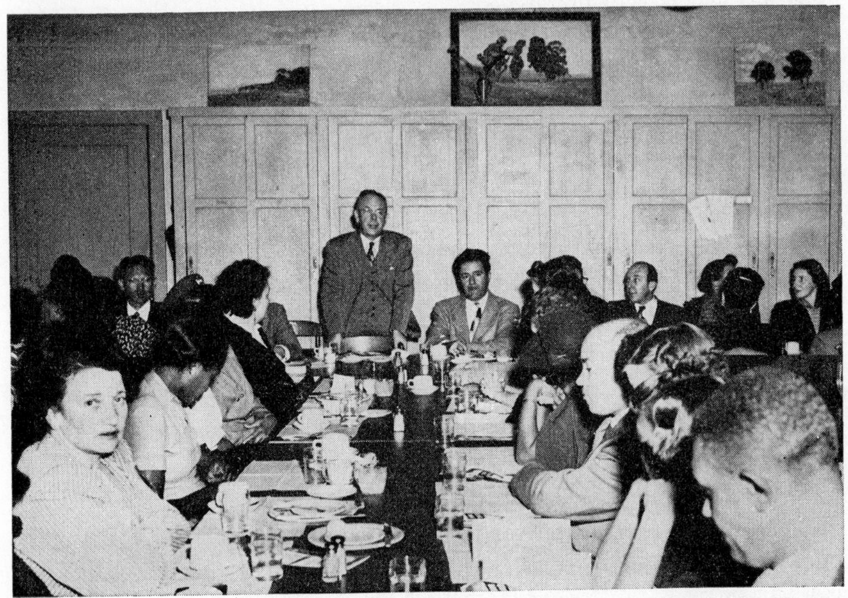

Fig. 17.3. The director of Health Education and Health Services Branch, Los Angeles City schools, talks to a community health council. (*Los Angeles City Health Department.*)

that welds together agencies and individuals into one group with united purposes.

The council is a representative group composed of members from the various agencies and organizations interested in community health. It brings together the health department, the voluntary agencies, the county medical and dental societies, the service clubs, women's clubs, parent-teacher associations, and other groups. It reaches the people directly by admitting citizens without group affiliation as members at large. It is a clearinghouse for the solution of community health problems.

The council may be called by a variety of names, such as "community health council," "health council," "health division of the community welfare council," "community health committee," and the like [15]; but its functions are the same regardless of what is is called.

The functions of a community health council, according to Lifson,[15] are to:

1. Coordinate as far as possible the thinking and planning of all organizations concerned with the public health.
2. Work to prevent overlapping and duplication.
3. Study health needs of the community through appraisals, inventories and other fact-finding activities.
4. Develop a community health program related to those needs.
5. Stimulate public interest in health problems and their solution.
6. Express itself with strength and authority on matters of health legislation to further sound measures, defeat objectionable ones.
7. Render to members common services in the field of statistics and research and community health education.

There is no reason for a council unless it has some specific task to perform. The health committee of the West Los Angeles Coordinating Council illustrates the actual work of a council. A new health officer was assigned to this district. The citizens and the health officer wanted to assess the health needs of West Los Angeles and to acquaint the people in the district with the health department's services, personnel, and needs. The West Los Angeles Coordinating Council assisted in setting up a health committee to function as a community health council. The group included representatives from the health department, Los Angeles County Tuberculosis and Health Association, Nora Sterry Elementary School, Emerson Junior High School, University Senior High School, University of California, Westwood Business Men's Association (including medical and dental representatives), parent-teacher association, Bureau of Public Assistance, and other community organizations, and citizens serving as members at large.

The group voted to make a survey of the area to determine the health needs of West Los Angeles, as previously cited. This survey was a first step in planning a community health program. Evaluation forms were developed. Available data on health needs were obtained from sources such as the vital statistics office of the health department. Additional information was obtained and evaluation instruments refined in a pilot study of 100 families. This study was carried on by the health committee with the assistance of health education students from the University of California. After the pilot study, plans were made for a large-scale

[15] S. S. Lifson, "The Role of the Community Health Council," *Public Health News*, July, 1948. (Reprints available.)

survey of 1,000 families as a sampling of the total community population. Volunteers were enlisted and trained to conduct house-to-house interviews. The survey was made. Considerable publicity in the local papers was given the health department and the survey itself. People were made aware of health department activities. Volunteer workers became part of the community health team. The findings of the study are now being analyzed and interpreted. It is known that a basis of planning for future action has been laid. The development of a total community health program has been initiated, and directions for next steps have been charted.

Evaluation of services and activities. Evaluation is the process of appraising the progress made toward the achievement of established purposes, objectives, or goals. Self-appraisal of community health program objectives is as important as the self-appraisals the individual makes to determine progress in improving his own health. People want to know how effective the community health program is and how well it is meeting the established health needs. Continuous evaluation of health services and activities makes it possible to utilize existing resources and brings to light the strengths and weaknesses, which stimulate improvement of the program. Evidence of progress is the best means of demonstrating to the public the values of a community health program.

Community appraisals are accomplished by persons making the evaluations, using inventories, schedules, survey forms, or questionnaires. One of the best community health appraisal forms is the American Public Health Association's *Evaluation Schedule,* with its accompanying *Guide to the Evaluation Schedule, Grading Standards,* and *Health Practice Indices,* all published by the association in 1947. Health-department personnel and lay citizens together can use these materials in determining the effectiveness of their program. The California State Department of Public Health has developed a community self-study form, *Inventory of Local Health Problems, Resources, and Facilities,* San Francisco, Calif., 1951. This form enables health personnel and lay citizens to determine how much health protection they have, what their problems are, and what available resources they have. Some communities prefer to develop their own evaluation instruments. For example, the citizens of Clinton County, Ohio, decided to make a survey. They developed their own questionnaire to discover their problems. The results of their survey are available in their publication of the Health Council of Clinton County's *Clinton County Health Survey,* Wilmington, Ohio, 1950. An excellent self-study guide for communities is the Hogg Foundation's *So You Want to Make a Community Study,* Austin, Tex., University of Texas Press, 1950.

Evaluation is one of the best means of interesting citizens in order to develop their understanding of the program, to awaken their concern about health affairs, and to stimulate action for an improved program. In 1951, the Missouri State Health Council published a one-page appraisal form called *Yardstick for Measuring Health Standards of Our County.* This survey form is designed to interest local people in learning more about the general health situation in their own communities or county. An evaluation form designed to appraise the effectiveness of the local health department is *How to Gauge Your Public Health Department,* published by the Health Publications Institute, Inc., Raleigh, N.C., 1951.

The need for local public health services. The type of community health program described above pertains to a local area such as a district, village, town, city, or county. It is estimated that: [16] "One third of the nation lives under substandard local health organization, ill-equipped to give basic minimum health protection at all times and to meet public health emergencies quickly and efficiently . . . ."

A committee of the American Public Health Association has proposed a plan by which adequate services may be provided: [17] "The 3,070 counties and their contained cities in the United States can be served by 1,197 units of local health administration."

Such a plan needs the support of agencies, professional associations, health councils, and citizens for it to become effective.

Health Programs of the Wider Community

The broad definition of a community presented in Chapter 16 included the state and the nation as community areas. These large geographical and governmental units constitute the wider community. The over-all public health structure includes the programs organized at the Federal, state, and local levels in order to promote and protect the health of the individual citizen and the group. Mountin and Flook compare the public health organization to a government building. The ground floor is composed of the local official and voluntary agencies and the private practitioners; the second floor includes the state official and voluntary agencies

[16] Haven Emerson and Martha Luginbuhl, "1,200 Local Public Health Departments for the United States," *American Journal of Public Health and the Nation's Health,* 35:898, September, 1945.

[17] *Ibid.*

and professional societies; and the third floor contains the national official and voluntary agencies and the professional societies [12].

Since each level of organization is working for the same purpose, that of improving the health of the individual and the group, an effective working interrelationship must exist, from the national level, through the state, to the local community, and vice versa.

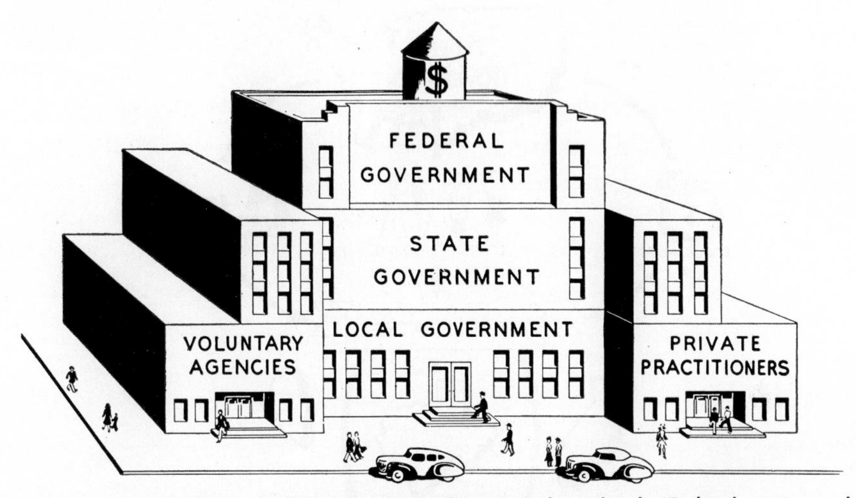

Fig. 17.4. The complete health structure is shown at three levels—Federal, state, and local. The local level shows coordinated activities among the official agency, the voluntary agencies, and the private practitioners. (*U.S. Public Health Service.*)

State Health Organization

The state department of public health plays the chief role in public health at the state level, for its responsibility is greater than that of other agencies. Its functions differ considerably from those of the local health department. The local health department is concerned with rendering direct services. The state health department, on the other hand, is furnishing advisory and consultant services. Some of its functions are regulatory, depending upon the specific state legal requirements. The state health department plays a vital role in administering financial assistance to the local health departments from both state and Federal sources. It fosters research projects which the local health department is unable to carry out. It serves an articulation function as the middleman between the Federal agencies and the local unit. It lends needed personnel to local units for special assignments. Also, it assumes active leadership in co-ordinating the various other agencies, voluntary and professional, functioning at the state level. Assisting the local health departments is its major responsibility [8].

The voluntary agencies and professional organizations operating at the state level, together with the other state governmental agencies, play a contributory and supplemental part in the state health program.

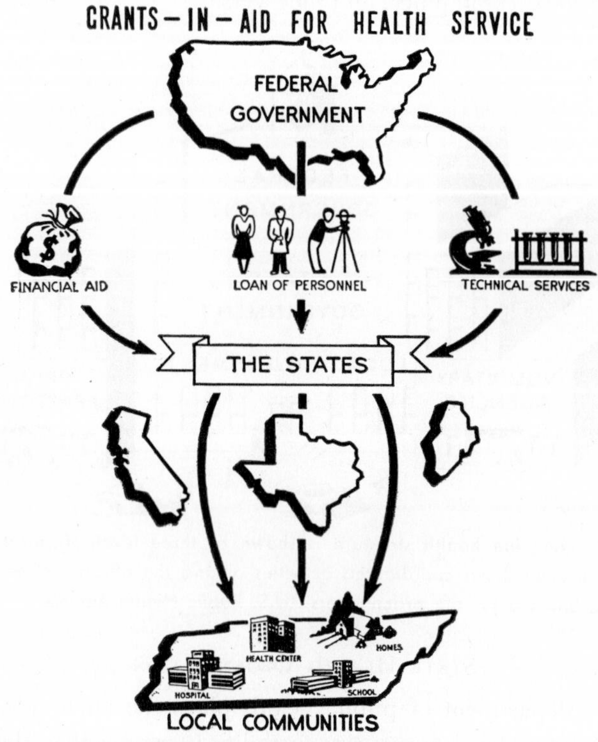

Fig. 17.5. Characteristic methods of health administration, showing Federal and state agencies assisting the local agencies. (*U.S. Public Health Service.*)

Many states have even more agencies interested and active in health work than is true in the local community. These range from the department of agriculture, with its extension services, to the state cancer society or the state medical society. As a result, a number of states have organized state health councils to plan, coordinate, and assist in developing health programs. Thirty-four state health councils are reported as active and functioning organizations [15].

National Health Organization

Official, voluntary, and professional health agencies and organizations are active also at the national level. The organization of these agencies is more complicated than at the lower levels, although recent organizational plans enacted by Congress are attempts to improve the organizational structure.

The Department of Health, Education, and Welfare. On Apr. 11, 1953, a Department of Health, Education, and Welfare became a legally established executive department. This gave new administrative status to Federal health activities under the direction of a Secretary with Cabinet rank. Mrs. Oveta Culp Hobby became the first Secretary of Health, Education, and Welfare, since she was President Eisenhower's appointee as Federal Security Administrator. Personnel in the new Department also includes an undersecretary, two assistant secretaries, and a Special Assistant Secretary on Health and Medical Affairs, who is a medical leader charged with the responsibility of reviewing health and medical progress.

All the functions of the Federal Security Agency were transferred to the new Department. The Federal Security Agency was composed of five main branches: (1) Public Health Service, (2) Office of Education, (3) Food and Drug Administration, (4) Social Security, and (5) Office of Vocational Rehabilitation. These now compose the Department of Health, Education, and Welfare.

The Federal government contributes to individual and group health in a variety of ways through its several agencies.

The United States Public Health Service. The chief public health agency in the Federal government is the Public Health Service. Its primary functions are to foster and conduct public health research through its research centers; conduct surveys and needed studies; collect and analyze vital statistics; aid in the development of health facilities; administer grants-in-aid to states; provide direct hospital and medical service for those authorized to receive care, such as coastguardmen; assist the state and local communities in developing complete public health programs, including health education; and administer health services for the protection of the nation, such as quarantine, immunization, and environmental sanitation.

Some 15,000 commissioned and civilian personnel compose the Public Health Service staff, consisting of physicians, dentists, research workers, sanitary engineers, pharmacists, nurses, public health educators, and others. To ensure a close, cooperative working relationship with states and local communities, Public Health Service personnel are stationed in regional offices throughout the country [12].

One example of the Public Health Service facilities is the National Institutes of Health located in Bethesda, Md. At present, there are seven Institutes devoted entirely to research in the medical and related sciences. These seven include the following: (1) National Microbiological Institute; (2) National Institute of Arthritis and Metabolic Diseases; (3) National Cancer Institute; (4) National Heart Institute; (5) National

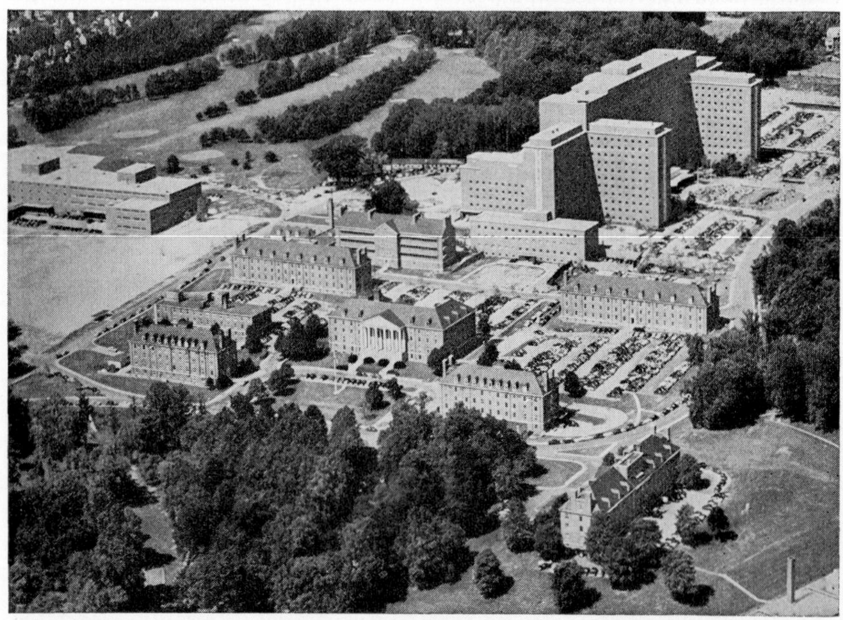

Fig. 17.6. Aerial photo of buildings of the National Institutes of Health, Bethesda, Md. The Clinical Center is the large building in the background. (*Washington Evening Star* photo, courtesy of U.S. Public Health Service.)

Institute of Dental Research; (6) National Institute of Mental Health; (7) National Institute of Neurological Diseases and Blindness. The purpose of the Institutes is to discover better methods for preventing, diagnosing, and treating serious diseases. Emphasis is placed today on research relating to the chronic diseases. An illustration of this is the current investigation by a research team of multiple sclerosis, a degenerative disease of the nervous system from which Lou Gehrig, baseball immortal, died at the age of thirty-seven. At present there is no treatment for the disease and the cause is not known.

Not all the research is carried on in the Institutes. Financial grants are administered by them for research projects in medical schools, universities, hospitals, and other research agencies. Several hundred fellowships are awarded each year as financial support from the Institutes to young scientists to ensure future research manpower [14].

The United States Office of Education. Although the Office of Education is not a direct Federal health agency, it makes an important contribution to public health. Emphasis is placed on school health education by promoting and improving school health programs throughout the country. Specialists in health education offer consultant services in school health to state officials, local school districts, and school health education personnel. The collection, interpretation, and reporting of data relating to school health programs throughout the country are a function of the Office. Studies on the types of health instruction and the extent, type, and organization of health services in the public schools are sample reports developed by specialists in health education. The Office also administers a grant-in-aid program for vocational education in health.

The Children's Bureau. This Bureau is one of several under the Social Security Administration, now a part of the Department of Health, Education, and Welfare. It administers vital health services for mothers and children through grants-in-aid. The Children's Bureau investigates and reports upon all matters relating to the health and welfare of children. It also works to extend and improve service for children in rural areas and in areas of special need. The Bureau staff is particularly interested in improved programs for crippled children. The Children's Bureau, the Office of Education, and the Public Health Service work cooperatively in promoting school health programs.

The Food and Drug Administration is discussed briefly in Chapter 12.

Professional societies. Some of the professional societies at the national level are the following: the American Medical Association, American Dental Association, American Public Health Association, American Hospital Association, American Association for Health, Physical Education and Recreation, American School Health Association, and Society of Public Health Educators.

National voluntary health agencies. The voluntary health agencies at the national level fulfill many of the functions that the state and local agencies do: education, service, and research are their primary concerns. However, some differences exist, since they serve at the national level and, in many instances, are the parent organizations. For example, the national agencies make every effort to strengthen the state and local agencies. They offer them advisory and consultant services. They promote in-service education of workers at the three levels. They prepare educational materials which are generally distributed to the public by the state and local organizations. Some of the functions of the national agencies are directed toward advancing themselves and "selling" their own organizations. They conduct and sponsor more research than is possible at the lower levels. They work to improve national legislation for health. In general, they strive for better health of the public.

The National Health Council. The coordinating body at the national level is the National Health Council. It provides the structure that welds together all efforts for health at the national level. Its aim is to "strengthen all health programs, governmental and voluntary, through joint planning and action of its members. It strives also to arouse greater citizen interest and greater citizen participation in the attainment and maintenance of physical and mental well-being for all." [18]

The functions of the National Health Council include promoting health education, serving as a clearinghouse for public health information, developing new state and local health councils and assisting old ones, promoting full-time local health departments, offering a consultant service on community health and other services to individuals and groups, and coordinating the activities of the national health agencies. This is the medium for community organization at the national level.

Summary

Community organization is necessary today in order to unite the individual members and groups of an area into one group with a common purpose, the developing or improving of a community health program. A functional health program at the local, state, and national levels comprises health services and educational activities organized and conducted by competent personnel.

Many opportunities exist for the citizen to participate actively in the community health program, thus assuming part of his civic responsibilities.

Suggested Activities

1. Make a study of your home community or the community in which you are living while attending college. Determine the physical setting, the racial patterns, the religious groups, the recreational and cultural pattern, the industrial pattern, and the social classes. Write a description of your community setting.

2. Join with other members of your class in surveying the health resources in your community. (*a*) What agencies and facilities are available? (*b*) What

[18] *The National Health Council, What It Is . . . What It Does.* New York: The National Health Council, 1952. (Pamphlet.)

health protection do you have? (*c*) What resources are needed to provide adequate health for all the people? (*d*) What are the major health problems? (*e*) What is being done to solve present-day problems? (*f*) How can additional services be obtained?

3. Visit one or more health resources in your community or state that interest you. For example, plan a trip to the health department, a voluntary agency, a hospital, a clinic, a health council, a county medical- or dental-society office, the schools, the service clubs, and the like. Write up your findings, and report to the class.

4. Develop a plan for improving the health of the community after you have conferred with community officials and citizens.

5. Analyze the ways and means by which you as a citizen can participate in working for community health. What community activities interest you now? Which activities seem to have future appeal to you as you settle down in the community of your choice? Review this chapter, and read references 19 and 20 for additional suggestions.

6. Present a sociodrama illustrating the functions of the community health council, the state health council, or the national health council.

7. Make a detailed study of the health activities of the Federal government. What recommendations for improving Federal activities do you propose?

8. Critically analyze the contribution of a voluntary health agency at the local, state, and national levels. Discuss the role of the voluntary agencies in present-day health activities. Are they essential? Should they be encouraged to develop? Do they need further coordination? What are your suggestions?

9. Evaluate the work of the National Health Council. Suggest recommendations for its future development.

10. Describe the interrelationships of health services and activities at the local, state, and Federal levels.

11. Preview, show, and discuss *So Much for So Little* (sound, 12 minutes), Public Health Service Film (description of a local health department).

Suggested Readings

1. A Report to the President by the President's Commission on the Health Needs of the Nation, *Building America's Health.* Vol. I, *Findings and Recommendations;* Vol. II, *America's Health Status, Needs and Resources.* Washington: Government Printing Office, 1952.

2. American Public Health Association, "The Local Health Department—Services and Responsibilities," *American Journal of Public Health and the Nation's Health,* 41:302–307, March, 1951.

3. Anderson, Gaylord, "Public Health—A Mandate from the People," *American Journal of Public Health and the Nation's Health,* 42:1367–1373, November, 1952.

4. Buell, Bradley, and associates, *Community Planning for Human Services.* New York: Columbia University Press, 1952.

5. Colcord, Joanna, rev. by Donald S. Howard, *Your Community.* New York: Russell Sage Foundation, 1947.

6. Emerson, Haven, and Martha Luginbuhl, "1,200 Local Public Health Departments for the United States," *American Journal of Public Health and the Nation's Health,* 35:898–904, September, 1945.

7. Gunn, S. M., and P. S. Platt, *Voluntary Health Agencies.* New York: The Ronald Press Company, 1945.

8. Hanlon, John, *Principles of Public Health Administration.* St. Louis: The C. V. Mosby Company, Medical Publishers, 1950.

9. Hiscock, Ira V., *Community Health Organization.* New York: Commonwealth Fund, Division of Publication, 1950.

10. Johns, Ray, and David F. Demarche, *Community Organization and Agency Responsibility.* New York: Association Press, 1951.

11. Kooz, Earl L., "Community Organization for Health: Practice and Precept," *Public Health Reports,* 68:86–87, January, 1953.

12. Mountin, Joseph W., and Evelyn Flook, "Guide to Health Organization in the United States," *Public Health Service Publication* 196. Washington: Government Printing Office, 1953.

13. Patterson, Raymond S., and Beryl J. Roberts, *Community Health Education in Action.* St. Louis: The C. V. Mosby Company, Medical Publishers, 1951.

14. U.S. Department of Health, Education, and Welfare, "The National Institutes of Health: Clinical Center," *Public Health Service Publication* 316. Washington: Government Printing Office, 1953.

Popular Readings

15. Lyon, Yolane, *Stepping Stones to a Health Council,* rev. ed. New York: National Health Council, 1952.

16. Maisel, Albert Q., "Your Neighbor's Health Is Your Business," *Public Affairs Pamphlet* 180. New York: National Health Council, 1952.

17. National Health Council, *Aids to Community Planning,* 3d ed. New York, 1952.

18. O'Connor, Basil, *America's Potential for Health.* New York: National Health Council, 1949.

19. Poston, Richard W., *Democracy Is You.* New York: Harper & Brothers, 1953.

20. Sanders, Irwin T., *Making Good Communities Better.* Lexington: University of Kentucky Press, 1950.

21. Stonorov, Oscar, and Louis I. Kahn, *You and Your Neighborhood.* New York: Revere Copper and Brass, Inc., 1944.

18. Solving International Health Problems

Health is a world-wide problem. The 2,500,000,000 persons living in an increasingly closer relationship with each other in the world-wide community provide ample evidence to substantiate this statement. Diseases have no respect for geographical boundaries between local neighborhoods or the nations of the world. As has been stated in Chapter 17, the public itself is responsible for its own healthful environment. In addition, the concept of health as something more than freedom from disease is being recognized, and a more positive outlook is developing among the peoples of the world. The significance of health status in relation to poverty and ignorance becomes increasingly evident as improvements in the health status of a group of people in respect to one of the factors results in a like improvement in the other factors.

Individuals in all nations of the world must become increasingly aware of the nature of world health problems in order to cooperate in solving these problems. College students may be able to make valuable contributions, now or in the future, to the solution of international health problems if they understand the factors involved. Such an understanding involves a consideration of the following questions: What is the significance of health in the world today? What are the outstanding health problems confronting the peoples of the world? What organizations are contributing to the solution of international health problems?

The Significance of Health in the World Today

No nation is free from the threat of epidemics while diseases are permitted to run rampant in other countries. Modern transportation has many advantages, but it also provides for the rapid movement of insect vectors, as well as human carriers, of many communicable diseases. Breakfast in England, lunch in North America, and back to England in time for tea is a demonstrated possibility, and even greater speeds are forecast for the near future as "jet," "rocket," and "atomic" become commonplace adjectives in a discussion of transportation. Such rapid movement adds immeasurably to the problem of controlling the spread of communicable diseases from one area of the world to another.

Health status influences and is influenced by other factors. The health status of the peoples of the world is allied closely with other factors. Calder illustrates this in a discussion of the construction of maps by United Nations organizations to show (1) the distribution of world hunger as determined by calorie intake, (2) ignorance as determined by number of illiterate persons, and (3) ill health as determined by the death rate of infants [1]. The similarity between the maps demonstrates clearly that these factors are aligned closely and that FAO (Food and Agriculture Organization), UNESCO (United Nations Educational, Scientific and Cultural Organization), and WHO (World Health Organization) are all concerned with the total problem of raising more than half the population of the world to decent standards of living and well-being.

Winslow [1] indicates a pattern which has persisted in relation to health: "The problems of poverty and disease in underdeveloped areas are complex and interrelated. Men and women in these lands are poor because they are sick, and sick because they are poor."

It is estimated that one-fifth of the human race who live in Europe, North America, and the British Commonwealth has an annual income of approximately $461 per person and an average life span of sixty-three years, while two-thirds of the human race who live in Africa, southeast Asia, the Pacific Islands, and Latin America have an annual income of about $41 per person and an average length of life of only thirty years [15].

What does health mean to the people of the world? The importance of health has been recognized by mankind for thousands of years. Calder [2] notes an ancient reference by Buddha to the desirability of health and comments about the attainment of health by the peoples of the world:

> *Arogya Parama Laba* ("health is the greatest blessing of all"). . . . Health may be the greatest blessing, but half of the people of the world do not know what it means. They know it only by its reverse as disease, ill-health and misery.

[1] C.-E. A. Winslow, "The Global Problem: Inequality of Opportunity," *Public Health Reports,* 67:318, April, 1952.

[2] Ritchie Calder, *The Lamp Is Lit: The Story of WHO,* p. 1. Geneva: World Health Organization, 1951.

They have no means to know that sense of well-being which is something quite different from not being ill. Health is not just the absence of disease.

No doctor can prescribe health; no government can ordain health by statute; no international agency can administer health. A community for instance, may provide houses; it cannot provide homes. A "home" is what a family makes of a house. So with health; all that a community, local, national or international can do is provide the means and the services—social conditions, public-health measures, sanitation, better treatment of diseases—by which the individual can enjoy the well-being and happiness which only he can create.

Unfortunately, there are too few healthy individuals who appreciate the health which they enjoy and too many individuals who never have the opportunity to experience the state of health suggested in the preceding statement.

As indicated in Chapter 1, the nations represented in the World Health Organization have agreed on a definition of health. They suggest that it is both a right and a duty of all individuals. Their concept of health is expressed in the following pattern: [3]

Health: "a state of *complete physical, mental and social well-being* and not merely the absence of disease or infirmity."

A right: "one of the *fundamental rights of every human being* without distinction of race, religion, political belief, economic or social condition."

A duty: "the health of ALL peoples is fundamental to the attainment of PEACE AND SECURITY and is *dependent upon the fullest co-operation of individuals and states.*"

The Development of World Organizations for Health

Many early efforts by nations to control disease and promote world health were doomed to failure because of the effect of control measures in limiting trade. However, in 1902 a permanent organization created for multilateral international action relating to public health was established by the nations in the Americas [13]. The meeting in Washington, D.C., of the First International Sanitary Conference of the American republics in that year resulted in the establishment of the Pan American Sanitary Bureau, which has contributed extensively to improvement of health conditions in the Americas.

The primary concern of the Pan American Sanitary Bureau was to control the spread of diseases between nations. In 1909 the International

[3] *World Health Organization: What It Is, What It Does, How It Works,* 5th ed., p. 1. Geneva: World Health Organization, 1951.

Office of Public Health was established, with headquarters in Paris, for the same purpose but on a world-wide scale. Forty-six countries were included in the membership of this organization.

The need for improving health conditions within, as well as between, countries was recognized, and the Rockefeller Foundation established an International Health Commission to aid in developing cooperative action for building up sound programs for disease control and health promotion within individual countries [13].

In 1923 the League of Nations, which was established following World War I, formed its Health Organization. This organization provided the first machinery for an effective approach to solving world-wide health problems. The accomplishments of the Health Organization of the League of Nations were outstanding until its functions were disrupted by World War II. The Service of Epidemiological Intelligence, which collected data on the prevalence and movement of communicable diseases and provided for extensive distribution of this information, was one of the most valuable functions of the League organization. Other services were provided by such groups as the Commission on Biological Standardization, the Malaria Commission, the Commission on Housing, and groups making nutrition studies.

The World Health Organization was developed from the background of international experiences with the Pan American Sanitary Bureau, the International Office of Public Health, the International Health Commission of the Rockefeller Foundation, and the League of Nations Health Organization.

At the United Nations meeting in San Francisco in 1945, delegations from Brazil and China introduced a resolution calling for a special meeting to establish an international health organization. The Economic and Social Council of the United Nations called for such a conference to meet in New York in July, 1946. At this New York meeting, the representatives of sixty-one nations drew up and adopted a constitution for the new organization. The representatives appointed an Interim Commission to function until the constitution was ratified by twenty-six nations. The Interim Commission was composed of representatives from sixteen nations selected by the conference.

The slow process of ratification by member nations delayed the final establishment of the organization but did not prevent the Interim Commission from functioning. In 1947 a cholera epidemic in Egypt provided an opportunity for international action, and the Commission accepted the challenge. Through the efforts of this world organization, some 32 tons of medical supplies was gathered from all over the world and rushed into Egypt to assist the Egyptian health workers in the vaccination and treatment program necessary to control the epidemic. One month after the onset of the epidemic it had spread throughout the country, and in a single day 1,000 new cases and 500 deaths were recorded [12]. In another six weeks the epidemic had been brought under control, and the battle was won. Many lives were saved and much misery was avoided as a result of the cooperation of many nations to assist the Egyptians.

Despite this evidence of the value of coordination of effort in solving health problems, the nations were slow in ratifying the constitution. The Interim Commission called a meeting for June 24, 1948, even though there were not enough signatory nations when the meeting date was set. With the stimulus of the call to meeting, many nations signed in order to be eligible for this first meeting of the World Health Assembly. On Apr. 7, 1948, the twenty-sixth nation signed the constitution, and as a result Apr. 7 is now celebrated each year as World Health Day. The United States became the forty-second nation to accept membership by ratifying the constitution on June 14, 1948. By the first meeting on June 24, fifty-four nations had ratified the constitution and by April, 1953, this number had grown to eighty-two.

Since the first meeting in 1948, the World Health Assembly has met each year for the purpose of planning and establishing over-all policies.

Officially, the World Health Organization was recognized on Sept. 1, 1948. The work of this organization in helping nations to solve their health problems has been outstanding. The function of the World Health Organization is discussed in greater detail later in the chapter.

Health Problems in the World Today

The theme for World Health Day on Apr. 7, 1952, was "Healthy surroundings make healthy people." The significance of this theme is better understood in the light of the comment by Brock Chisholm,[4] first director-general of the World Health Organization: "Despite the magnificent progress made by medical science, three out of every four men, women and children in the world still suffer from diseases spread by unsafe water supplies, unsanitary excreta disposal, uncontrolled insects and rodents, and inadequate protection of milk and other foods."

Chisholm [5] suggests that "The major health problem of the world today

[4] Brock Chisholm, "World Health Day," *United Nations Bulletin,* 12:304, Apr. 1, 1952.

[5] "The World's Health," *The Quotarian,* December, 1951, p. 10.

is not death; it is chronic and repeated infection and infestation whereby millions of people become social liabilities rather than instruments of social progress and welfare."

He also reports the following facts relative to health status: (1) there is only 1 native doctor in the whole of Ethiopia; (2) somewhere in the world someone dies of tuberculosis every 7 seconds; (3) before the WHO campaign to control malaria in Greece, 4 out of 5 Greeks were malaria victims, and on an average 30 days per person per year were lost because of this one disease; (4) there are 4½ million square miles of land lying fallow in Africa alone primarily because of African sleeping sickness spread by the tsetse fly; (5) there is evidence in some countries that 60 to 80 per cent of the population is syphilitic [11].

The shortage of trained health personnel is a serious problem in the underdeveloped areas of the world. A report on the conditions in southeast Asia includes the information that Afghanistan has 100 doctors for 16 million people, 1 midwife to 100,000 population in some districts, 1 public health officer for each million people, and 1 hospital bed for 3,000 people [9].

The regional director for the southeast Asia regional office of the World Health Organization in a report on health conditions in Afghanistan, Burma, Ceylon, India, Indonesia, and Thailand summarizes the health problem in his area in relation to several factors: (1) there are nearly 500 million people in an area three-fourths as large as the United States; (2) 80 per cent of the population is illiterate; (3) the average annual income is approximately $50; (4) the average per capita expenditure on health is no more than 20 cents; (5) birth rates are between 25 and 40 per 1,000 population; (6) death rates are between 15 and 20 per 1,000 population; (7) the population of India has increased approximately 23 million during a 5-year period; (8) the expectation of life is between 25 and 35 years; (9) the infant mortality rate averages 150 per 1,000 population and goes over 300 in some areas; (10) malaria claims over 100 million new cases and more than 1 million deaths per year; (11) it is estimated that in India there are 2½ million cases of tuberculosis resulting in ½ million deaths each year [9].

Maternal and infant mortality rates are considered to be a good index of the state of health in a community. In highly developed areas maternal death rates are less than 1 per 1,000 live births, while in underdeveloped areas they are as high as 5 to 10 per 1,000. Infant mortality rates vary from below 30 to above 300 per 1,000 live births.

Statistical information is not available for all nations, but the data presented in Table 17 illustrate the great differences in chances for survival in the different nations. The wide variation in health status of the peoples of the world suggests the need for active international cooperation to assist the less fortunate to improve their health status.

Chisholm,[6] in a speech on the fifth anniversary of the World Health Organization, stressed this need for cooperation: "The lesson is simple

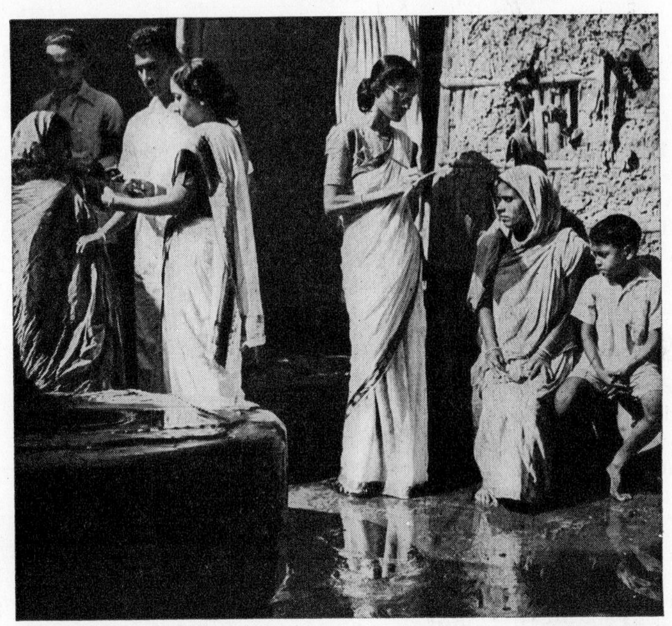

Fig. 18.1. Plague-control team, led by an Indian woman doctor, interviews slum dwellers and inoculates potential victims with antiplague vaccine. (*By permission of World Health Organization.*)

and clear; if sickness and poverty go hand in hand, so also do health and prosperity. And the way to world health and prosperity is through international action, for the evil we fight is the enemy of us all—and in this battle there can be no neutrals."

The World Health Organization at Work

Fortunately, the leaders of the World Health Organization have realized that this group cannot solve the health problems of nations by sending in an army of workers to kill insects, immunize individuals, or provide penicillin injections. Improvements in health status of the peoples of the

[6] "Health Is Wealth," *United Nations Bulletin,* 14:244, Apr. 1, 1953.

Table 17. Chances per 1,000 of Survival through Specified Periods of Life for Males and Females in Various Countries *

Country	Calendar year	Males			Females		
		From birth to age 15	From age 15 to Age 45	From age 15 to Age 65	From birth to age 15	From age 15 to Age 45	From age 15 to Age 65
North and South America:							
United States:							
White	1949	955	928	663	965	957	793
Nonwhite	1949	928	838	480	942	865	554
British Honduras	1944–1948	770	729	423	797	748	514
Canada	1947	928	926	696	945	938	768
Jamaica	1945–1947	832	808	480	846	815	574
Mexico	1940	660	700	388	671	742	454
Trinidad and Tobago	1945–1947	872	816	451	887	817	522
Europe:							
Denmark	1941–1945	926	927	729	942	934	753
England and Wales	1949	950	939	684	961	948	788
France	1946–1948	916	904	654	935	928	765
Malta and Gozo	1946	816	910	631	832	906	668
The Netherlands	1947–1949	950	950	775	961	958	809
Norway	1945–1948	941	913	745	956	941	808
Sweden	1941–1945	946	918	728	959	933	772
Oceania:							
Australia	1946–1948	952	934	679	963	948	777
New Zealand	1947	959	943	717	967	953	791
Asia and Africa:							
Ceylon	1945–1947	758	793	483	742	736	482
Japan	1949–1950	880	835	560	889	853	641
Union of South Africa, European	1945–1947	936	916	635	948	932	735

* Basic data from *United Nations Demographic Yearbook*, 1951, and reports of various countries; data for selected countries from Metropolitan Life Insurance Co. *Statistical Bulletin*, March, 1952, p. 4.

world cannot be imposed upon them from outside. Rather, they must be the result of the combined efforts of an enlightened population assisted by trained personnel and equipment from other nations if necessary.

Some of the underlying philosophy of the World Health Organization is expressed in the following statement: [7]

[7] Calder, *op. cit.*, pp. 2–6.

WHO, therefore, is not an international system of medicine. It is not just an outsize medical college to produce better doctors or more nurses (though both are important); a learned society, which brings experts together; a repository of facts about the world's ailments, or a consulting room for the treatment of the sick. It is concerned with the Whole Man; his body, his brain, his emotions; with the child even before he is born and with the mother who gives him birth; with the family of which he is a part; with the community in which he will live and work; with the amenities of life and with the conditions which will enable him to develop as an individual and as a personality the better to play his part in a healthy world society. . . .

WHO argues that, with all of the help and experience which advanced medical thinking and practice can offer, health services must emerge and grow and cannot be imposed, even by most enlightened authority. A demonstration team, however successful in eradicating a disease, or diseases, from an area is no substitute for the social services and local measures which must succeed them.

With such an enlightened underlying philosophy the World Health Organization has undertaken the task of providing assistance in improving the health status of the peoples of the world.

Organizational structure of the World Health Organization. The organizational structure of the World Health Organization is illustrated in Figure 18.2. Leadership of WHO is vested in the Health Assembly, which meets annually. The Assembly is composed of representative delegations from each of the member nations. This body is responsible for determining the policies and setting the guide lines for the WHO program.

The executive board is composed of eighteen members selected by the Health Assembly. This group is responsible for putting into effect the decisions reached by the Health Assembly and for initiating emergency action which is necessary between meetings of the Assembly. This technical and nonpolitical group meets at least twice each year.

The working section of WHO is the Secretariat, headed by the director-general. This group is composed of both technical and administrative personnel.

The functions of WHO are allocated to the regional offices of the organization as much as is possible, with the Geneva headquarters serving to coordinate all the activities of the regional offices and the many divisions shown in the structural chart.

Activities of the World Health Organization. The activities of WHO are numerous and varied. Some of the activities are of a general nature for the benefit of all member nations, while other activities are more specific in order to assist a particular nation in solving a health problem. The activities are carried on by the several divisions shown in Fig. 18.2.

Advisory Services. The function of the Department of Advisory Services is to assist countries in the development of health administration. Its purpose is accomplished by such means as public health demonstration teams, through the functions of consultants from professional training centers, and by granting fellowships.

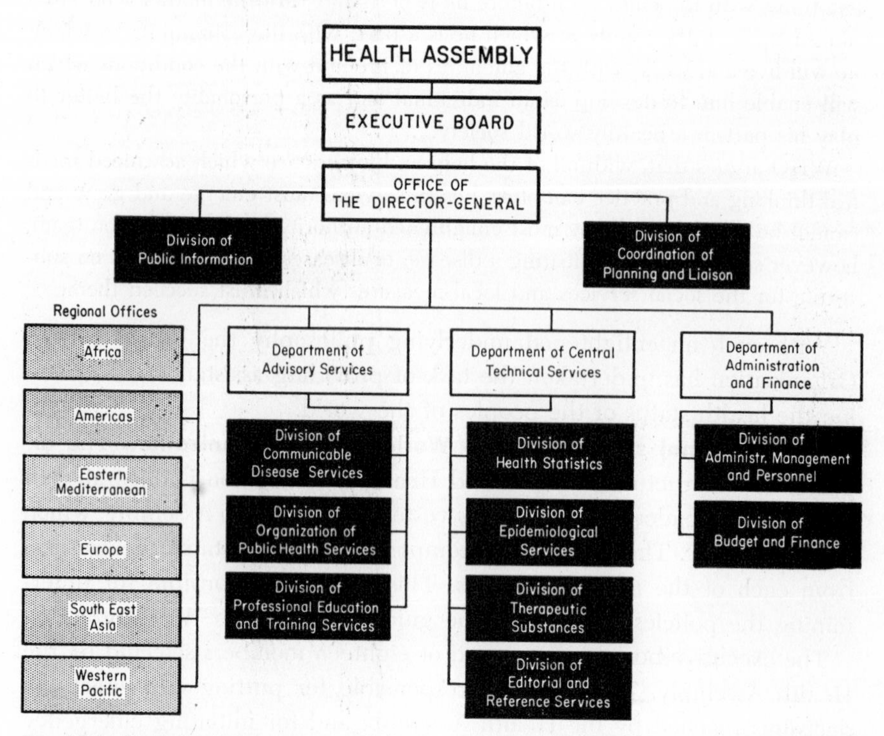

Fig. 18.2. Organizational structure of the World Health Organization. (*By permission of World Health Organization.*)

The demonstration teams and consultants reach many individuals directly and many others indirectly, as is illustrated in a report on WHO: [8]

Demonstrations often result in emulation. For example, in the battle against malaria, WHO control projects gave protection to 1½ million people in 1951. But the total number of people protected by the methods which WHO demonstrated was more than 50 million.

Thus the direct action of WHO, through international administration, inspired similar action by individual countries 33 times greater. At the same time, schemes begun or planned in various countries envisaged the ultimate protection of no fewer than 450 million people.

[8] *World Health Organization: What It Is, What It Does, How It Works, op. cit.,* pp. 2–3.

The benefits resulting from functions carried on by Advisory Services is illustrated by malaria-control campaigns carried on in Greece and Bengal. In Greece, the control measures used to eliminate the mosquitoes which transmit malaria resulted in many other improvements, including (1) an increase in the average gross income for families in the malaria districts from $196.34 to $385.15, (2) a 67 per cent increase in the area

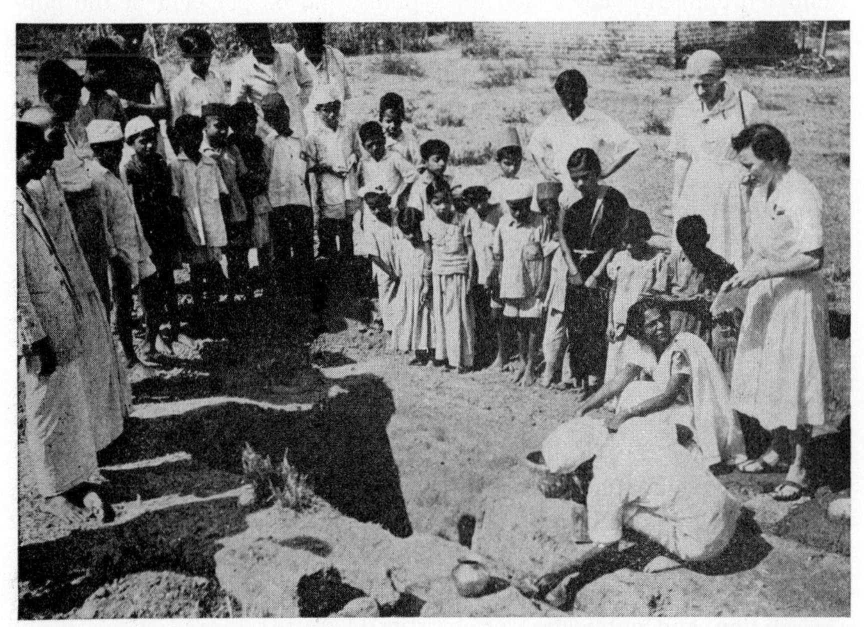

Fig. 18.3. Children at a Malnad (India) school take an intense interest in the construction of a new "deep-hole" latrine, part of a school health program being developed with help from members of the WHO-UNICEF malaria-control team operating in the Malnad area. (*By permission of United Nations.*)

under cultivation, (3) a reduction in the incidence of fly-borne typhoid and dysentery, (4) an increase in egg output through elimination of pests afflicting hens, and (5) a 15 to 20 per cent increase in milk output by elimination of flies which decreased the vitality of cattle [1, 16]. In Bengal, the control program not only reduced malaria but resulted in an increase of 543 pounds of rice per acre per year because the farmers were able to work more effectively [1].

Some other benefits afforded by Advisory Services include the following: (1) A malaria control campaign in Ceylon was started in September of 1946, and by the end of 1947 the country's death rate was decreased from 22 to 14$\frac{3}{10}$ per 1,000 population as a result of a decrease in malaria deaths and other causes as well. (2) WHO in cooperation with UNICEF (United Nations International Children's Emergency Fund) and the Scandinavian Red Cross societies worked with the governments of European countries to tuberculin-test over 20 million children and young adults and to vaccinate with BCG the 15 million who were found to be negative. (3) The entire population in the Ghund Valley in India was examined clinically and tested for syphilis, and 65 per cent of the population was found to be positive; yet five months after penicillin treatment no new cases had occurred. (4) Yaws has been virtually eliminated as a result of penicillin treatment measures in Haiti, Thailand, and Indonesia [1].

Central Technical Services. The functions of Central Technical Services Department produce results less spectacular than the activities of the Advisory Services Department but equally significant.

The contributions of Technical Services include (1) publishing the first international pharmacopeia, which contains formulae for making up medicines to ensure uniform strength of the preparations in the different nations; (2) standardizing biological substances such as the antibiotics, serums, and vitamins in order to provide an added margin of safety in treatment of diseases in the various nations; (3) the broadcasting of up-to-the-minute information relative to epidemic diseases to all national health services as well as to ships at sea and to aircraft in flight; (4) maintaining a library service available to the various nations and publishing materials for world-wide distribution, and (5) the collection, interpretation, and publication of statistics [1, 2, 16].

Among the publications of WHO are the *Bulletin of the World Health Organization, International Digest of Health Legislation, Chronicle of the World Health Organization, Weekly Epidemiological Record,* and *Monthly Epidemiological and Statistical Report.*

Cooperation with other international agencies. The program of the World Health Organization is carried on in close cooperation with other international agencies whenever the opportunity arises. An example of this joint policy is the cooperative program for tuberculin testing and BCG vaccination between WHO and UNICEF, which was mentioned earlier in the chapter.

Keeney [9] illustrates the magnitude of the combined projects which are being undertaken in the following statement: "In Asia, the World Health

[9] S. M. Keeney, "Two Cooperative Projects of WHO and UNICEF," *Public Health Reports,* 68:606, June, 1953.

Organization and the United Nations International Children's Emergency Fund (UNICEF) work hand in hand on 50 projects in 15 countries in which UNICEF has invested $20,000,000 in supplies and WHO is supplying 100 professional personnel, to mass campaigns where the foreign technical personnel may be only 5 per cent of the project."

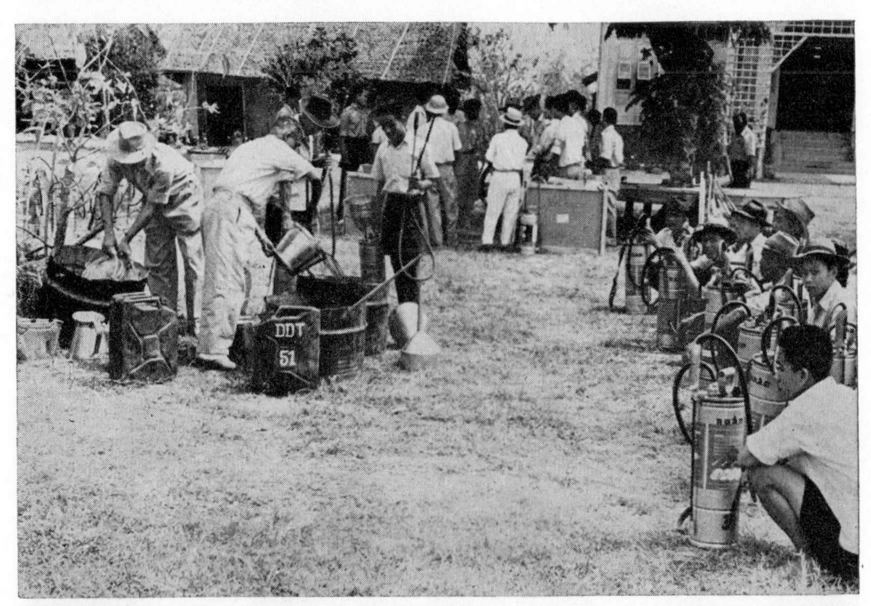

Fig. 18.4. Malaria control demonstration in Thailand by a team from the World Health Organization. (*By permission of United Nations.*)

WHO also has cooperated with UNICEF in venereal-disease-control programs, with the Food and Agricultural Organization in plans to increase the amount of land under cultivation through disease-control programs, and with the International Labour Organization in problems associated with industrial hygiene.

Some of the additional sources of funds for international activities in health include the United Nations Expanded Program for Technical Assistance to Underdeveloped Countries, the Technical Assistance Program of the United States (Truman's Point Four), the British Commonwealth Technical Assistance Plan (the Colombo plan), the CARE Organization of the United States of America, national and religious relief and welfare organizations, the International Committee of the Red Cross, and the League of Red Cross Societies.

Bilateral International Health Programs of the United States

In addition to the multilateral international health programs, which pool the resources of all the nations, there are many agreements between two nations to assist in solving the health problems of one or both of the countries. The bilateral programs in which the United States has participated with other nations are in addition to the activities of WHO but are planned in cooperation with this international organization.

Cooperation to improve health in the Americas. Within a month after the bombing of Pearl Harbor, the foreign ministers of the American

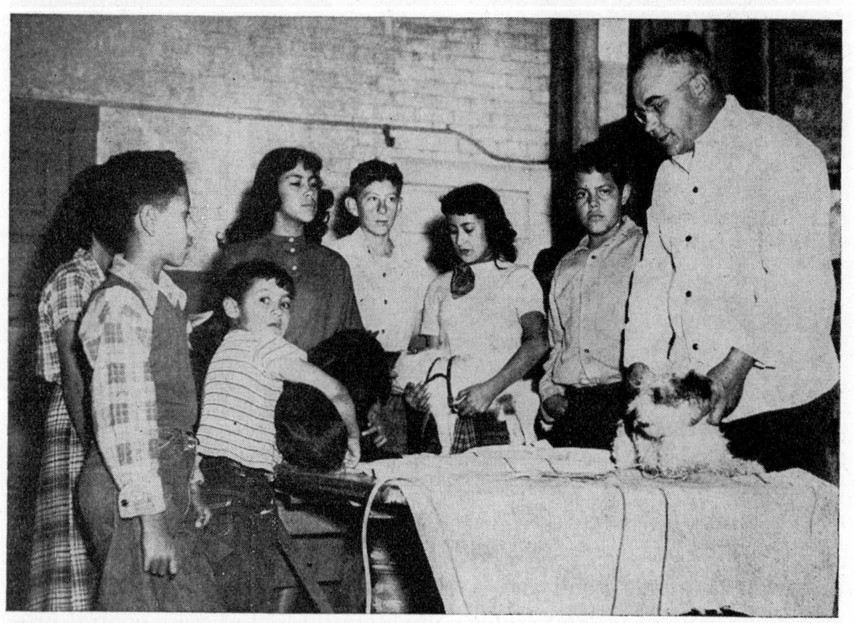

Fig. 18.5. The Pan American Sanitary Bureau, Regional Office of the World Health Organization, is cooperating with United States and Mexican government public health officials in a rabies-control campaign along the Mexican border. (*By permission of World Health Organization.*)

republics called for cooperation among the republics on health and sanitation programs. The United States Office of the Coordinator of Inter-American Affairs undertook a cooperative health program in eighteen of the Latin-American countries with emphasis in the following four areas: [10]

[10] Henry Van Zile Hyde, "International Health: Bilateral International Health Programs of the United States," *American Journal of Public Health*, 41:1474, December, 1951.

1. The development of local health services through health centers.
2. Sanitation of the environment, with particular emphasis on water supply, sewage disposal, and insect control.
3. The training and full-time employment of professional public health workers.
4. Education of the public in health matters.

The progress of this program, carried out during the first nine years after 1942 by joint services within the ministry of health of cooperating governments, includes 201 water-supply systems constructed; 74 sewage systems constructed; 121 health centers operated; 342 other health facilities provided, including hospitals, nursing schools, laboratories, markets, and public laundries; 1,302 Latin-American professional persons assisted with advanced training in public health; technical and financial aid to schools of public health in Mexico, Santiago, and São Paulo; and, 240 local training courses provided at subprofessional levels [8].

Cooperative programs outside the Americas. In 1944 the United States and Liberia undertook a bilateral health program to assist the latter in developing health services and medical facilities. This marked the advent of the United States Public Health Service in a bilateral international phase of health work. In addition to aiding in controlling malaria and smallpox, one of the most noteworthy accomplishments is the effect of the total program in increasing the annual health budget of Liberia tenfold during the first seven years of the program [8].

The recognition of the threat of communism in areas where filth, disease, and human misery were prevalent has resulted in the development of additional bilateral international programs. The work of the United States Public Health Service Mission to Greece has been an outstanding development as a result of this attempt to forestall communism. The Public Health Service Mission subsequently became the public health division of the ECA (Economic Cooperation Administration) Mission to Greece. Turkey, southeast Asia, and the Philippines have more recently been the host to ECA missions which include medical-care and sanitation programs in their undertakings.

One of the bilateral programs has been administered through the TCA (Technical Cooperation Administration) by the Department of State as part of President Truman's Point Four program. Point Four programs in Iran and Lebanon are under way, and plans are being made for additional programs in other countries in the Near East and South Asia.

Summary

Health is an important individual problem. In addition, it is a community problem of world-wide scope. Individuals in all nations of the world must assume added responsibilities for assisting others to attain that quality of life which enables them to live effectively.

The World Health Organization has made many contributions to the improvement of health status of individuals and countries. Continued cooperation between the World Health Organization and other organizations working for the improvement of the health status of peoples is essential in order to make additional advances in the battle for healthful living.

Suggested Activities

1. Compare the health status of one of the underprivileged nations of the world with that of the United States. Note comparative improvements which have been made during the last half-century.
2. Construct a world map, and by using the *Weekly Epidemiological Record,* published by the World Health Organization, keep a record of the location and movement of serious disease problems in the world.
3. Write to the Pan American Sanitary Bureau, Regional Office of the World Health Organization, 1501 New Hampshire Ave., Washington 6, for information regarding activities of WHO in the Americas.
4. Plan to celebrate World Health Day, Apr. 7, on your campus. Prepare illustrative material to use on bulletin boards to inform other students about world health. If foreign students attend your school, organize a panel discussion of world health problems by representatives of different nations.

Suggested Readings

1. Calder, Ritchie, *The Lamp Is Lit: The Story of the World Health Organization.* Geneva: World Health Organization, 1951.
2. Chisholm, Brock, "International Health: The Role of WHO, Past, Present, and Future," *American Journal of Public Health,* 41:1460–1463, December, 1951.
3. Chisholm, Brock, "The Right to Health," *United Nations Bulletin,* 11:445–446, December, 1951.
4. Dublin, Louis I., *The Facts of Life from Birth to Death.* New York: The Macmillan Company, 1951.
5. Halverson, Wilton L., "Summary of Activities of the World Health Organization," *The Annual,* 1950, pp. 8–12, Western Branch American Public Health Association.
6. Halverson, Wilton L., "World Health Organization," *Life and Health,* 64: 6–7, June, 1949.

7. "Health Is Wealth," *United Nations Bulletin,* 14:244–245, Apr. 1, 1953.

8. Hyde, Henry Van Zile, "International Health: Bilateral International Health Programs of the United States," *American Journal of Public Health,* 41:1473–1476, December, 1951.

9. Mani, Chandra, "International Health: Application of WHO Programs and Policies in a Region," *American Journal of Public Health,* 41:1469–1472, December, 1951.

10. Soper, Fred L., "International Health: Some Aspects of WHO's Programs in the Americas," *American Journal of Public Health,* 41:1464–1468, December, 1951.

11. "The World's Health," *The Quotarian,* December, 1951.

12. United Nations Department of Public Information, *Everyman's United Nations,* 3d ed., pp. 339–344. New York, 1952.

13. Winslow, C.-E. A., "International Health," *American Journal of Public Health,* 41:1455–1459, December, 1951.

14. Winslow, C.-E. A., "The Cost of Sickness and the Price of Health," *Monograph Series, No.* 7. Geneva: World Health Organization, 1951.

15. Winslow, C.-E. A., "The Global Problem: Inequality of Opportunity," *Public Health Reports,* 67:318, April, 1952.

16. *World Health Organization: What It Is, What It Does, How It Works,* 5th ed. Geneva: World Health Organization, 1951.

In conclusion: *Mens sana in corpore sano in societate sana.*

Index

I

X

Y

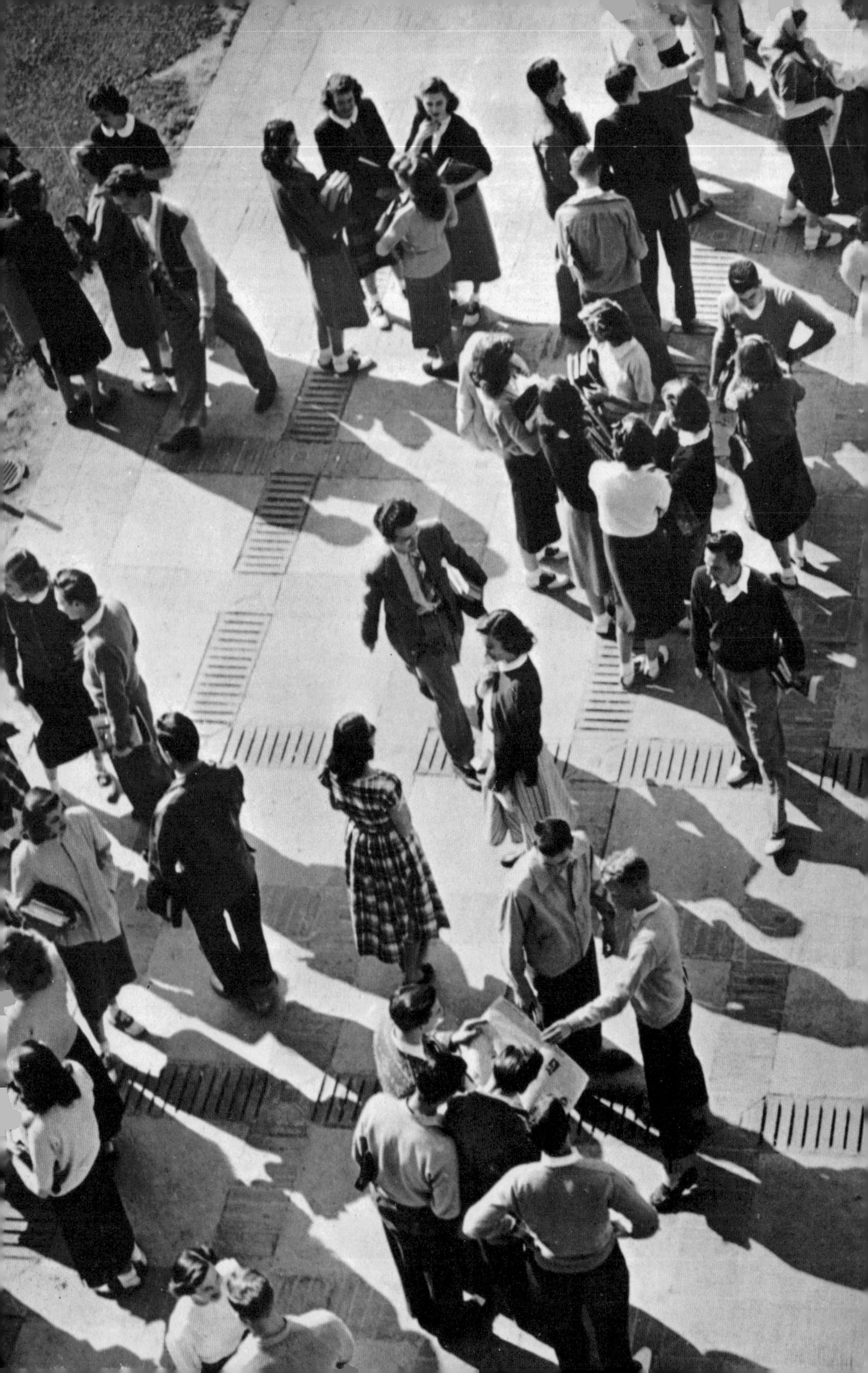